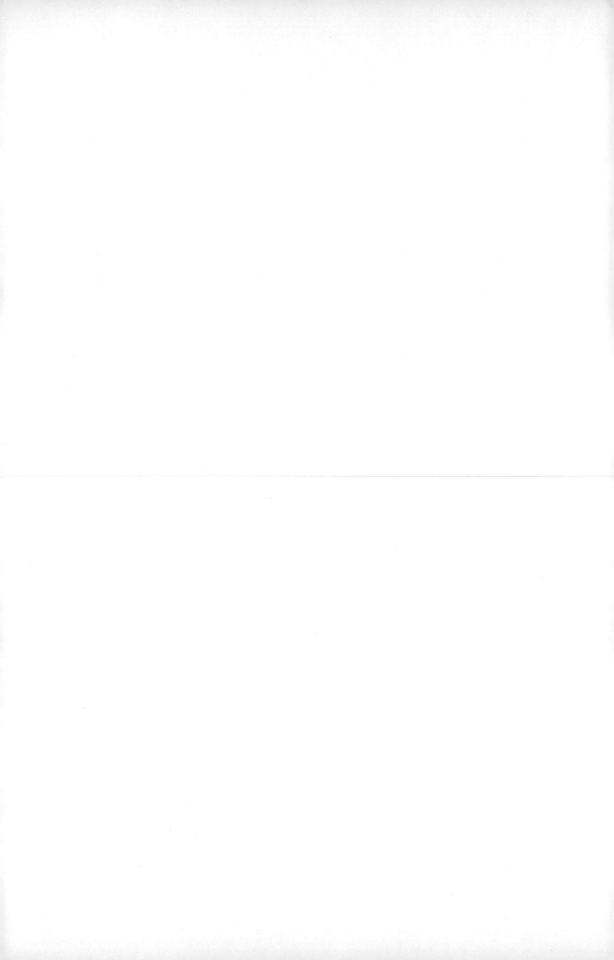

Breast Imaging Essentials

Editors

YIMING GAO
SAMANTHA L. HELLER

RADIOLOGIC CLINICS
OF NORTH AMERICA

www.radiologic.theclinics.com

Consulting Editor
FRANK H. MILLER

July 2024 • Volume 62 • Number 4

ELSEVIER

1600 John F. Kennedy Boulevard • Suite 1800 • Philadelphia, Pennsylvania, 19103-2899

http://www.theclinics.com

RADIOLOGIC CLINICS OF NORTH AMERICA Volume 62, Number 4
July 2024 ISSN 0033-8389, ISBN 13: 978-0-443-13087-8

Editor: John Vassallo (j.vassallo@elsevier.com)
Developmental Editor: Malvika Shah

Radiologic Clinics of North America (ISSN 0033-8389) is published bimonthly by Elsevier Inc., 360 Park Avenue South, New York, NY 10010-1710. Months of issue are January, March, May, July, September, and November. Periodicals postage paid at New York, NY and additional mailing offices. Subscription prices are USD 561 per year for US individuals, USD 100 per year for US students and residents, USD 643 per year for Canadian individuals, USD 754 per year for international individuals, USD 100 per year for Canadian students/residents, and USD 315 per year for international students/residents. For institutional access pricing please contact Customer Service via the contact information below. To receive student and resident rate, orders must be accompanied by name of affiliated institution, date of term and the signature of program/residency coordinatior on institution letterhead. Orders will be billed at individual rate until proof of status is received. Foreign air speed delivery is included in all *Clinics* subscription prices. All prices are subject to change without notice. **POSTMASTER:** Send address changes to *Radiologic Clinics of North America*, Elsevier Health Sciences Division, Subscription Customer Service, 3251 Riverport Lane, Maryland Heights, MO63043. **Customer Service: Telephone: 1-800-654-2452** (U.S. and Canada); **1-314-447-8871** (outside U.S. and Canada). **Fax: 1-314-447-8029. E-mail: journalscustomerservice-usa@elsevier.com (for print support); journalsonlinesupport-usa@elsevier.com (for online support)**.

Reprints. For copies of 100 or more of articles in this publication, please contact the Commercial Reprints Department, Elsevier Inc., 360 Park Avenue South, New York, New York 10010-1710. Tel.: +1-212-633-3874; Fax: +1-212-633-3820; E-mail: reprints@elsevier.com.

Radiologic Clinics of North America also published in Greek Paschalidis Medical Publications, Athens, Greece.

Radiologic Clinics of North America is covered in *MEDLINE/PubMed (Index Medicus), EMBASE/Excerpta Medica, Current Contents/Life Sciences, Current Contents/Clinical Medicine, RSNA Index to Imaging Literature, BIOSIS, Science Citation Index,* and *ISI/BIOMED*.

Contributors

CONSULTING EDITOR

FRANK H. MILLER, MD, FACR, FSAR, FSABI
Lee F. Rogers, MD Professor of Medical
Education, Chief, Body Imaging Section,
Medical Director, MRI, Professor, Department
of Radiology, Northwestern Memorial Hospital,
Northwestern University Feinberg School of
Medicine, Chicago, Illinois, USA

EDITORS

YIMING GAO, MD, FSBI
Associate Professor, Department of Radiology,
New York University School of Medicine, New
York, New York, USA

SAMANTHA L. HELLER, PhD, MD, FSBI
Professor, Department of Radiology, New York
University School of Medicine, New York, New
York, USA

AUTHORS

BEATRIZ ELENA ADRADA, MD, FSBI
Professor, Department of Breast Imaging, The
University of Texas MD Anderson Cancer
Center, Houston, Texas, USA

SHADI AMINOLOLAMA-SHAKERI, MD, FSBI
Professor and Breast Radiology Division Chief,
Department of Radiology, University of
California Davis, Sacramento, California, USA

DEBBIE L. BENNETT, MD
Associate Professor, Department of Breast
Imaging, Mallinckrodt Institute of Radiology,
Washington University in St. Louis School of
Medicine, St Louis, Missouri, USA

ASHA A. BHATT, MD
Associate Member, Moffitt Cancer Center,
Tampa, Florida, USA

ARIANNA BUCKLEY, MD
Assistant Professor, Department of Breast
Imaging, Mallinckrodt Institute of Radiology,
Washington University in St. Louis School of
Medicine, St Louis, Missouri, USA

SONA A. CHIKARMANE, MD
Associate Chair of Professional Development,
Assistant Professor of Radiology, Harvard
Medical School, Breast Imaging Division,
Department of Radiology, Brigham and
Women's Hospital, Boston, Massachusetts,
USA

VICTORIA DOMONKOS, MD
Resident Physician, Department of Radiology,
The Ottawa Hospital, University of Ottawa,
Ottawa, Ontario, Canada

J. KEVIN DUNBAR, MBChB, MPH, FFPH
Regional Head of Screening Quality Assurance
Service (SQAS) - South, NHS England,
England, United Kingdom

KAITLIN M. FORD, MD
Breast Imaging Fellow, Department of
Radiology, University of California Davis,
Sacramento, California, USA

ERIC KIM, MD
Clinical Assistant Professor, Department of
Radiology, New York University Grossman
School of Medicine, New York, New York, USA

JIN YOU KIM, MD, PhD
Associate Professor, Department of Radiology,
Medical Research Institute, Pusan National
University Hospital, Pusan National University
School of Medicine, Busan, Republic of Korea

MICHELLE V. LEE, MD
Professor, Department of Breast Imaging,
Mallinckrodt Institute of Radiology,
Washington University in St. Louis School of
Medicine, St Louis, Missouri, USA

ALANA A. LEWIN, MD
Clinical Assistant Professor, Department of
Radiology, New York University Grossman
School of Medicine, New York University
Langone Health, Laura and Isaac Perlmutter
Cancer Center, New York, New York, USA

**GERALD LIP, MB BCH, BAO (Ireland), MRCS
(Ireland), FRCR (London)**
Clinical Director, Northeast of Scotland Breast
Screening Programme, Consultant
Radiologist, NHS Grampian, Vice Chair, RCR
British Society of Breast Radiology, National
Innovation Fellow, Chief Scientists Office,
Aberdeen Royal Infirmary, Aberdeen, Scotland,
United Kingdom; North East Scotland Breast
Screening Service, Aberdeen Royal Infirmary,
Aberdeen, United Kingdom

VALENTINA LONGO, MD
Breast Radiologist, Department of Bioimaging,
Radiation Oncology and Hematology, UOC of
Radiodiagnostica Presidio Columbus,
Fondazione Policlinico Universitario A. Gemelli
IRCSS, Rome, Italy

KATHRYN P. LOWRY, MD
Associate Professor, Department of Radiology,
University of Washington School of Medicine,
Fred Hutchinson Cancer Center, Seattle,
Washington, USA

RITSE M. MANN, MD, PhD
Breast Radiologist, Department of Imaging,
Radboud University Medical Center, Nijmegen,
the Netherlands; Department of Radiology, The
Netherlands Cancer Institute, Amsterdam, the
Netherlands

**MARIANA AFONSO MATIAS, MD, PG Cert
Med Leadership, PG Cert Med Education**
Breast Clinician, Breast Unit, Leeds Teaching
Hospital NHS Trust, Level 1 Chancellor Wing,
St James Hospital, Leeds, United Kingdom

BETHANY NIELL, MD, PhD
Senior Member, Moffitt Cancer Center,
Professor, Department of Oncologic Sciences,
University of South Florida, Tampa, Florida,
USA

SAVANNAH C. PARTRIDGE, PhD
Professor, Department of Radiology, University
of Washington, Affiliate Member, Fred
Hutchinson Cancer Center, Seattle,
Washington, USA

MIRAL M. PATEL, MD
Associate Professor, Department of Breast
Imaging, The University of Texas MD Anderson
Cancer Center, Houston, Texas, USA

KIMBERLY M. RAY, MD
Associate Clinical Professor, Department of
Radiology and Biomedical Sciences, University
of California, San Francisco, UCSF Medical
Center, San Francisco, California, USA

JEAN M. SEELY, MD, FRCPC
Head of Breast Imaging Section, Professor,
Department of Radiology, Clinician
Investigator, The Ottawa Hospital, University of
Ottawa, Ottawa, Ontario, Canada

**NISHA SHARMA, MBChB, BSc (Hons),
MRCP, FRCR, MSc**
Director of Breast Screening and Clinical Lead
for Breast Imaging, Breast Unit, Leeds
Teaching Hospital NHS Trust, Level 1
Chancellor Wing, St James Hospital, Leeds,
United Kingdom

SHARON SMITH, MD
Resident Physician, Breast Imaging Division,
Department of Radiology, Brigham and
Women's Hospital, Boston, Massachusetts,
USA

RAMAN VERMA, MD, FRCPC
Breast Imaging Section, Assistant Professor,
Department of Radiology, Radiologist, The
Ottawa Hospital, University of Ottawa, Ottawa,
Ontario, Canada

LOUISE S. WILKINSON, BA, BM, BCh, FRCR
Consultant Radiologist, Oxford Breast Imaging
Centre, Churchill Hospital, Headington,
Oxford, United Kingdom

CASE C. ZUIDERVELD, BS
Medical Student, University of Washington
School of Medicine, Seattle, Washington, USA

Contents

> Interval breast cancers are not detected at routine screening and are diagnosed in the interval between screening examinations. A variety of factors contribute to interval cancers, including patient and tumor characteristics as well as the screening technique and frequency. The interval cancer rate is an important metric by which the effectiveness of screening may be assessed and may serve as a surrogate for mortality benefit.

> The goal of screening is to detect breast cancers when still curable to decrease breast cancer–specific mortality. Breast cancer screening in the United States is routinely performed with digital mammography and digital breast tomosynthesis. This article reviews breast cancer doubling time by tumor subtype and examines the impact of doubling time on breast cancer screening intervals. By the article's end, the reader will be better equipped to have informed discussions with patients and medical professionals regarding the benefits and disadvantages of the currently recommended screening mammography intervals.

> Fibrocystic changes are commonly seen in clinically symptomatic patients and during imaging workup of screening-detected findings. The term "fibrocystic changes" encompasses a broad spectrum of specific benign pathologic entities. Recognition of classically benign findings of fibrocystic changes, including cysts and layering calcifications, can prevent unnecessary follow-ups and biopsies. Imaging findings such as solid masses, nonlayering calcifications, and architectural distortion may require core needle biopsy for diagnosis. In these cases, understanding the varied appearances of fibrocystic change aids determination of radiologic–pathologic concordance. Management of fibrocystic change is typically conservative.

> Breast density refers to the amount of fibroglandular tissue relative to fat on mammography and is determined either qualitatively through visual assessment or

quantitatively. It is a heritable and dynamic trait associated with age, race/ethnicity, body mass index, and hormonal factors. Increased breast density has important clinical implications including the potential to mask malignancy and as an independent risk factor for the development of breast cancer. Breast density has been incorporated into breast cancer risk models. Given the impact of dense breasts on the interpretation of mammography, supplemental screening may be indicated.

Breast MR imaging is a complementary screening tool for patients at high risk for breast cancer and has been used in the diagnostic setting. Normal enhancement of breast tissue on MR imaging is called breast parenchymal enhancement (BPE), which occurs after administration of an intravenous contrast agent. BPE varies widely due to menopausal status, use of exogenous hormones, and breast cancer treatment. Degree of BPE has also been shown to influence breast cancer risk and may predict treatment outcomes. The authors provide a comprehensive update on BPE with review of the recent literature.

Breast cancer risk prediction models based on common clinical risk factors are used to identify women eligible for high-risk screening and prevention. Unfortunately, these models have only modest discriminatory accuracy with disparities in performance in underrepresented race and ethnicity groups. The field of artificial intelligence (AI) and deep learning are rapidly advancing the field of breast cancer risk prediction with the development of mammography-based AI breast cancer risk models. Early studies suggest mammography-based AI risk models may perform better than traditional risk factor-based models with more equitable performance.

Hereditary breast cancers are manifested by pathogenic and likely pathogenic genetic mutations. Penetrance expresses the breast cancer risk associated with these genetic mutations. Although BRCA1/2 are the most widely known genetic mutations associated with breast cancer, numerous additional genes demonstrate high and moderate penetrance for breast cancer. This review describes current genetic testing, details the specific high and moderate penetrance genes for breast cancer and reviews the current approach to screening for breast cancer in patients with these genetic mutations.

Practice Advances

Breast MR imaging and contrast-enhanced mammography (CEM) are both techniques that employ intravenously injected contrast agent to assess breast lesions. This approach is associated with a very high sensitivity for malignant lesions that typically exhibit rapid enhancement due to the leakiness of neovasculature. CEM may be readily available at the breast imaging department and can be performed on the spot. Breast MR imaging provides stronger enhancement than the x-ray-based techniques and offers higher sensitivity. From a patient perspective, both modalities have their benefits and downsides; thus, patient preference could also play a role in the selection of the imaging technique.

Considering the high cost of dynamic contrast-enhanced MR imaging and various contraindications and health concerns related to administration of intravenous gadolinium-based contrast agents, there is emerging interest in non-contrast-enhanced breast MR imaging. Diffusion-weighted MR imaging (DWI) is a fast, unenhanced technique that has wide clinical applications in breast cancer detection, characterization, prognosis, and predicting treatment response. It also has the potential to serve as a non-contrast MR imaging screening method. Standardized protocols and interpretation strategies can help to enhance the clinical utility of breast DWI. A variety of other promising non-contrast MR imaging techniques are in development, but currently, DWI is closest to clinical integration, while others are still mostly used in the research setting.

This article highlights the recent publications and changing trends in practice regarding management of high-risk lesions of the breast. Traditional management has always been a surgical operation but this is recognized as overtreatment. It is recognized that overdiagnosis is inevitable but what we can control is overtreatment. Vacuum-assisted excision is now established as an alternative technique to surgery for further sampling of these high-risk lesions in the United Kingdom. Guidelines from the United Kingdom and Europe now recognize this alternative pathway, and data are available showing that vacuum-assisted excision is a safe alternative to surgery.

Practice Challenges

Abbreviated breast MR (AB-MR) imaging is a relatively new breast imaging tool, which maintains diagnostic accuracy while reducing image times compared with full-protocol breast MR (FP-MR) imaging. Breast imaging audits involve calculating individual and organizational metrics, which can be compared with established benchmarks, providing a standard against which performance can be measured. Unlike FP-MR imaging, there are no established benchmarks for AB-MR imaging but studies demonstrate comparable performance for cancer detection rate, positive predictive value 3, sensitivity, and specificity with T2. We review the basics of performing an audit, including strategies to implement if benchmarks are not being met.

This article describes an approach to planning and implementing artificial intelligence products in a breast screening service. It highlights the importance of an in-depth understanding of the end-to-end workflow and effective project planning by a multidisciplinary team. It discusses the need for monitoring to ensure that performance is stable and meets expectations, as well as focusing on the potential for inadvertantly generating inequality. New cross-discipline roles and expertise will be needed to enhance service delivery.

Effective patient communication is paramount in breast radiology, where standardized reporting and patient-centered care practices have long been established. This communication profoundly affects patient experience, well-being, and adherence to medical advice. Breast radiologists play a pivotal role in conveying diagnostic findings and addressing patient concerns, particularly in the context of cancer diagnoses. Technological advances in radiology reporting, patient access to electronic medical records, and the demand for immediate information access have reshaped radiologists' communication practices. Innovative approaches, including image-rich reports, visual timelines, and video radiology reports, have been used in various institutions to enhance patient comprehension and engagement.

RADIOLOGIC CLINICS OF NORTH AMERICA

THE CLINICS ARE AVAILABLE ONLINE!
Access your subscription at:
www.theclinics.com

PROGRAM OBJECTIVE

The objective of the *Radiologic Clinics of North America* is to keep practicing radiologists and radiology residents up to date with current clinical practice in radiology by providing timely articles reviewing the state of the art in patient care.

TARGET AUDIENCE

Practicing radiologists, radiology residents, and other healthcare professionals who provide patient care utilizing radiologic findings.

LEARNING OBJECTIVES

Upon completion of this activity, participants will be able to:
1. Describe the clinical symptoms seen in fibrocystic changes.
2. Discuss the clinical integration of artificial intelligence for breast imaging.
3. Recognize relatively new breast imaging tools that maintain diagnostic accuracy while reducing cost.

ACCREDITATION

The Elsevier Office of Continuing Medical Education (EOCME) is accredited by the Accreditation Council for Continuing Medical Education (ACCME) to provide continuing medical education for physicians.

The EOCME designates this journal-based CME activity for a maximum of 13 *AMA PRA Category 1 Credit*(s)™. Physicians should claim only the credit commensurate with the extent of their participation in the activity.

All other healthcare professionals requesting continuing education credit for this enduring material will be issued a certificate of participation.

DISCLOSURE OF CONFLICTS OF INTEREST

The EOCME assesses conflict of interest with its instructors, faculty, planners, and other individuals who are in a position to control the content of CME activities. All relevant conflicts of interest that are identified are thoroughly vetted by EOCME for fair balance, scientific objectivity, and patient care recommendations. EOCME is committed to providing its learners with CME activities that promote improvements or quality in healthcare and not a specific proprietary business or a commercial interest.

The planning committee, staff, authors, and editors listed below have identified no financial relationships or relationships to products or devices they or their spouse/life partner have with commercial interest related to the content of this CME activity:

Beatriz Elena Adrada, MD, FSBI; Shadi Aminololama-Shakeri, MD, FSBI; Debbie L. Bennett, MD; Asha A. Bhatt, MD; Arianna Buckley, MD; Sona A. Chikarmane, MD; Victoria Domonkos, MD; J. Kevin Dunbar, MBChB, MPH, FFPH; Kaitlin M. Ford, MD; Yiming Gao, MD, FSBI; Samantha L. Heller, PhD, MD, FSBI; Eric Kim, MD; Jin You Kim, MD, PhD; Kothainayaki Kulanthaivelu; Michelle V. Lee, MD; Alana A. Lewin, MD; Michelle Littlejohn; Valentina Longo, PhD; Kathryn P. Lowry, MD; Mariana Afonso Matias, MD; Frank H. Miller, MD, FACR, FSAR, FSABI; Bethany Niell, MD, PhD; Miral M. Patel, MD; Kimberly M. Ray, MD; Jean M. Seely, MDCM, FCRPC; Malvika Shah; Sharon Smith, MD; John Vassalo; Raman Verma, MD, FRCPC; Louise S. Wilkinson, BM, BCh, FRCR; Case C. Zuiderveld

The planning committee, staff, authors, and editors listed below have identified financial relationships or relationships to products or devices they or their spouse/life partner have with commercial interest related to the content of this CME activity:

Gerald Ka Tuck Lip, MB BCH BAO, MRCS, FRCR: *Speaker*: Bayer, Hologic, Inc., GE Healthcare

Ritse. M. Mann, MD, PhD: *Researcher*: Siemens Healthineers, Bayer, Beckton & Dickinson, ScreenPoint Medical, Koning Medical, Lunit, Inc., PA Imaging; *Consultant*: Siemens Healthineers, Bayer, Beckton & Dickinson, ScreenPoint Medical; *Advisor*: Siemens Healthineers, Bayer, Beckton & Dickinson, ScreenPoint Medical, Koning Medical, PA Imaging; *Speaker:* Siemens Healthineers, Bayer, Beckton & Dickinson, ScreenPoint Medical; *Royalties*: Elsevier, Inc.

Savannah C. Partridge, PhD: *Advisor*: Guerbet LLC; *Researcher*: GE Healthcare, Philips Healthcare

Nisha Sharma, MBChB, BSc (Hons), MRCP, FRCR, MSc: *Speaker*: BD, Hologic, Inc.

UNAPPROVED/OFF-LABEL USE DISCLOSURE

The EOCME requires CME faculty to disclose to the participants:
1. When products or procedures being discussed are off-label, unlabelled, experimental, and/or investigational (not US Food and Drug Administration [FDA] approved); and
2. Any limitations on the information presented, such as data that are preliminary or that represent ongoing research, interim analyses, and/or unsupported opinions. Faculty may discuss information about pharmaceutical agents that is outside of FDA-approved labelling. This information is intended solely for CME and is not intended to promote off-label use of these medications. If you have any questions, contact the medical affairs department of the manufacturer for the most recent prescribing information.

TO ENROLL
To enroll in the *Radiologic Clinics of North America* Continuing Medical Education program, call customer service at 1-800-654-2452 or sign up online at http://www.theclinics.com/home/cme. The CME program is available to subscribers for an additional annual fee of USD 340.00.

METHOD OF PARTICIPATION
In order to claim credit, participants must complete the following:
1. Complete enrolment as indicated above.
2. Read the activity.
3. Complete the CME Test and Evaluation. Participants must achieve a score of 70% on the test. All CME Tests and Evaluations must be completed online.

CME INQUIRIES/SPECIAL NEEDS
For all CME inquiries or special needs, please contact elsevierCME@elsevier.com.

Preface
Breast Imaging Essentials

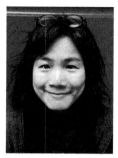
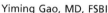

Yiming Gao, MD, FSBI   Samantha L. Heller, PhD, MD, FSBI
Editors

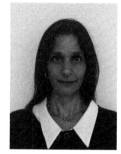

We welcome you to this collection of "Breast Imaging Essentials." We hope these articles will offer a fresh take on foundational knowledge and provide tools to understand cutting-edge advances in breast cancer imaging.

The collection is divided into four thematic sections: *Basics Revisited, Understanding Risk, Practice Advances,* and *Practice Challenges.* In the section on *Basics Revisited*, we tackle the nature and significance of interval cancers in understanding screening outcomes. In the second article, we take an in-depth look at tumor doubling time and its impact on how we optimize screening intervals. The final article in this section offers a clinically focused perspective on fibrocystic change, a commonly encountered but poorly understood entity.

In the section on *Understanding Risk*, we offer an update on breast cancer biomarkers and their role in risk prediction. In the first article, we explore recent developments in breast density assessment and implications for cancer detection and risk stratification. The second article focuses on background parenchymal enhancement both as a perceptive challenge on MR imaging and as a biomarker for short-term and long-term risk. The next review delves into the promises and challenges of using artificial intelligence (AI) for breast cancer risk assessment. The last article of the section discusses the nature of intermediate- to high-risk genetic mutations and reviews guidelines for appropriate testing and imaging approaches at the patient level.

Next, in *Practice Advances*, we take a close look at advanced imaging techniques. First, we compare abbreviated MR imaging and contrast-enhanced mammography, providing an analysis of strengths and limitations. This is followed by an in-depth discussion of noncontrast MR imaging with DWI, which is a valuable adjunct to conventional MR imaging techniques. The work also focuses on leveraging noncontrast techniques as potential screening alternatives. The third article in this section offers an international perspective on nonsurgical management of high-risk lesions.

Our final section on *Practice Challenges* addresses current and evolving issues in the clinical

Radiol Clin N Am 62 (2024) xiii–xiv
https://doi.org/10.1016/j.rcl.2024.01.003
0033-8389/24/© 2024 Published by Elsevier Inc.

realm. The first review offers a thoughtful consideration of how to perform an abbreviated MR imaging audit based on conventional MR imaging standards. In the second article, we consider the complex issues surrounding the implementation of AI in the clinical world and offer a framework with which to navigate them. In the final article, we explore how emerging technological innovations have and will transform the way we communicate with our patients.

Many thanks to the authors, who gave their time and expertise for this project. We are delighted to offer this wonderful collection to you, and we hope you learn as much as we have.

DISCLOSURE

None.

Yiming Gao, MD, FSBI
Department of Radiology, New York University
School of Medicine, New York, NY, USA

Samantha L. Heller, PhD, MD, FSBI
Department of Radiology, New York University
School of Medicine, New York, NY, USA

E-mail addresses:
yiming.gao@nyulangone.org (Y. Gao)
Samantha.Heller@nyulangone.org (S.L. Heller)

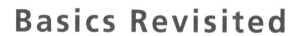

Basics Revisited

Interval Cancers in Understanding Screening Outcomes

Kimberly M. Ray, MD

KEYWORDS

• Interval cancer • Screening • Mammography • Tomosynthesis • MR imaging • Ultrasound

KEY POINTS

- Interval cancers are not detected at screening and are diagnosed in the interval between routine screening examinations.
- The interval cancer rate is affected by patient and tumor characteristics as well as the screening technique and interval.
- The interval cancer rate may serve as a surrogate endpoint for mortality in the assessment of new screening techniques.

INTRODUCTION

Screening mammography has been shown to reduce breast cancer mortality through the detection of disease during its asymptomatic, preclinical phase. However, up to 15% to 30% of cancers may be missed at routine screening.[1] An interval breast cancer is defined as a cancer that is diagnosed, typically on the basis of clinical signs or symptoms, after a normal screening examination, during the interval before the next routine screen. Interval cancers have been shown to be associated with more aggressive biology and higher mortality rates compared to screen-detected cancers.[2,3] Consequently, the interval cancer rate (ICR) is an important metric by which the effectiveness of screening may be assessed, and the ICR may serve as a surrogate marker for the mortality benefit of screening.[4]

RISK FACTORS FOR INTERVAL BREAST CANCERS

Studies have shown that among interval breast cancers, 20% to 25% are missed at screening mammography due to interpretive error as these cancers are detectable on blinded retrospective review. Strategies to minimize these avoidable false negatives include attention to good mammographic technique, comparison with prior studies, awareness of the subtle mammographic signs of malignancy, and avoidance of satisfaction of search error.[5–8]

For the remaining 75% to 80% of interval cancers that are not detectable on prior screening examinations, there are many possible predisposing factors that relate to patient and tumor characteristics as well as screening technique and regimens. An understanding of how these various factors may contribute to screening failure is necessary in order to develop strategies for improvement.

Patient Characteristics

Dense breast tissue is a known limitation of mammography due to its potential to mask underlying cancer. A population-based study of American women showed that mammographic sensitivity was 87% for women with fatty breasts and progressively declined with increasing density to 62.9% in women with extremely dense breasts.[9] Since younger age is correlated with breast density, the latter is a major contributor to screening failure in

Department of Radiology and Biomedical Sciences, University of California, San Francisco, UCSF Medical Center, 1825 4th Street, L3185, Box 4034, San Francisco, CA 94107, USA
E-mail address: Kimberly.ray@ucsf.edu

Radiol Clin N Am 62 (2024) 559–569
https://doi.org/10.1016/j.rcl.2023.12.012

young women. However, because overall breast cancer incidence increases with age, the false-negative rate of mammography in women with dense breasts also increases steadily with age.[10]

Supplemental screening techniques may improve cancer detection in women with dense breasts. However, as will be discussed later, supplemental screening on the basis of breast density alone or in combination with other risk factors remains controversial and requires weighing of the risks and benefits.

Higher rates of interval breast cancers have also been shown to correlate with family history of breast cancer, particularly in mutation carriers, for whom mammography has proved to be markedly limited.[11,12] This is likely due to a combination of biologically aggressive disease in this population and higher breast density given the younger age at disease onset.

Patients with a personal history of breast cancer who are treated with breast conserving surgery continue to be at elevated risk for local recurrence in the ipsilateral or contralateral breast at a rate of 0.5% to 1% per year.[13,14] Early detection of second breast cancers through mammographic screening has been shown to improve survival outcomes.[15] However, mammographic sensitivity is decreased in this population, likely due in part to the difficulty of assessing for recurrence in the setting of post-surgical changes. Mammography has been shown to be especially limited in women with personal history who are 50 years or younger at diagnosis and those with extremely dense breasts.[16]

Tumor Characteristics

Tumor characteristics may also contribute to mammography failure. Infiltrating lobular carcinoma (ILC) often presents a perceptual challenge and may be more often missed at screening owing to its infiltrative growth pattern, presenting as subtle asymmetry or architectural distortion rather than a discrete mass.[17–19] Consequently, ILC is overrepresented among false negatives at screening mammography and more likely than other histologic subtypes to present as a symptomatic interval cancer at a more advanced stage.[20,21]

Tumor growth rates also influence screen detection. Screening is inherently biased toward the detection of slower growing cancers. This is referred to as length bias, whereby tumors with slow to intermediate growth rates that have a longer preclinical phase or sojourn time, will be more amenable to screen detection. In contrast, very fast growing tumors may arise in the interval

between screening examinations and thereby evade detection. In keeping with these observations, studies have reported higher expression of markers of cellular proliferation among interval cancers such as Ki-67 index and S-phase fraction.[22–24]

Further studies have shown that interval cancers more often exhibit poor prognostic features compared to screen-detected cancers such as larger tumor size and higher nuclear grade, higher rates of nodal metastases, and more advanced disease stage.[25–27] Compared to screen-detected cancers, interval cancers are more often triple-negative or human epidermal growth factor receptor 2 (HER2) overexpressing,[28,29] subtypes that are both biologically more aggressive compared to estrogen receptor positive, luminal subtypes (**Fig. 1**). As expected, interval cancers have been shown to have worse survival outcomes compared to cancers detected at screening.[2,30]

STRATEGIES TO REDUCE INTERVAL CANCERS

There are 2 basic approaches to reducing the interval cancer rate (ICR). The first is to reduce the screening interval, which should enable the detection of more tumors with faster growth rates. The second entails an improvement in the sensitivity of screening with newer technology such as digital breast tomosynthesis as well as adjuncts to mammography including ultrasound and MR imaging. As will be discussed, the ICR is an important surrogate measure of the benefit of new and/or supplemental screening tests.

Screening Intervals

Studies based on biennial screening have reported interval cancers representing 17% to 30% of total cancers as compared to 14.7% for annual screening and 32% to 38% for triennial screening.[1,31] Data from population screening show interval cancer rates less than 0.8 cancers/1000 screens in annual screening programs and 0.8 to 2.1 cancers/1000 screens in biennial screening programs, with the majority of interval cancers arising in year 2 of a biennial interval.[1]

In a single study from Canada in which 148,575 women were screened with digital mammography, the ICR was 0.89/1000 for those screened annually versus 1.45/1000 for women screened biennially.[32] Therefore, it has been observed that efforts to increase adherence to annual screening would be an effective way to decrease interval cancers.[33]

Because there is a range of cancer growth rates at any age, annual screening offers the greatest benefit and has been shown to reduce ICR in all

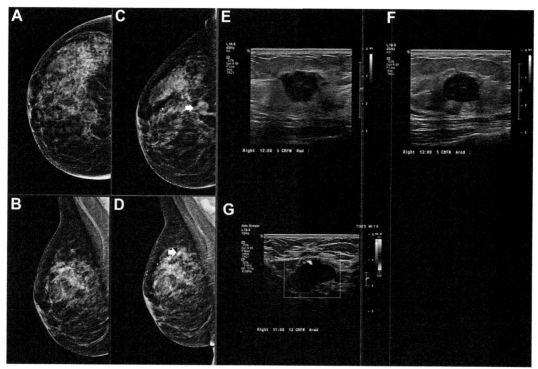

Fig. 1. A 67-year-old female patient with heterogeneously dense breasts who had a negative screening digital breast tomosynthesis examination (*A, B*; only 2D images of the right breast shown). Six months later, she reported a palpable right upper central breast lump and diagnostic mammography (*C, D*) showed a new irregular mass (*arrows*). Ultrasound images (*E, F*) showed an irregular, hypoechoic mass with angular margins and an enlarged right axillary lymph node (*G*). Pathology showed invasive ductal carcinoma, estrogen and progesterone receptor negative, human epidermal growth factor receptor 2 positive, with axillary nodal metastasis.

age groups.[34] However, younger women have been shown on average to have higher rates of rapidly growing tumors, as evidenced by the shorter average lead time for cancer detection in younger women.[35,36] Analysis of data from the Swedish Two-County Trial and Breast Cancer Detection Demonstration Project (BCDDP) showed that the lead time for mammography screening in women aged 40 to 49 years is approximately 2 years, as compared to 3.5 years in women over 50 years of age.[35,36] In order for screening to be maximally effective, the screening interval should be less than half of the lead time.[36,37] Therefore, for women aged 40 to 49, annual screening is especially critical for reducing breast cancer mortality. Studies have shown the ICR to be significantly lower in women age 40 to 49 years when comparing annual versus biennial or triennial screening intervals.[38–40]

INTERVAL CANCER RATE AS SURROGATE MARKER FOR ASSESSING NEWER TECHNOLOGIES

Mammography is the only screening modality to be validated by randomized control trial (RCTs) that use mortality as their endpoint. Absent proof of mortality benefit, establishing the value of a new screening test is challenging and subject to various biases (**Table 1**). Finding cancers earlier may not necessarily alter their natural history and delay the time of death (lead time bias). Finding additional cancers is not necessarily beneficial because some cancers may be so indolent that they do not pose a significant health threat (overdiagnosis). Nevertheless, it is necessary to rely on surrogate measures to assess newer technologies since randomized trials require such large populations and lengthy follow-up that the technologies may be obsolete by trial completion.[4,41]

The biological behavior of cancers detected or prevented by a screening test can provide valuable clues to the efficacy of that test. For example, the ICR has been proposed as a surrogate measure for mortality since interval cancers are by definition progressive (therefore not overdiagnosed) and associated with more aggressive biology and worse prognosis.[4,42] If the ICR is reduced through the application of a screening test, then a mortality benefit is likely.

Table 1
Potential biases in assessing the effectiveness of a screening test

Screening Outcome Measure	Bias	Source of Bias
Finding cancer at an earlier stage	Lead time bias	Finding cancer at an earlier stage may not alter the disease outcome (delay the time of death). However, survival time appears to be prolonged due to earlier diagnosis.
Finding cancers with better prognosis	Length bias	Tumors with slow to intermediate growth rates that have a longer preclinical phase are more likely to be detected through screening. These cancers may have better survival outcomes than those that are clinically detected.
Finding more cancers	Overdiagnosis	Some indolent cancers may not have lethal potential, especially in older patients and/or those with competing comorbidities.

CANDIDATE SCREENING TECHNIQUES FOR REDUCING THE INTERVAL CANCER RATE
Digital Breast Tomosynthesis

Digital breast tomosynthesis (DBT) has been shown to reduce screening recall rates and increase invasive cancer detection compared to screening with digital mammography (DM) alone.[43] In the absence of RCTs assessing mortality as an endpoint, it is unknown whether the improved cancer detection with DBT may translate into mortality benefit. Some series have shown that the additional cancers detected at DBT predominantly reflect the biologically less aggressive, luminal A subtype that is more likely to present as a small spiculated mass,[44–47] raising the question of whether their earlier detection is of clinical benefit. One way to determine if the cancers detected at DBT are likely to impact mortality is to assess the ICR .[42]

Several prospective European trials and retrospective US observational studies have addressed the effect of DBT on the ICR relative to conventional digital mammography.[48–55] None of these studies has demonstrated a statistically significant reduction in the ICR in women undergoing DBT screening. An Italian RCT reported 70% increased cancer detection rate for DBT relative to DM, yet there was no significant difference in the rate of interval cancers or advanced cancers at subsequent screening round.[49] Investigators for the Malmo Breast Tomosynthesis Screening Trial compared the ICR for trial subjects that underwent DBT plus DM to controls randomly selected from the screening population undergoing DM alone.[55] Although there was a statistically significant lower ICR in the DBT arm relative to controls (1.6 vs 2.8 per 1000), the populations compared had different screening intervals. After controlling for age, which

determines the screening interval in the Swedish screening program, the difference in ICR was no longer statistically significant.

A major limitation of studies to date in assessing ICR with DBT is that they have all been underpowered to detect statistically significant differences given that interval cancers are rare events.[56] Durand and colleagues reported one of the largest US studies on ICR including over 380,000 examinations, but estimated they would require a sample size of more than 2.2 million to show a difference in ICR of 0.1 per 1000 women with DBT at 80% power.[53] The ongoing Tomosynthesis Mammographic Imaging Screening trial (TMIST) has a target enrollment of 129,000 women, and therefore may also lack sufficient power to demonstrate any reduction in ICR, although other surrogate markers such as advanced cancer rates will also be investigated.[57]

Kerlikowske and colleagues performed a large US retrospective cohort study using data from the Breast Cancer Surveillance Consortium (BCSC) database, which is composed of 5 registries representative of the US population.[58] Results of 504,427 women undergoing 1,379,089 screening mammograms 2011 to 2018 were reported. During the follow-up period, 0.57 symptomatic interval invasive cancers per 1000 DBT examinations and 0.61 per 1000 DM examinations were detected within 12 months of screening. The ICR was not significantly different for DBT and DM overall or when stratified based on breast density or BCSC 5-year risk.

Houssami and colleagues performed a meta-analysis of 4 prospective, population-based European studies comparing interval cancers in DBT versus DM screening.[42] There was no significant difference in the ICR between modalities, but there was a statistically significant reduction in the rate of axillary node-positive interval cancers in the DBT-screened group. This observation suggests that despite its lack of effect on the ICR, DBT may potentially downstage breast cancer at diagnosis and could potentially reduce the rate of advanced stage cancer on long-term follow-up, which would be expected to yield a mortality benefit.

Ultrasound

Ultrasound (US) has been studied as adjunct to screening mammography, primarily for women with dense breast tissue. Corsetti and colleagues performed a retrospective cohort study comparing women with dense breasts and negative screening mammography that underwent supplemental US screening (n = 7224) to women with non-dense breasts (n = 12,504) who underwent mammography alone.[59] An additional 4.4 cancers per 1000 screens were detected in the US arm. The interval cancer rate in women with dense breasts who underwent supplemental US screening was similar to that for women with non-dense breasts receiving mammography alone (1.1 vs 1.0 per 1000). As the ICR would be expected to be higher in the absence of supplemental screening based on prior studies,[10] the investigators suggested that supplemental US screening might help overcome the limitations of breast density.

The ACRIN 6666 trial prospectively evaluated the performance of mammography alone versus in combination with hand-held screening US over 3 annual screening rounds in 2662 women with dense breasts and intermediate breast cancer risk.[60] Fifty-four percent of study participants had a personal history of breast cancer. Mammography and US examinations were interpreted independently. Supplemental US resulted in an additional 4.3 cancers per 1000 screens, the majority of which were node-negative invasive cancers. The interval cancer rate was 1.2 per 1000. Interval cancers accounted for only 8% of all cancers in the trial, comparing favorably with the 15% ICR for annual mammography screening reported in the literature for an unselected patient population.[31] However, this was at the cost of higher false-positive rates. On incidence screens, the rate of biopsy recommendation remained high at 5%, with a cancer yield of only 7.4%.

Song and colleagues reported the performance of US surveillance in women with and without a personal history of breast cancer who had negative mammography.[61] Despite a higher incremental cancer detection rate (2.88 vs 0.53 per 1000) in women with versus without personal history, the ICR remained higher for women with personal history (1.50 vs 0.53 per 1000). Among women with personal history, the ICR was higher in those age < 50 years than age ≥ 50 years (3.86 vs 0.25) and in women with dense relative to fatty breasts (2.58 vs 0). Therefore, the authors cautioned that supplemental breast US screening may not be sufficiently effective for younger women aged < 50 years with personal history of breast cancer.

In the J-START (Japan Strategic Anti-cancer Randomized Trial) trial, women 40 to 49 years were assigned to undergo screening with mammography alone versus in combination with handheld US.[62] Women with history of breast cancer in the past 5 years were excluded. Fifty-eight percent of women in the study had dense breasts. Supplemental US resulted in a statistically significant increase in the cancer detection rate (CDR) from 3.3 to 5 per 1,000, with a higher proportion of stage 0 and 1 cancers in the intervention group. There was an accompanying statistically significant reduction in the ICR from 1.0 to 0.5 per 1,000, which remained significant after subgroup analysis stratified by breast density.[63]

Lee and colleagues performed a retrospective cohort study using data from 2 Breast Cancer Surveillance Consortium (BCSC) registries that reflect US community practice.[64] A total of 3386 women who underwent 6081 concurrent screening mammography and ultrasonography examinations were compared to a risk-matched control group that underwent mammography alone. Women with personal history of breast cancer were excluded. Nearly three-quarters of the women undergoing screening ultrasound had dense breasts, half were younger than 50 years, and over half had low or average BCSC 5-year risk scores. There were no statistically significant differences in either the cancer detection rates (5.4 vs 5.5 per 1000) or interval cancer rates (1.5 vs 1.9 per 1000) for screening with mammography alone or in combination with ultrasound. However, significantly higher false-positive biopsy and short interval follow-up rates as well as lower positive predictive value (PPV) of biopsy were noted for screening ultrasound. The authors acknowledged that their lower risk population included women with non-dense breasts and their small number of total cancers may have limited their ability to detect significant differences in CDR and ICR. In addition, their outcomes reflected the performance of community practices, which may differ from that of screening trial centers.

Taken together, studies of supplemental US screening suggest that it may modestly reduce the ICR in select patient populations. However, this is at the cost of a higher false-positive follow-up and biopsy recommendation rate. More evidence is needed to define the patient selection criteria that would yield the greatest benefit from screening US.

Breast MR imaging

Hereditary breast cancer

MR imaging screening has been primarily investigated in women with elevated breast cancer risk. Relative to women of average risk, those with BRCA1 or BRCA2 mutations are estimated to have a greater than 60% lifetime risk of developing breast cancer, with younger age of disease onset and faster tumor growth rates.[65] With routine annual screening mammography, interval cancer rates for BRCA carriers range from 35% to 50%, with invasive tumor size larger than 1 cm in 40% to 78% and regional nodal metastases in 20% to 56% of patients.[12,66] Because of the inadequate performance of mammography alone in this patient population, international screening guidelines recommend MR imaging surveillance for women with hereditary breast cancer risk.[65,67,68] A substantial body of evidence supports the use of MR imaging in this patient population, and the impact of MR imaging on the ICR serves as an important surrogate measure of its effectiveness.

A systematic review by Warner and colleagues pooled data from 11 prospective studies that screened women at very high risk for breast cancer using a combination of mammography and MR imaging, with or without ultrasound and clinical breast examination.[69] Reported sensitivity of combined mammography and MR imaging ranged from 80% to 100%, compared to 25% to 59% with mammography alone. More than half of the cancers were in situ or smaller than 1 cm and rates of axillary nodal metastasis were 12% to 21%. The interval cancer rate was less than 10% in studies with more than 1 round of screening. False-positive (FP) rates were highest in the first year, with a gradual decline in subsequent years, reaching equivalence to mammography after 4 years.

A more recent meta-analysis of 1951 women with BRCA1/2 mutations from 6 prospective MR imaging screening studies, which included 345 women with a personal history of breast or ovarian cancer, showed that MR imaging had higher sensitivity than mammography (85.3% vs 39.6%, $P < .001$), although MR imaging had lower specificity (84.7% vs 93.6%, $P = .01$).[70] The interval cancer rate was 12.5%.

Additional performance measures of MR imaging screening, when viewed in conjunction with the reduction in the ICR, lend support to the hypothesis that MR imaging improves long-term outcomes in BRCA mutation carriers. Observational studies have shown a downward shift in the stage of breast cancers detected by MR imaging.[71,72]

Furthermore, annual MR imaging screening has led to significantly decreased rates of advanced-stage and node-positive breast cancer at 6 years of follow-up.[73] BRCA2 carriers who were diagnosed with early stage disease at MR imaging have shown improved 10-year survival.[74] Therefore, although mortality data are lacking, the downstaging of disease with MR imaging screening, a subsequent reduction in the rate of interval and advanced cancers and improved survival outcomes all strongly suggest that a mortality benefit is likely.

Breast MR imaging has also been studied in women at elevated risk due to a family history of breast cancer. The FaMRIsc multicenter, RCT in the Netherlands, enrolled women 30 to 55 years with lifetime risk of at least 20% due to family history, but without any known genetic mutation.[75] Women were randomized to annual breast MR imaging and biennial mammography or annual mammography alone. Relative to the mammography only arm, the CDR in the MR imaging arm increased from 2.0 to 8.2 per 1000 for invasive cancer, and the ICR declined from 0.6 to 0.3 per 1000. Downstaging of disease was also observed in the MR imaging arm with smaller median tumor size (9 mm vs 17 mm), and lower rates of nodal metastasis (17 vs 63%). Therefore, the pattern of outcomes for those with familial risk is similar to mutation carriers, although the magnitude of the benefit is smaller.

Personal history of breast cancer

MR imaging surveillance of women with a personal history of breast cancer has been recommended given their elevated risk status and the suboptimal sensitivity of mammography, particularly in those with dense breasts and/or young age at presentation.[16,76] Retrospective studies of MR imaging surveillance have shown similar rates of cancer detection but significantly lower rates of false-positives in women with a personal history of breast cancer compared to those without such history as well as compared to mutation carriers or those with family history of breast cancer.[60,77]

Cho and colleagues reported on a prospective, multicenter trial that compared annual mammography alone or in combination with supplemental ultrasound or MR imaging in a cohort of 754 women with history of breast cancer at age ≤50 years.[78] Participants underwent 3 annual MR imaging screenings in addition to mammography and US, with independent readings. The addition of MR imaging to mammography led to an incremental cancer yield of 3.8 per 1000 and increased sensitivity from 52.9% to 100%. By comparison, the addition of ultrasound to mammography increased sensitivity to 82.4% and all US-detected cancers were also detected by MR imaging. Most detected cancers were stage 0 or 1 and node negative. There were no interval cancers. By comparison, a prior study reported 7.5 interval cancers per 1000 women with personal history of breast cancer before age 50 who underwent mammography screening, suggesting that MR imaging could effectively lower the ICR in this patient population.[16] However, compared with mammography alone, the addition of MR imaging increased the recall rate (4.4% to 13.8%), biopsy rate (from 0.5% to 2.7%), and short-term follow-up rate (from 3.6% to 10.2%), which led to decreased specificity (from 96% to 87%).

The ACRIN 6666 trial enrolled women with dense breasts who were at intermediate risk for breast cancer, with over half having a personal history of breast cancer.[60] Study patients underwent a single round of MR imaging screening after 3 annual rounds of mammography and ultrasound screening. The cancer yield of MR imaging was the same for women with or without a personal history, although the false-positive rate was lower for the former. Similar to the study by Cho and colleagues,[78] the incremental cancer yield of MR imaging was higher than US, with a single prevalence round of MR imaging screening yielding 14.7 additional cancers per 1000 relative to mammography plus US. Cho and colleagues reported a much lower supplemental yield of MR imaging (3.8 per 1000), which likely reflects patient selection; in their study, 91.9% of patients had preoperative MR imaging and those at highest risk of recurrence (positive surgical margins or omission of postoperative radiotherapy) were excluded from the study. Data regarding the impact of MR imaging on the ICR in the ACRIN study are not available.

Supplemental magnetic resonance screening for dense breasts

Given the higher likelihood of screening failure in women with dense breasts and the elevated risk conferred by density, breast MR imaging has also undergone evaluation as a tool for supplemental screening in women with dense breasts. In the Dutch DENSE RCT, supplemental screening with MR imaging versus mammography alone was compared in women with extremely dense breasts and no additional risk factors.[79] Prevalence screening with MR imaging yielded an incremental CDR of 16.5 per 1000 and a corresponding large reduction in the interval cancer rate from 5.0 to 0.8 per 1000. Of note, the study employed a biennial screening interval, which likely accounted for the high baseline ICR, especially since a greater

proportion of interval cancers will arise during the second year. Therefore, the results may not be generalizable to annual screening. Study investigators noted that the high recall rate of 94.9 per 1000 screenings on MR imaging was concerning, although the biopsy PPV of 26.3% was comparable to mammography.

Compared to the J-START ultrasound screening trial, the incremental cancer detection rate of MR imaging was much higher for the DENSE trial (16.5 vs 3.3 per 1000) and the reduction in ICR was much greater (−4.2 vs −0.5 per 1000). However, the breast cancer incidence is likely to differ between the 2 trial populations, Japanese women aged 40 to 49 years versus Dutch women aged 50 to 75 years. In addition, the baseline interval-cancer rates were much lower in the J-START trial (1.0 vs 5.0), which may be related to a lower breast cancer incidence, the shorter 1-year screening interval, as well as the inclusion of all breast density categories.

The ECOG-ACRIN 1141 Trial investigated the performance of abbreviated breast MR imaging (Ab-MRI) relative to DBT in women of average risk with dense breasts.[80] Ab-MRI has been shown to have equivalent diagnostic performance to full protocol MR imaging and has been proposed as a cost-effective supplemental screening technique for women with dense breasts. MR imaging and DBT were performed concurrently but interpreted independently. The invasive cancer detection rate per 1000 was 11.8 for abMRI vs 4.8 for DBT. No interval cancers were found at 1 year follow-up. The sensitivity of Ab-MRI was significantly higher than that of DBT (95.7% vs 39.1%) and its specificity was significantly lower (86.7% vs 97.4%), although there was no significant difference in biopsy PPV (19.0% vs 35.5%). The relatively reduced specificity for MR imaging compared to DBT may partly be attributable to the availability of prior comparison examinations only for DBT.

SUMMARY

Interval breast cancers represent clinically progressive disease that evades screen detection. Such cancers tend to be biologically aggressive and are associated with worse clinical outcomes. Therefore, the ICR is an important measure of the effectiveness of screening and can be used as a surrogate for the mortality benefit of new or supplemental screening techniques. For screening mammography, annual screening is associated with a lower ICR than biennial screening.

Among candidate technologies for supplemental screening, MR imaging is associated with the largest reduction in the ICR and is recommended for high-risk screening, particularly in gene mutation carriers. Among women of intermediate and average risk, outcomes data are much more limited regarding alternative or supplemental techniques, including DBT, US, and MR imaging. Both US and MR imaging have been shown to reduce the ICR in the setting of RCTs involving select patient populations that limit generalizability of their results. For women of average risk undergoing annual mammography screening, the baseline ICR is low, and most studies evaluating the added benefit of DBT have been underpowered to demonstrate statistically significant reductions in the ICR.

A reduction in the ICR is highly suggestive of, but not mandatory for the prediction of a mortality benefit. Other surrogate endpoints also need to be considered. The prevention of advanced stage disease through earlier detection is also strongly correlated with a reduction in mortality. In many of the studies reviewed here, there is evidence that MR imaging, US, and to a lesser extent DBT, result in downstaging of disease at diagnosis. With MR imaging, a corresponding reduction in advanced cancers has also been shown on subsequent screening rounds, which is a compelling indicator of benefit, even in the setting of a modest decrease in ICR. Additional studies employing a combination of these surrogate endpoints are needed to further define the relative benefits and risks of different screening approaches for specific patient populations.

CLINICS CARE POINTS

- Factors that increase the risk of interval breast cancers include higher breast density, younger age, genetic or familial risk, and personal history of breast cancer.

- Annual screening mammography is associated with lower interval cancer rates than biennial screening.

- Supplemental screening with breast MR imaging has been shown to lower the ICR, particularly for gene mutation carriers.

DISCLOSURE

The author has nothing to disclose.

REFERENCES

1. Houssami N, Hunter K. The epidemiology, radiology and biological characteristics of interval breast cancers in population mammography screening. NPJ Breast Cancer 2017;3:12.
2. Domingo L, Blanch J, Servitja S, et al. Aggressiveness features and outcomes of true interval cancers: comparison between screen-detected and symptom-detected cancers. Eur J Cancer Prev 2013;22:21–8.
3. Niraula S, Biswanger N, Hu P, et al. Incidence, characteristics, and outcomes of interval breast cancers compared with screening-detected breast cancers. JAMA Netw Open 2020;3(9):e2018179.
4. Irwig L, Houssami N, Armstrong B, et al. Evaluating new screening tests for breast cancer. BMJ 2006; 332(7543):678–9.
5. Harvey JA, Fajardo LL, Innis CA. Previous mammograms in patients with impalpable breast carcinoma: Retrospective vs blinded interpretation. AJR 1993; 161:1167–72.
6. Sickles EA. Mammographic features of 300 consecutive nonpalpable breast cancers. AJR 1986;146(4): 661–3.
7. Hofvind Solveig, Geller Berta, Skaane Per. Mammographic features and histopathological findings of interval breast cancers. Acta Radiol 2008;49(9): 975–81.
8. Brenner RJ. Brenner RJ False-negative mammograms. Medical, legal, and risk management implications. Radiol Clin North Am 2000;38(4):741–57.
9. Carney PA, Miglioretti DL, Yankaskas BC, et al. Individual and combined effects of age, breast density, and hormone replacement therapy use on the accuracy of screening mammography. Ann Intern Med 2003;138(3):168–75.
10. Kerlikowske K. The mammogram that cried Wolfe. N Engl J Med 2007;356:297–300.
11. Nguyen TL, Li S, Dite GS, et al. Interval breast cancer risk associations with breast density, family history and breast tissue aging. Int J Cancer 2020; 147(2):375–82.
12. Komenaka IK, Ditkoff BA, Joseph KA, et al. The development of interval breast malignancies in patients with BRCA mutations. Cancer: Interdisciplinary International Journal of the American Cancer Society 2004;100(10):2079–83.
13. Kreike B, Hart AAM, van de Velde T, et al. Continuing risk of ipsilateral breast relapse after breast-conserving therapy at long-term follow-up. Int J Radiat Oncol Biol Phys 2008;71:1014–21.
14. Gao X, Fisher SG, Emami B. Risk of second primary cancer in the contralateral breast in women treated for early-stage breast cancer: a population-based study. Int J Radiat Oncol Biol Phys 2003;56: 1038–45.
15. Lu WL, Jansen L, Post WJ, et al. Impact on survival of early detection of isolated breast recurrences after the primary treatment for breast cancer: a meta-analysis. Breast Cancer Res Treat 2009;114:403–12.

16. Houssami N, Abraham LA, Miglioretti DL, et al. Accuracy and outcomes of screening mammography in women with a personal history of early-stage breast cancer. JAMA 2011;305(8):790–9.

17. Holland R, Hendriks JHCL, Mravunac M. Mammographically occult breast cancer: a pathologic and radiologic study. Cancer 1983;52:1810–9.

18. Ma L, Fishell E, Wright B, et al. Case–control study of factors associated with failure to detect breast cancer by mammography. J Natl Cancer Inst 1992;84:781–5.

19. Sickles EA. The subtle and atypical mammographic features of invasive lobular carcinoma. Radiology 1991;153:25–6.

20. Hilleren DJ, Andersson IT, Lindholm K, et al. Invasive lobular carcinoma: mammographic findings in a 10-year experience. Radiology 1991 Jan;178(1):149–54.

21. Krecke KN, Gisvold JJ. Invasive lobular carcinoma of the breast: mammographic findings and extent of disease at diagnosis in 184 patients. AJR 1993;161:957–60.

22. Vitak B, Stal O, Manson JC, et al. Interval cancers and cancers in non-attenders in the Ostergotland Mammographic Screening Programme. Duration between screening and diagnosis, S-phase fraction and distant recurrence. Eur J Cancer 1997;33:1453–60.

23. Crosier M, Scott D, Wilson RG, et al. Differences in Ki67 and c-erbB2 expression between screen-detected and true interval breast cancers. Clin Cancer Res 1999;5:2682–8.

24. Kirsh VA, Chiarelli AM, Edwards SA, et al. Tumor characteristics associated with mammographic detection of breast cancer in the Ontario Breast Screening Program. J Natl Cancer Inst 2011;103:942–50.

25. Meshkat B, Prichard RS, Al-Hilli Z, et al. A comparison of clinical-pathological characteristics between symptomatic and interval breast cancer. Breast 2015;24:278–82.

26. Weber RJ, van Bommel RMG, Louwman MW, et al. Characteristics and prognosis of interval cancers after biennial screen-film or full-field digital screening mammography. Breast Cancer Res Treat 2016;158:471–83.

27. Burrell HC, Sibbering DM, Wilson AR, et al. Screening interval breast cancers: mammographic features and prognosis factors. Radiology 1996;199(3):811–7.

28. Domingo L, Sala M, Servitja S, et al. Phenotypic characterization and risk factors for interval breast cancers in a population-based breast cancer screening program in Barcelona, Spain. Cancer Causes Control 2010;21:1155–64.

29. Rayson D, Payne JI, Abdolell M, et al. Comparison of clinical-pathologic characteristics and outcomes of true interval and screen-detected invasive breast cancer among participants of a Canadian breast screening program: a nested case-control study. Clin Breast Cancer 2011;11:27–32.

30. Porter GJR, Evans AJ, Burrell HC, et al. Interval breast cancers: prognostic features and survival by subtype and time since screening. J Med Screen 2006;13(3):115–22.

31. Henderson LM, Miglioretti DL, Kerlikowske K, et al. Breast cancer characteristics associated with digital versus film-screen mammography for screen-detected and interval cancers. AJR Am J Roentgenol 2015;205:676–84.

32. Seely JM, Peddle SE, Yang H, et al. Breast density and risk of interval cancers: the effect of annual versus biennial screening mammography policies in Canada. Can Assoc Radiol J 2022;73(1):90–100.

33. Friedewald SM, Grimm LJ. Digital breast tomosynthesis and detection of interval invasive and advanced breast cancers. JAMA 2022 Jun 14;327(22):2198–200.

34. Moorman SEH, Pujara AC, Sakala MD, et al. Annual screening mammography associated with lower stage breast cancer compared with biennial screening. AJR 2021;217:40–7.

35. Moskowitz M. Breast cancer: age-specific growth rates and screening strategies. Radiology 1986;161(1):37–41.

36. Tabar L, Faberberg G, Day NE, et al. What is the optimum interval between mammographic screening examinations? An analysis based on the latest results of the Swedish two-county breast cancer screening trial. Br J Cancer 1987;55(5):547–51.

37. Kopans DB. Breast imaging. 3rd edition. Philadelphia, PA: Lippincott; 2007. p. 129–35.

38. Klemi PJ, Toikkanen S, Rasanen O, et al. Mammography screening interval and the frequency of interval cancers in a population-based screening. Br J Cancer 1997;75:762–6.

39. Miglioretti DL, Zhu W, Kerlikowske K, et al. Breast cancer surveillance consor-tium. breast tumor prognostic characteristics and biennial vs annual mammography, age, and menopausal status. JAMA Oncol 2015;1:1069–77.

40. White E, Miglioretti DL, Yankaskas BC, et al. Biennial versus annual mam-mography and the risk of late-stage breast cancer. J Natl Cancer Inst 2004;96:1832–9.

41. Yaffe M. What should the burden of proof be for acceptance of a new breast-cancer screening technique? Lancet 2004;364:1111–2.

42. Houssami N, Hofvind S, Soerensen AL, et al. Interval breast cancer rates for digital breast tomosynthesis versus digital mammography population screening: An individual participant data meta-analysis. EClinicalMedicine 2021;34:100804.

43. Marinovich ML, Hunter KE, Macaskill P, et al. Breast cancer screening using tomosynthesis or mammography: a meta-analysis of cancer detection and recall. J Natl Cancer Inst 2018;110(9):942–9.

44. Skaane P, Bandos AI, Niklason LT, et al. Digital mammography versus digital mammography plus tomosynthesis in breast cancer screening: the oslo tomosynthesis screening trial. Radiology 2019;291(1):23–30.

45. Caumo F, Romanucci G, Hunter K, et al. Comparison of breast cancers detected in the Verona screening program following transition to digital breast tomosynthesis screening with cancers detected at digital mammography screening. Breast Cancer Res Treat 2018;170(2):391–7.

46. Conant EF, Barlow WE, Herschorn SD, et al. Association of digital breast tomosynthesis vs digital mammography with cancer detection and recall rates by age and breast density. JAMA Oncol 2019;5(5):635–42.

47. Johnson K, Zackrisson S, Rosso A, et al. Tumor characteristics and molecular subtypes in breast cancer screening with digital breast tomosynthesis: the malmö breast tomosynthesis screening trial. Radiology 2019;293(2):273–81.

48. Hovda T, Holen AS, Lang K, et al. Interval and consecutive round breast cancer after digital breast tomosynthesis and synthetic 2D mammography versus standard 2D digital mammography in BreastScreen Norway. Radiology 2020;294:256–64.

49. Pattacini P, Nitrosi A, Giorgi Rossi P, et al. A randomized trial comparing breast cancer incidence and interval cancers after tomosynthesis plus mammography versus mammography alone. Radiology 2022;303:256–66.

50. Skaane P, Sebuodegard S, Bandos AI, et al. Performance of breast cancer screening using digital breast tomosynthesis: results from the prospective population-based Oslo Tomosynthesis Screening Trial. Breast Cancer Res Treat 2018;169:489–96.

51. Bahl M, Gaffney S, McCarthy AM, et al. Breast cancer characteristics associated with 2D digital mammography versus digital breast tomosynthesis for screening detected and interval cancers. Radiology 2018;287:49–57.

52. Conant EF, Zuckerman SP, McDonald ES, et al. Five consecutiveyears of screening with digital breast tomosynthesis: outcomes by screening year and round. Radiology 2020;295:285–93.

53. Durand MA, Friedewald SM, Plecha DM, et al. False-negative rates of breast cancer screening with and without digital breast tomosynthesis. Radiology 2021;298:296–305.

54. McDonald ES, Oustimov A, Weinstein SP, et al. Effectiveness of digital breast tomosynthesis compared with digital mammography: outcomes analysis from 3 years of breast cancer screening. JAMA Oncol 2016;2:737–43.

55. Johnson K, Lang K, Ikeda DM, et al. Interval breast cancer rates and tumor characteristics in the prospective population-based Malmo Breast Tomosynthesis Screening Trial. Radiology 2021;299:559–67.

56. Monticciolo DL. Digital breast tomosynthesis: a decade of practice in review. JACR 2023;20(2):127–33.

57. National Cancer Institute. TMIST Study Comparing Digital Mammograms (2-D) with Tomosynthesis Mammograms (3-D). What are the goals of TMIST? Available at: https://www.cancer.gov/about-cancer/treatment/clinical-trials/nci-supported/tmist#what-are-the-goals-of-tmist, Accessed 27 August 2023.

58. Kerlikowske K, Su Y, Sprague BL, et al. Association of screening with digital breast tomosynthesis vs digital mammography with risk of interval invasive and advanced breast cancer. JAMA 2022;327(22):2220–30.

59. Corsetti V, Houssami N, Ghirardi M, et al. Evidence of the effect of adjunct ultrasound screening in women with mammography-negative dense breasts: interval breast cancers at 1 year follow-up. Eur J Cancer 2011;47:1021–6.

60. Berg WA, Zhang Z, Lehrer D, et al. Detection of breast cancer with addition of annual screening ultrasound or a single screening MRI to mammography in women with elevated breast cancer risk. JAMA 2012;307:1394–404.

61. Song SE, Cho N, Chang JM, et al. Diagnostic performances of supplemental breast ultrasound screening in women with personal history of breast cancer. Acta Radiol 2018;59:533–9.

62. Ohuchi N, Suzuki A, Sobue T, et al. Sensitivity and specificity of mammography and adjunctive ultrasonography to screen for breast cancer in the Japan Strategic Anti-cancer Randomized Trial (J-START): a randomised controlled trial. Lancet 2016;387(10016):341–8.

63. Harada-Shoji N, Suzuki A, Ishida T, et al. Evaluation of adjunctive ultrasonography for breast cancer detection among women aged 40-49 years with varying breast density undergoing screening mammography: a secondary analysis of a randomized clinical trial. JAMA Netw Open 2021;4(8):e2121505.

64. Lee JM, Arao RF, Sprague BL, et al. Performance of screening ultrasonography as an adjunct to screening mammography in women across the spectrum of breast cancer risk. JAMA Intern Med 2019;179(5):658–67.

65. NCCN. Genetic/familial high-risk assessment: breast, ovarian, and pancreatic. NCCN clinical practice guidelines in oncology. version 3.2023 ed. https://www.nccn.org/guidelines/guidelines-detail?category=2&id=1503.

66. Brekelmans CT, Seynaeve C, Bartels CC, et al. Effectiveness of breast cancer surveillance in

BRCA 1/2 gene mutation carriers and women with high familial risk. J Clin Oncol 2001;19:924–30.

67. Monticciolo DL, Newell MS, Moy L, et al. Breast cancer screening for women at higher-than-average risk: updated recommendations from the ACR. J Am Coll Radiol 2023;S1546-1440(23):00334.

68. Mann RM, Balleyguier C, Baltzer PA, et al. European society of breast imaging (EUSOBI). breast MRI: EUSOBI recommendations for women's information. Eur Radiol 2015;25:3669–78.

69. Warner E, Plewes DB, Shumak RS, et al. Comparison of breast magnetic resonance imaging, mammography, and ultrasound for surveillance of women at high risk for hereditary breast cancer. J Clin Oncol 2001;19:3524–31.

70. Phi XA, Houssami N, Obdeijn IM, et al. Magnetic resonance imaging improves breast screening sensitivity in BRCA mutation carriers age $\geq$ 50 years: evidence from an individual patient data meta-analysis. J Clin Oncol 2015;33:349–56.

71. Bick U, Engel C, Krug B, et al, German Consortium for Hereditary Breast and Ovarian Cancer GC-HBOC. High-risk breast cancer surveillance with MRI: 10-year experience from the German consortium for hereditary breast and ovarian cancer. Breast Cancer Res Treat 2019;175(1):217–28.

72. Guindalini RSC, Zheng Y, Abe H, et al. Intensive surveillance with biannual dynamic contrast-enhanced magnetic resonance imaging downstages breast cancer in BRCA1 mutation carriers. Clin Cancer Res 2019;25(6):1786–94.

73. Warner E, Hill K, Causer P, et al. Prospective study of breast cancer incidence in women with a BRCA1 or BRCA2 mutation under surveillance with and without magnetic resonance imaging. J Clin Oncol 2011;29: 1664–9.

74. Evans DG, Harkness EF, Howell A, et al. Intensive breast screening in BRCA2 mutation carriers is associated with reduced breast cancer specific and all cause mortality. Hered Cancer Clin Pract 2016;14:8.

75. Saadatmand S, Geuzinge HA, Rutgers EJT, et al. MRI versus mammography for breast cancer screening in women with familial risk (FaMRIsc): a multicentre, randomised, controlled trial. Lancet Oncol 2019;20(8):1136–47.

76. Monticciolo DL, Newell MS, Moy L, et al. Breast cancer screening in women at higher-than-average risk: recommendations from the ACR. J Am Coll Radiol 2018;15:408–14.

77. Lehman CD, Lee JM, DeMartini WB, et al. Screening MRI in women with a personal history of breast cancer. J Natl Cancer Inst 2016;108(3):djv349.

78. Cho N, Han W, Han BK, et al. Breast cancer screening with mammography plus ultrasonography or magnetic resonance imaging in women 50 years or younger at diagnosis and treated with breast conservation therapy. JAMA Oncol 2017;3:1495–502.

79. Bakker MF, de Lange SV, Pijnappel RM, et al. Supplemental MRI screening for women with extremely dense breast tissue. N Engl J Med 2019;381(22):2091–210.

80. Comstock CE, Gatsonis C, Newstead GM, et al. Comparison of abbreviated breast MRI vs digital breast tomosynthesis for breast cancer detection among women with dense breasts undergoing screening. JAMA 2020;323(8):746–56.

Tumor Doubling Time and Screening Interval

Asha A. Bhatt, MD[a],[*], Bethany Niell, MD, PhD[a],[b]

KEYWORDS

• Tumor doubling time • Sojourn time • Breast cancer screening • Screening intervals

KEY POINTS

- Sojourn time refers to the duration of time a woman is asymptomatic (clinically occult) but the breast cancer is detectable by mammography.
- An optimal breast cancer screening interval maximizes detection of malignancies during the sojourn time.
- To screen detect a faster growing tumor (short tumor volume doubling time) before the malignancy becomes clinically evident, a shorter screening interval must be used. For slower growing tumors, a longer screening interval may still detect malignancies before the tumors become clinically apparent.

INTRODUCTION

The American Cancer Society (ACS) predicts that there will be a greater than 297,000 cases of invasive ductal carcinoma and 55,000 cases of ductal carcinoma in situ diagnosed in 2023 alone.[1] The aim of breast cancer screening is to detect tumors when small and node negative to decrease breast cancer–associated mortality and morbidity. The goal of this article is to help readers understand the concept of tumor doubling time and its impact upon optimizing the timing of screening mammography intervals.

SCREENING BASICS—UNDERSTANDING THE TIMELINE FOR BREAST CANCER GROWTH

To evaluate an optimal interval for breast cancer screening, one must understand the timeline of breast cancer growth on detection. This timeline spans the development of the first malignant cells, the growth required for the tumor to reach the threshold of detection by imaging and the point at which the cancer becomes detectable by clinical examination. Imaging examinations performed for cancer screening should detect malignancy in the preclinical stage before the tumor becomes clinically evident. Screen-detected cancers are typically at an earlier stage compared to tumors identified on clinical breast examination.

First malignant cells (imaging occult) → Cancer detectable by imaging (clinically occult) → Cancer detected clinically.

In the above timeline, sojourn time is the duration of the preclinical screen-detectable phase, or the time in which a woman is asymptomatic (clinically occult) but the breast cancer is detectable by mammography.[2]

[Key Point: Sojourn time refers to the duration of time a woman is asymptomatic (clinically occult) but the breast cancer is detectable by mammography.]

Sojourn time is directly influenced by tumor doubling time.

TUMOR DOUBLING TIME

The National Cancer Institute defines tumor doubling time as the "the amount of time it takes for 1 cell to divide or for a group of cells (such as a tumor) to double in size. The doubling time is different for different kinds of cancer cells or tumors."[3] Breast cancer tumor volume doubling

[a] Moffitt Cancer Center, 12902 Magnolia Drive, Tampa, FL 33612, USA; [b] Department of Oncologic Sciences, University of South Florida, 12901 Bruce B. Downs Boulevard MDC 44. Tampa, FL 33612, USA
* Corresponding author.
E-mail address: Asha.Bhatt@moffitt.org

Radiol Clin N Am 62 (2024) 571–580
https://doi.org/10.1016/j.rcl.2023.12.011

time (TVDT) can guide treatment decisions and predict prognosis.

Various models have been proposed to predict tumor growth patterns. These include power law, exponential, generalized logistic, Gompertz, Bertalanffy–Putter, and Mendelsohn models.[4–7] However, there is no consensus on the growth pattern that solid tumors exhibit.[4] Exponential growth calculations are one of the more commonly used methods for in vivo studies to predict breast cancer growth.[8]

SERIAL MAMMOGRAMS AS A METHOD TO ESTIMATE BREAST CANCER DOUBLING TIME

Serial mammograms demonstrate that TVDTs are significantly different for benign and malignant breast masses (Table 1). In a study, lesions with a TVDT greater than 4 years were 11 times more likely to be benign whereas lesions with a TVDT of less than 1 year were 6 times more likely to be an invasive malignancy.[9]

Serial mammograms may also evaluate the various histologic features of breast malignancies and TVDT. Higher tumor grade and lack of estrogen receptor (ER) expression have been associated with shorter TVDTs (rapid growth rates) (see Table 1).[10] This study showed that Ki-67 protein was one of the strongest predictors of growth rate. It also showed that lobular carcinomas had a significantly longer TVDT compared with ductal subtypes (431 vs 236 days).[11]

The sensitivity of mammography increases with greater tumor size. In a modeling study, Wang and colleagues showed an increase in sensitivity from 0% to 85% for tumors ranging from 2 to 20 mm in size. The estimated sensitivity at 5, 10, 15, and 50 mm for tumors was 35%, 65%, 78%, and 97%, respectively.[12] Compared to tumors with short TVDT, slower growing malignancies (longer TVDT) are more likely to be detected on serial mammograms, so approaches dependent on sequential mammograms may yield artificially low growth rates.[13] Estimating TVDT by mammography is further complicated by dense glandular tissue which may obscure tumors.

BREAST ULTRASOUND AS A METHOD TO ESTIMATE BREAST CANCER DOUBLING TIME

The cross-sectional imaging capabilities of breast ultrasound may be better suited to accurately predict TVDT.[14] An average TVDT of 8 months for invasive breast cancers was described by Ryu.[14] For triple- negative tumors, Ryu showed a 2.4-fold and 1.6-fold shorter TVDT (103 $\pm$ 43 days) compared to ER-positive (241 $\pm$ 166 days) and human epidermal growth factor receptor 2 (HER2)-positive (162 $\pm$ 60 days) tumors, respectively. Interestingly, ER-positive tumors showed an increase in TVDT with increasing tumor size whereas TVDT remained constant in HER2-positive and triple-negative tumors.[14] Another study by Lee and colleagues, demonstrated that triple negative cancers have the shortest TVDT (fastest growth rates) followed by HER2-positive breast cancers.[15]

IS TVDT DIFFERENT FOR BREAST CANCER GENE MUTATION CARRIERS COMPARED TO AVERAGE RISK PATIENTS?

Invasive malignances of BReast CAncer gene (BRCA) mutation carriers have TVDTs which are approximately half of the TVDTs detected in non-carrier females (48 days vs 84 days).[16] The malignances in BRCA mutation carriers were more often higher grade (64% were grade 3 compared to 32% for non-carriers) and showed a higher mean mitotic count (23 vs 4) than the non-carriers.[16] The higher incidence of interval cancers in BRCA mutation carriers may be related to the shorter tumor doubling times noted in mutation carriers compared to sporadic cancers.[17]

Tumor Doubling Time by Age

TVDT is shorter in younger women. Women younger than 50 years of age have a median doubling time of 80 days compared to 157 days in women 50 to 70 years of age (Table 2).[18] Similar findings were demonstrated when comparing women younger than age 60 (145 days) compared to over 60 (185 days).[10] Another study noted that

Table 1 Tumor volume doubling time for benign versus malignant masses	
Type of Lesion	TVDT (mo)
Benign (n=40)	30
Invasive cancer (n=28) 90% IDC, 10% ILC	10

Table 2 Age and median tumor volume doubling time from Peer at al (1993)[18]	
Age	Median TDT (d)
< 50	80 (2.6 mo)
50–70	157(5.2 mo)
>70	188 (6.3 mo)

Table 3
Tumor characteristics and TVDT determined by ultrasound and mammography from various studies.[11,14,15,19,21]

Tumor Characteristic	Doubling Time (DT) (d)[a]
Triple negative	
Lee et al. n = 67	69 ± 62
Nakashima et al. n = 28	178 ± 178
Ryu et al. n = 17	103 ± 43
Zhang et al. n = 18	127 ± 48
HER2+ and HR −	
Lee et al. n = 22	80 ± 71
Nakashima et al. n = 13	123 ± 123
Ryu et al. n = 12	162 ± 60
Zhang et al. n = 10	184 ± 71
HR +	
HER2 −	
Lee et al. n = 204	396 ± 71
Nakashima et al. n = 209	267 ± 267
Zhang et al. n = 29	257 ± 185
HER2 + or −	
Lee et al. n = 30	333 ± 70
Ryu et al. n = 37	241 ± 166
HER2 +	
Nakashima et al. n = 15	238 ± 238
Zhang et al. n = 12	211 ± 116
Grade 1	
Fornvik et al. n = 8	296 (Range 147–531)
Lee et al. n = 39	587 ± 69
Ryu et al. n = 13	204 ± 149
Zhang et al. n = 15	225 ± 143
Grade 2	
Fornvik et al. n = 16	352 (Range 139–749)
Lee et al. n = 155	379 ± 71
Ryu et al. n = 25	230 ± 179
Zhang et al. n = 42	201 ± 156
Grade 3	
Fornvik et al. n = 7	105 (Range 46–157)
Lee et al. n = 129	94 ± 63
Ryu et al. n = 28	154 ± 0.8
Zhang et al. n = 12	169 ± 90
Ki-67 < 14%	
Lee et al. n = 250	276 ± 68
Ryu et al. n = 56	205 ± 146
Zhang et al. n = 33	224 ± 136

Table 3
(continued)

Tumor Characteristic	Doubling Time (DT) (d)[a]
Ki-67 ≥ 14%	
Lee et al. n = 73	78 ± 62
Ryu et al. n = 10	114 ± 78
Zhang et al. n = 36	145 ± 87

[a] mean ± SD.

women less than 52 years of age had mean and SD TVDT of 167 ± 89 days whereas those 52 or greater had TVDT of 225 ± 109 days.[19]

HAS THERE BEEN A CHANGE IN TVDT OVER TIME?

Despite the interval increase in breast cancer incidence, Dahan and colleagues showed that tumor doubling time has remained stable over the past 80 years.[20] Published tumor volume doubling time estimates (**Table 3**) remain valid and may still be used to determine optimal breast cancer screening intervals.

IMPACT OF TUMOR VOLUME DOUBLING TIME ON SCREENING INTERVAL

Recommendations for screening intervals should be based on the length of the sojourn time which is partially dependent upon tumor growth rates (**Fig. 1**).[22] An ideal breast cancer screening interval maximizes detection of malignancies during the sojourn time. The detection of malignancy during the sojourn time is maximized by screening at an interval that is no more than half the sojourn time.[23]

[Key point: An optimal breast cancer screening interval maximizes detection of malignancies during the sojourn time.]

Faster growing tumors have shorter sojourn times than slower growing tumors. To screen detect a faster growing tumor (short TVDT) before the malignancy becomes clinically evident, a shorter screening interval must be used. Longer screening intervals increase interval cancers, because fewer cancers are detected during the sojourn time (**Fig. 2**). For slower growing tumors, a longer screening interval may still detect malignancies before the tumors become clinically apparent (**Fig. 3**).

[Key Point: To screen detect a faster growing tumor (short TVDT) before the malignancy becomes clinically evident, a shorter screening interval must be used. For slower growing tumors, a longer

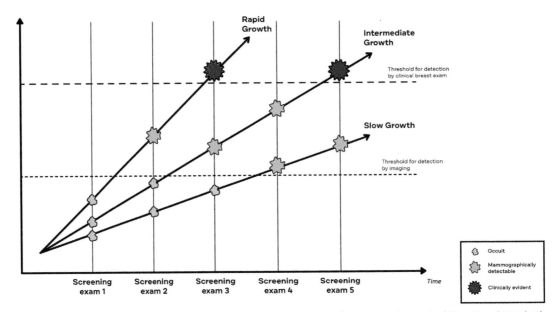

Fig. 1. Impact of screening interval on screen-detected malignancies by tumor volume doubling time (TVDT). The lower horizontal dashed line indicates the threshold for cancer detection (below this *line* can be defined as being mammographically occult). The second horizontal dashed line indicates the threshold for cancer detection by palpation (below this *line* can be defined as being clinically occult). The vertical lines represent screening intervals.

screening interval may still detect malignancies before the tumors become clinically apparent.]

Screening Mammography Intervals

Screening decreases breast cancer mortality and morbidity.[24–27] Different breast cancer screening guidelines exist in the United States and around the world.[28] Screening recommendations for average risk women vary by medical professional organizations (**Table 4**).

The major areas of variability across the recommendations include the age at which one should start screening, the age to stop screening, and the screening mammography interval. The following section will focus on the benefits and risks for various screening intervals.

ANNUAL, BIENNIAL, OR TRIENNIAL SCREENING IN AVERAGE RISK WOMEN— BENEFITS AND RISKS

Annual (once every year) and biennial (once every 2 years) are the 2 most common recommendations for screening mammography in the United States. Biannual mammography (every 6 months) and triennial (every 3 years) are not currently recommended within the United States. Each interval results in a different balance of benefits and risks.

According to Cancer Intervention and Surveillance Modeling Network (CISNET) models, the greatest median breast cancer mortality reduction is from annual screening (2D or 3D) in women aged 40 to 79.[25,35,36] Annual screening results in 37% mortality reduction and 217 life years gained whereas biennial screening results in only 30% mortality reduction and 165 life years gained (**Table 5**).[25,35] Annual screening for women aged 40 to 74 results in a 71% improvement in mortality reduction compared to biennial screening for women 50 to 74 year old.[25] For women younger than age 50, mortality is significantly reduced by screening intervals which are less 24-month (RR, 0.82 [95% CI, 0.72–0.94]) compared with intervals that are 24 months or longer (RR, 1.04 [95% CI, 0.72–1.52]).[27] When comparing triennial versus biennial screening for women aged 50 to 74, the breast cancer deaths averted per 100 women screened are similar at 3.4 to 5.1 versus 4.1 to 6.5, respectively.[36] In women with non-dense breasts, triennial screening results in a median of 1.6–2 fewer breast cancer deaths averted per 1000 screened, compared to biennial screening (RR=2).[36] Annual screening maximizes mortality reduction regardless of breast density when compared to longer screening intervals.[36]

Compared to biennial screening, annual screening mammography is associated with the detection of lower grade malignancies, smaller tumor sizes, fewer late or advanced stage cancers, and fewer interval cancers.[27,34,37–41] Late and

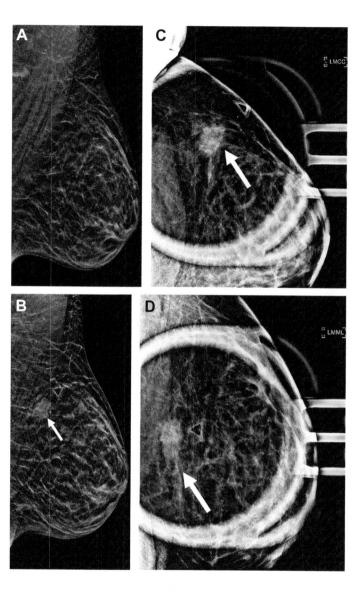

Fig. 2. Mammograms from a patient with a rapidly growing (short TVDT) malignancy. (*A*) mediolateral oblique(MLO) screening mammogram of the left breast from November 2020 demonstrates no mammographic evidence of malignancy. (*B*) MLO diagnostic mammogram of the left breast from May 2021 demonstrates a new mass with associated calcifications (*arrow*) that corresponds to the area of clinical concern. (*C*) May 2021 cranial caudal (CC) and (*D*) ML spot magnification mammograms demonstrate a mass with associated fine pleomorphic calcifications (*arrow*). Histology revealed a triple negative invasive cancer.

advanced stage cancers are defined as cases with positive lymph nodes or metastasis.[42] Biennial screening results in 44% of cancers detected at later stages compared to only 24% for women undergoing annual mammography.[41] Data from the Breast Cancer Surveillance Consortium (BCSC) demonstrate that premenopausal women who underwent biennial screening had a significantly increased risk of stage IIb or higher tumors (RR=1.28, [95% CI, 1.01–1.63], P=.040), tumors larger than 15 mm (RR=1.21 [95% CI,1.07–1.37], P=.002), and tumors with less-favorable prognostic characteristics (RR=1.11 [95% CI, 1.00–1.22], P=.047).[39] Younger women typically develop more aggressive tumors with shorter TVDT. For women aged 40 to 49, biennial screening results in a larger proportion of late-

stage diagnoses compared to annual screening (28% vs 21%).[38] BCSC data also demonstrate that postmenopausal women using hormone therapy (HT) who underwent biennial screening had a borderline significant increase in risk of tumors >15 mm (RR=1.13, [95% CI, 0.98–1.31], P=.087), positive lymph nodes (RR=1.18, [95% CI, 0.98–1.42], P=.089), and tumors with less-favorable prognosis (RR=1.12, [95% CI, 1.00–1.25], P=.053).[39] Additionally, BCSC data showed that postmenopausal women not using HT also had an increase in risk of tumors >15 mm (RR=1.11, [95% CI, 1.00–1.22], P=.045).[39]

Compared to longer screening intervals, annual screening mammography decreases interval cancers.[27,34] Interval cancers are tumors which are clinically detected between screening rounds.

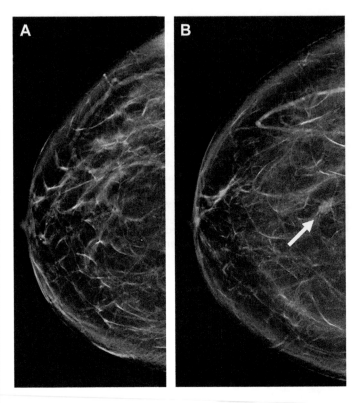

Fig. 3. Screening mammogram images from a woman with a slow growing (long TVDT) malignancy. (*A*) CC view from November 2018 screening mammogram with no mammographic evidence of malignancy. (*B*) CC view from November 2022 screening mammogram shows a new asymmetry (*arrow*). Histology revealed a grade 1 invasive ductal carcinoma.

Table 4
Screening interval recommendations for average risk women by 6 medical professional organizations in the United States[29–34]

Organization	Age to Start	Screening Interval Recommendation	Age to Stop Screening
United States Preventive Services Task Force	40	Biennial	74
American College of Obstetricians and Gynecologist	offer at 40, no later than 50	Annual or Biennial	75, then shared decision
American cancer society	45, option to start at 40	Annual for 45–54 Can switch to Biennial after age 55	Screening should continue if a woman is in good health and is expected to live at least 10 more years
National Comprehensive Cancer Network	40	Annual	Not stated
American College of Radiology and Society of Breast Imaging	40	Annual	No limit, tailor to the individual

Table 5
Estimated benefits of biennial and annual screening tomosynthesis adapted from Cancer Intervention and Surveillance Modeling Network(Median lifetime benefits and range across 6 models)[35]

	Biennial				Annual			
Age range	40–74	40–79	50–74	50–79	40–74	40–79	50–74	50–79
% Mortality reduction	30	33.3	25.4	28	37	41.7	30.6	34.5
Breast Cancer deaths averted	8.2	8.9	6.7	7.6	10.3	11.5	8.6	9.8
Life years gained	165.2	173.9	120.8	129.3	216.6	229.7	155.6	173.2
QALYs Gained	116.8	124.2	86.1	91.7	146.1	154.3	109	118.4

The proportion of interval cancers increases with the length of the screening interval (30% with annual, 40.6% with biennial, and 44.3% with triennial screening).[37] A retrospective review of women diagnosed with breast cancer demonstrates similar results; patients who underwent annual screening had a lower percentage of interval cancers (10.5%) compared to biennial (37.5%) or biennial and triennial (33.3%).[41] Another retrospective review demonstrated that the percentage of interval cancers in women undergoing annual screening was approximately half that of women who elected to undergo biennial screening.[43] In women with dense breasts, annual screening decreases interval cancers 63/70,814 (ICR 0.89/1000, [95% CI, 0.67–1.11]) compared to biennial screening 225/77,761 (ICR 1.45/1000 (annualized), [95% CI, 1.19–1.72]).[44]

Using data from a retrospective review of positive mammograms, Michaelson and colleagues created a mathematical model to predict the probability of metastasis as a function of tumor size. Annual screening decreased the incidence of metastatic disease by 33% compared to 14% and 7% in biennial and triennial screening schedules, respectively.[13]

Annual mammography increases false-positive recalls and false-positive biopsies compared to longer screening intervals (**Table 6**). For a woman aged 40 to 49, the likelihood of a false-positive recall and false-positive biopsy are greater than a woman over age 50, whereas the likelihood of a missed breast cancer diagnosis is lower. A woman aged 40 to 49 who undergoes annual screening mammography will experience a false-positive mammogram once every 10 years, a false-positive biopsy once every 149 years, and a missed breast cancer once every 1000 years.[25] A woman aged 60 to 69 who undergoes annual screening mammography will experience a false-positive screening mammogram once every 12.7 years, a false-positive biopsy once every 196 years, and a missed breast cancer once every 714 years.[25] The cumulative probability of a false-positive recall after 10 years of screening with full-field digital mammography with biennial exams is 38.1% and 56.3% for annual examinations.[45] Irrespective of screening interval, the probability of being recalled from screening mammography decreases with each subsequent mammogram (false-positive recall rate probability of 16.3% at the first mammogram and 9.6% at subsequent mammogram).[46]

Table 6
Estimated risks of biennial and annual screening tomosynthesis adapted from Cancer Intervention and Surveillance Modeling Network (median lifetime harms and range across 5 models)[35]

	Biennial				Annual			
Age range	40–74	40–79	50–74	50–79	40–74	40–79	50–74	50–79
False positive screens	1540 (1520–1551)	1624 (1601–1636)	1021 (1003–1027)	1105 (1084–1113)	2423 (2385–2446)	2595 (2550–2621)	1543 (1513–1557)	1716 (1678–1733)
Benign biopsies	210 (207–212)	222 (219–223)	148 (146–149)	160 (157–161)	281 (276–283)	301 (295–304)	192 (188–194)	212 (208–214)
Over-diagnosed cases	12 (4–33)	14 (6–37)	10 (4–29)	12 (6–34)	19 (5–45)	23 (7–52)	16 (5–39)	19 (7–46)

Overdiagnosis is less impacted by screening interval especially in women with low competing risks of mortality. Due to heterogeneity in study methodology and design rigor, published estimates of breast cancer over diagnosis vary widely from 0% to 54%.[26,27] Evaluation of BCSC data shows that for women 50 to 74 who undergo biennial screening, 15.4% (95% uncertainty interval, 9.4% to 26.5%) of screen-detected cancer cases were estimated to be overdiagnosed.[47] Estimates adjusted for lead time in the European-based population screening programs, show lower estimates, ranging from 1% to 10%.[48] In the Swedish Two-County trial and the Breast Screening Program in England, overdiagnosis estimates are 4.3 and 2.3 per 1000 women screened, respectively. However, the benefits in terms of numbers of deaths prevented are approximately double at 8.8 and 5.7 per 1000 women screened.[49] For a 40-year-old woman, it is estimated that her risk of overdiagnosis is approximately 0.1% due to her life expectancy and low mortality.[50] CISNET models (**table 6**) show low overdiagnosis estimates for invasive cancer whether screening is done biennially in women aged 50 to 74 year old or annually in women aged 40 to 74 year old (10 vs 19).[51]

SUMMARY

More aggressive tumors have shorter tumor volume doubling times. Tumor volume doubling time impacts sojourn time. Sojourn time refers to the duration of time a woman is asymptomatic (clinically occult) but the breast cancer may be detectable by screening mammography. An optimal breast cancer screening interval maximizes detection of malignancies during the sojourn time. To screen detect a faster growing tumor (short TVDT) before the malignancy becomes clinically evident, a shorter screening interval must be used. For slower growing tumors, a longer screening interval may still detect malignancies before the tumors become clinically apparent. Longer screening intervals increase interval cancers because fewer cancers are detected during the sojourn time.

CLINICS CARE POINTS

- Compared to biennial screening, annual screening mammography is associated with smaller tumor sizes, fewer late or advanced stage cancers, and fewer interval cancers.

- Annual mammography increases false-positive recalls and false-positive biopsies compared to longer screening intervals.
- Irrespective of screening interval, the probability of being recalled from screening mammography decreases with each subsequent mammogram.

DISCLOSURE

The authors have nothing to disclose.

REFERENCES

1. Breast Cancer Statistics | How Common Is Breast Cancer? | American Cancer Society. Accessed July 20, 2023. https://www.cancer.org/cancer/types/breast-cancer/about/how-common-is-breast-cancer.html
2. Aarts AMWM, Duffy SW, Geurts SME, et al. Test sensitivity of mammography and mean sojourn time over 40 years of breast cancer screening in Nijmegen (The Netherlands). J Med Screen 2019; 26(3). https://doi.org/10.1177/0969141318814869.
3. Definition of doubling time - NCI Dictionary of Cancer Terms - NCI. Accessed July 3, 2023. https://www.cancer.gov/publications/dictionaries/cancer-terms/def/doubling-time
4. Gerlee P. The model muddle: In search of tumor growth laws. Cancer Res 2013;73(8):2407–11.
5. Renner-Martin K, Brunner N, Kühleitner M, et al. On the exponent in the Von Bertalanffy growth model. PeerJ 2018;2018(1). https://doi.org/10.7717/PEERJ.4205/SUPP-2.
6. Hart D, Shochat E, Agur Z. The growth law of primary breast cancer as inferred from mammography screening trials data. Br J Cancer 1998;78(3):382.
7. Heesterman BL, Bokhorst JM, De Pont LMH, et al. Mathematical Models for Tumor Growth and the Reduction of Overtreatment. J Neurol Surg B Skull Base 2019;80(1):72.
8. Talkington A, Durrett R. Estimating tumor growth rates in vivo. Bull Math Biol 2015;77(10):1934.
9. Sadeghipour N, Tseng J, Anderson K, et al. Tumor volume doubling time estimated from digital breast tomosynthesis mammograms distinguishes invasive breast cancers from benign lesions. Eur Radiol 2023;33(1):429–39.
10. MacInnes EG, Duffy SW, Simpson JA, et al. Radiological audit of interval breast cancers: Estimation of tumour growth rates. Breast : official journal of the European Society of Mastology 2020;51:114.
11. Förnvik D, Lång K, Andersson I, et al. Estimates of breastcancer growth rate from mammograms and its relation to tumour characteristics. Radiat Protect Dosim 2016;169(1):151–7.

12. Wang J, Gottschal P, Ding L, et al. Mammographic sensitivity as a function of tumor size: A novel estimation based on population-based screening data. Breast 2021;55:69–74.

13. Michaelson JS, Halpern E, Kopans DB. Breast Cancer: Computer Simulation Method for Estimating Optimal Intervals for Screening1. Radiology 1999;212(2):551–60. R99AU49551.

14. Ryu EB, Chang JM, Seo M, et al. Tumour volume doubling time of molecular breast cancer subtypes assessed by serial breast ultrasound. Eur Radiol 2014;24(9):2227–35.

15. Lee SH, Kim YS, Han W, et al. Tumor growth rate of invasive breast cancers during wait times for surgery assessed by ultrasonography. Medicine (Baltim) 2016;95(37):e4874.

16. Tilanus-Linthorst MMA, Kriege M, Boetes C, et al. Hereditary breast cancer growth rates and its impact on screening policy. Eur J Cancer 2005;41(11):1610–7.

17. Grassmann F, He W, Eriksson M, et al. Interval breast cancer is associated with other types of tumors. Nat Commun 2019;10(1). https://doi.org/10.1038/S41467-019-12652-1.

18. Peer PG, van Dijck JA, Hendriks JH, et al. Age-dependent growth rate of primary breast cancer. Cancer 1993;71(11):3547–51.

19. Zhang S, Ding Y, Zhu Q, et al. Correlation Factors Analysis of Breast Cancer Tumor Volume Doubling Time Measured by 3D-Ultrasound. Med Sci Monit 2017;23:3147.

20. Dahan M, Hequet D, Bonneau C, et al. Has tumor doubling time in breast cancer changed over the past 80 years? A systematic review. Cancer Med 2021;10(15):5203.

21. Nakashima K, Uematsu T, Takahashi K, et al. Does breast cancer growth rate really depend on tumor subtype? Measurement of tumor doubling time using serial ultrasonography between diagnosis and surgery. Breast Cancer 2019;26(2):206–14.

22. Moskowitz M. Breast cancer: age-specific growth rates and screening strategies. Radiology 1986;161(1):37–41.

23. Kopans DB. "Chapter 4: Screen for Breast Cancer." Breast Imaging. Philadelphia, PA: Lippincott Williams & Wilkins; 2005.

24. Mandelblatt JS, Cronin KA, Bailey S, et al. Effects of mammography screening under different screening schedules: model estimates of potential benefits and harms. Ann Intern Med 2009;151(10):738.

25. Hendrick RE, Helvie MA. United States preventive services task force screening mammography recommendations: Science ignored. Am J Roentgenol 2011;196(2). https://doi.org/10.2214/AJR.10.5609/ASSET/IMAGES/02_10_5609_01.

26. Marmot MG, Altman DG, Cameron DA, et al. The benefits and harms of breast cancer screening: an independent review. Br J Cancer 2013;108(11):2205–40.

27. Myers ER, Moorman P, Gierisch JM, et al. Benefits and Harms of Breast Cancer Screening: A Systematic Review. JAMA 2015;314(15):1615–34.

28. Ren W, Chen M, Qiao Y, et al. Global guidelines for breast cancer screening: A systematic review. Breast 2022;64:85–99.

29. A Q, JS L, RA M, et al. Screening for Breast Cancer in Average-Risk Women: A Guidance Statement From the American College of Physicians. Ann Intern Med 2019;170(8):547–60.

30. Oeffinger KC, Fontham ETH, Etzioni R, et al. Breast Cancer Screening for Women at Average Risk: 2015 Guideline Update From the American Cancer Society. JAMA 2015;314(15):1599–614.

31. Baker JL, Bennett DL, Bonaccio E, et al. NCCN Guidelines Version 1.2023 Breast Cancer Screening and Diagnosis Continue NCCN Guidelines Panel Disclosures. Published online 2023. Accessed July 28, 2023. https://www.nccn.org/home/member-

32. Pearlman M, Jeudy M, Chelmow D. Breast Cancer Risk Assessment and Screening in Average-Risk Women. Obstet Gynecol 2017;130(1):E1–16.

33. Recommendation: Breast Cancer: Screening United States Preventive Services Taskforce. Available at: https://www.uspreventiveservicestaskforce.org/uspstf/recommendation/breast-cancer-screening. Accessed July 28, 2023.

34. Monticciolo DL, Newell MS, Hendrick RE, et al. Breast Cancer Screening for Average-Risk Women: Recommendations From the ACR Commission on Breast Imaging. J Am Coll Radiol 2017;14(9):1137–43.

35. Trentham-Dietz A, Christina Hunter Chapman M, Jinani Jayasekera M, et al. Breast Cancer Screening With Mammography: An Updated Decision Analysis for the U.S. Preventive Services Task Force.; 2023. www.ahrq.gov

36. Trentham-Dietz A, Kerlikowske K, Stout NK, et al. Tailoring breast cancer screening intervals by breast density and risk for women 50 and older: Collaborative modeling of screening outcomes. Ann Intern Med 2016;165(10):700.

37. Kerlikowske K, Zhu W, Hubbard RA, et al. Outcomes of screening mammography by frequency, breast density, and postmenopausal hormone therapy. JAMA Intern Med 2013;173(9):807–16.

38. White E, Miglioretti DL, Yankaskas BC, et al. Biennial versus annual mammography and the risk of late-stage breast cancer. J Natl Cancer Inst 2004;96(24):1832–9.

39. Miglioretti DL, Zhu W, Kerlikowske K, et al. Breast Tumor Prognostic Characteristics and Biennial vs Annual Mammography, Age, and Menopausal Status. JAMA Oncol 2015;1(8):1069–77.

40. Eby PR. Evidence to Support Screening Women Annually. Radiol Clin North Am 2017;55(3):441–56.

41. Moorman SEH, Pujara AC, Sakala MD, et al. Annual Screening Mammography Associated With Lower Stage Breast Cancer Compared With Biennial Screening. AJR Am J Roentgenol 2021;217(1):40–7.

42. Breast Cancer Staging | ACS. Accessed August 26, 2023. https://www.facs.org/for-patients/home-skills-for-patients/breast-cancer-surgery/breast-cancer-types/breast-cancer-staging/

43. Hunt KA, Rosen EL, Sickles EA. Outcome analysis for women undergoing annual versus biennial screening mammography: a review of 24,211 examinations. AJR Am J Roentgenol 1999;173(2):285–9.

44. Seely JM, Peddle SE, Yang H, et al. Breast Density and Risk of Interval Cancers: The Effect of Annual Versus Biennial Screening Mammography Policies in Canada. Can Assoc Radiol J 2022;73(1):90–100.

45. Ho TQH, Bissell MCS, Kerlikowske K, et al. Cumulative Probability of False-Positive Results After 10 Years of Screening With Digital Breast Tomosynthesis vs Digital Mammography. JAMA Netw Open 2022;5(3):E222440.

46. Hubbard RA, Kerlikowske K, Flowers CI, et al. Cumulative probability of false-positive recall or biopsy recommendation after 10 years of screening mammography: a cohort study. Ann Intern Med 2011;155(8):481–92.

47. Ryser MD, Lange J, Inoue LYT, et al. Estimation of Breast Cancer Overdiagnosis in a U.S. Breast Screening Cohort. Ann Intern Med 2022;175(4):471.

48. Puliti D, Duffy SW, Miccinesi G, et al. Overdiagnosis in mammographic screening for breast cancer in Europe: A literature review. J Med Screen 2012;19(SUPPL. 1):42–56.

49. Duffy SW, Tabar L, Olsen AH, et al. Absolute numbers of lives saved and overdiagnosis in breast cancer screening, from a randomized trial and from the Breast Screening Programme in England. J Med Screen 2010;17(1):25.

50. Hendrick RE. Obligate overdiagnosis due to mammographic screening: A direct estimate for U.S. women. Radiology 2018;287(2):391–7.

51. Monticciolo DL, Helvie MA, Edward Hendrick R. Current issues in the overdiagnosis and overtreatment of breast cancer. Am J Roentgenol 2018;210(2):285–91.

Fibrocystic Change

Debbie L. Bennett, MD*, Arianna Buckley, MD, Michelle V. Lee, MD

KEYWORDS

- Fibrocystic change • Fibrocystic breast disease • Cyst • Benign breast disease • Mastalgia
- Breast pain

KEY POINTS

- Fibrocystic changes reflect a spectrum of specific benign pathologic conditions in the breast, ranging from cysts to proliferative changes with atypia.
- Clinical symptoms of fibrocystic changes include palpable mass and breast pain.
- Although there are classically benign imaging findings associated with cysts and layering calcifications, some imaging findings of fibrocystic change are nonspecific (solid mass, nonlayering calcifications, and architectural distortion) and require biopsy for definitive diagnosis.
- Management of breast pain associated with fibrocystic change includes reassurance and nonpharmacologic measures.

INTRODUCTION

Fibrocystic change is a general, nonspecific term that refers to a spectrum of benign histopathologic processes in the breast. Fibrocystic change is very common, clinically affecting up to 50% of women, and seen histologically in up to 90% of women.[1] Fibrocystic change was previously termed "fibrocystic breast disease" or "cystic mastopathy."[2] Pathologists now describe the specific benign histopathologic finding.[3] Understanding the spectrum of fibrocystic change can aid the breast imager in image interpretation and management decisions.

Fibrocystic changes are generally classified into 3 groups: nonproliferative, proliferative without atypia, and proliferative with atypia (**Box 1**).[4,5] Nonproliferative entities are the most common (70%), followed by proliferative lesions without atypia (27%), and proliferative lesions with atypia (3%–4%).[4,5]

Each of these groups is associated with varying levels of risk of subsequent breast cancer development, with the highest relative risk associated with proliferative changes with atypia (**Table 1**).[5,6] These lesions are generally considered risk indicators rather than precursor lesions. The risk remains elevated for more than 15 years and is higher for women diagnosed at a younger age (<45 years).[5,7]

INCIDENCE AND PRESENTATION

Fibrocystic changes begin in women in their 20s and become more common in their 30s and 40s, peaking at age 43.[8] Cysts increase in incidence after age of 40 years and peak at age of 50 years. The incidence of both fibrocystic changes and cysts decreases in women thereafter.[8]

Factors associated with fibrocystic changes include nulliparity in premenopausal women and use of hormone replacement therapy in postmenopausal women.[8] There is no association between the use of oral contraceptives and fibrocystic change. Obesity (body mass index >30) is associated with a significantly decreased risk of fibrocystic change and cysts.[8] Elevated breast density is associated with proliferative changes with atypia,[9] which may be related to decreased involutional change in women with dense breasts.[10]

Patients with fibrocystic changes may present with clinical symptoms such as palpable abnormality, pain, or nipple discharge.[11] Many patients report "lumpy" breasts with multiple palpable areas or pain in both breasts.[12,13] Because fibrocystic changes typically respond to variations in estrogen and progesterone levels, symptoms

Department of Breast Imaging, Mallinckrodt Institute of Radiology, Washington University in St. Louis School of Medicine, 510 South Kingshighway Boulevard, Box 8131, St Louis, MO, USA
* Corresponding author.
E-mail address: Debbie.bennett@wustl.edu

Radiol Clin N Am 62 (2024) 581–592
https://doi.org/10.1016/j.rcl.2023.12.008
0033-8389/24/© 2024 Elsevier Inc. All rights reserved.

Box 1
Spectrum of histologic diagnoses in fibrocystic change

Nonproliferative changes

　Cysts

　Fibrosis

　Apocrine metaplasia

　Mild epithelial/ductal hyperplasia

　Columnar cell change

　Fibroadenoma

Proliferative changes without atypia

　Usual ductal hyperplasia, moderate or florid

　Adenosis

　Sclerosing adenosis

　Radial scar

　Papilloma

Proliferative changes with atypia

　ADH

　ALH

Hartmann LC, Sellers TA, Frost MH, et al. Benign breast disease and the risk of breast cancer. N Engl J Med. Jul 21 2005;353(3):229-37.

tend to fluctuate throughout the menstrual cycle.[14,15]

Cysts may rupture and become inflamed as material within the cyst is released into the adjacent stroma. This can result in a long-standing cyst being newly palpable, as the adjoining breast tissue may feel firmer due to inflammation.[12]

Asymptomatic patients may be incidentally diagnosed with fibrocystic changes from screening

Table 1
Relative risk of breast cancer development associated with type of fibrocystic changes

	Relative Risk (95% Confidence Interval)
Nonproliferative changes	
Hartmann, 2005	1.27 (1.15–1.41)
Dyrstad, 2015	1.17 (0.94–1.47)
Proliferative changes without atypia	
Hartmann, 2005	1.88 (1.66–2.12)
Dyrstad, 2015	1.76 (1.58–1.95)
Proliferative changes with atypia	
Hartmann, 2005	4.24 (3.26–5.41)
Dyrstad, 2015	3.93 (3.24–4.76)

examinations. Fibrocystic changes are also found incidentally during the removal of breast tissue for other reasons (eg, reduction mammoplasty).[16]

NORMAL ANATOMY AND IMAGING TECHNIQUE

Fibrocystic changes develop from the terminal ductal lobular unit (TDLU) of the breast parenchyma. The TDLU is the functional unit of the breast from which most pathologic conditions develop. Cells in the TDLU are hormonally responsive and subject to normal cycles of development and involution during puberty, pregnancy, lactation, and menopause. Hormonally responsive changes also occur during each menstrual cycle. Fibrocystic changes are thought to reflect the imbalance of normal development and involution,[3] leading to both proliferative and nonproliferative lesions. The incidence of fibrocystic changes peaks at the time of menopause-related involutional changes (late 30s–40s).[3]

Anatomic Considerations

Fibrocystic changes fall into 1 of 3 main pathophysiologic pathways of development: dilatation of ducts and acini with associated epithelial metaplasia, epithelial proliferation, and proliferation of ducts and acini.

As tissue involution occurs and terminal ducts become obstructed, the accumulation of fluid within the terminal duct structures (ducts and acini) leads to the formation of cysts.[17] Cysts are hypothesized to result from an imbalance of the normal homeostasis of fluid secretion and resorption.[17] Metaplasia of the epithelial lining can occur during cyst formation. Apocrine metaplasia describes the transformation of the normal breast epithelial cells into cells resembling apocrine sweat glands and is common in benign cysts.[18] Stromal fibrosis is characterized by the proliferation of stroma with obliteration and atrophy of the acini and ducts.[19]

Epithelial proliferation is termed usual ductal hyperplasia when the cells lining the acini and ducts are more numerous but otherwise seem close to normal epithelium. Columnar cell lesions involve dilated and enlarged acini with proliferation of columnar epithelium; flat epithelial atypia describes columnar cell lesions with cytologic atypia.[20] Proliferation of acini in the TDLU is called adenosis. Sclerosing adenosis is a specific type of benign adenosis that is surrounded by fibrosis that compresses and distorts the acini.[21]

When the proliferation of epithelial cells is clonal with abnormal architecture, the lesion is termed atypical ductal hyperplasia (ADH). ADH is pathologically similar to ductal carcinoma in situ (DCIS) but distinguished by its small volume.[22] Atypical lobular hyperplasia (ALH) results from the proliferation of dyshesive epithelial cells that distort and distend the acini. ALH is less extensive than lobular carcinoma in situ (LCIS).[23,24]

Diagnostic Protocols

Palpable masses may be identified by the patient or clinical provider. Although benign findings are more commonly described as mobile, soft, and with discrete margins, physical examination is generally not able to distinguish a cyst from a solid mass.[25–27] Diagnostic imaging is therefore indicated for women presenting with palpable masses.

The American College of Radiology appropriateness criteria for initial imaging of palpable breast masses categorizes patients by age into those younger than 30 years, 30 to 39 years, and 40 years and older.[28] Ultrasound should be used as the initial imaging test for younger patients. Older patients should begin with diagnostic mammogram with ultrasound used as a complementary imaging test.

For patients with a screen-detected finding, standard institutional protocols should be followed. Ultrasound can be considered for initial evaluation of a mass if the margins are definitively circumscribed on digital breast tomosynthesis images.[29] Otherwise, diagnostic mammography with spot compression views can be performed. Magnification views should be obtained to evaluate calcifications.

Histopathology and Imaging Findings

Because the spectrum of pathologies seen with fibrocystic changes is so broad, the imaging findings are also varied and often nonspecific. There are 2 general categories of imaging findings of fibrocystic changes—those associated with cysts (nonproliferative changes) and those associated with epithelial hyperplasia and proliferation.[30] Often the 2 types of imaging findings are seen together (Fig. 1A-D).

Cysts are typically oval, circumscribed masses. They are often multiple and bilateral and may fluctuate in size over time. Although the fluid content of cysts typically results in low-density masses mammographically, ultrasound provides definitive diagnosis of breast cysts and distinguishes them from benign-appearing solid masses (Fig. 2A, B).[31]

Breast cysts may be simple, complicated, or clustered.[32] A simple cyst is anechoic with an imperceptible wall and is entirely fluid-filled.[32] A complicated cyst is similar to a simple cyst but has homogeneous low-level internal echoes because of either hemorrhagic or proteinaceous debris (Fig. 2C).[33] Clustered microcysts are a collection of simple cysts, each small, without discrete solid component (Fig. 2D, E).[33] Apocrine metaplasia is typically seen as a new or enlarging lobular or microlobulated mass or as new or increased calcifications.[34]

On MR imaging, cysts are round or oval, circumscribed, nonenhancing masses. Typically, cysts demonstrate high signal on T2-weighted images and low signal intensity on T1-weighted images but these characteristics can be variable when the cyst fluid contains protein or hemorrhage (Fig. 3A, B). Occasionally, a thin rim of uniform enhancement may be seen with inflammatory cysts.[35,36] The internal rim of the cyst should remain smooth with inflammatory cysts.

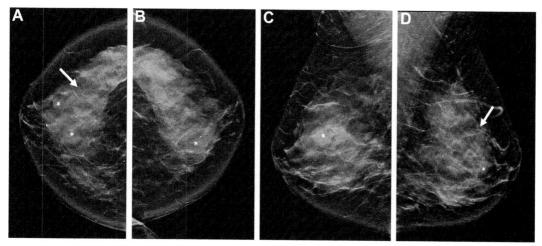

Fig. 1. Bilateral CC (*A, B*) and MLO (*C, D*) screening mammogram images in a 44-year-old woman demonstrate scattered round calcifications (*arrow*) and oval, low-density masses (*asterisk*) in both breasts. These findings are typical for fibrocystic change and are often seen together.

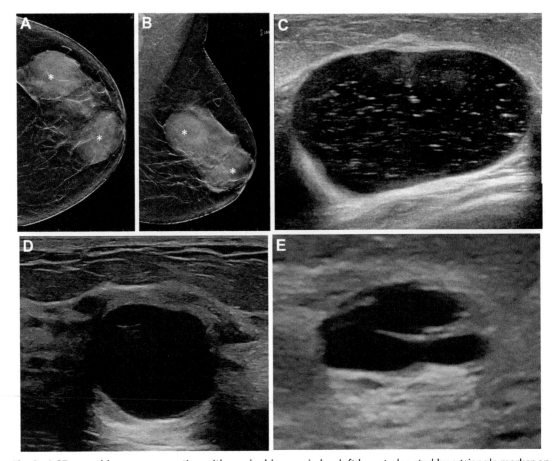

Fig. 2. A 37-year-old woman presenting with a palpable mass in her left breast, denoted by a triangle marker on CC (*A*) and MLO (*B*) mammogram images. Multiple oval masses were seen on mammogram (*asterisk*). The area of palpable concern corresponded with a complicated cyst with internal mobile debris (*C*). Multiple other benign simple cysts (*D*) and clusters of cysts (*E*) were also noted.

Fibrocystic changes related to epithelial hyperplasia and proliferative changes typically present with calcifications on mammography. These are usually diffuse, round, and bilateral (see **Fig. 1**A, B).[35] Classically benign milk of calcium presents as layering calcifications on a true lateral view, as they reflect sedimented calcium within cysts (**Fig. 4**A–D).[37]

Calcifications associated with fibrocystic changes may be grouped, unilateral, amorphous, or coarse heterogeneous and may require stereotactic biopsy (**Fig. 5**A–F).[38,39] Calcifications associated with ADH tend to more closely resemble DCIS but are smaller in volume. ALH and LCIS are not typically associated with calcifications and are an incidental finding in 0.5% to 3.8% of breast biopsies.[23,24]

Less commonly, fibrocystic changes may present as architectural distortion, requiring biopsy

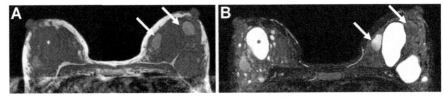

Fig. 3. T1-weighted, nonfat-saturated (*A*) and fluid-sensitive (STIR) (*B*) axial MR images of both breasts in a 39-year-old woman undergoing high-risk screening show multiple oval, circumscribed masses of varying T1 and T2 signal intensity in both breasts. Simple fluid is seen in some of the cysts as T1-hypointense and T2-hyperintense (*asterisk*). Others are hyperintense on T1-weighted imaging and dark on T2-weighted imaging, consistent with cysts with hemorrhagic or proteinaceous debris (*arrows*). These cysts also demonstrate fluid levels. STIR, short tau inversion recovery.

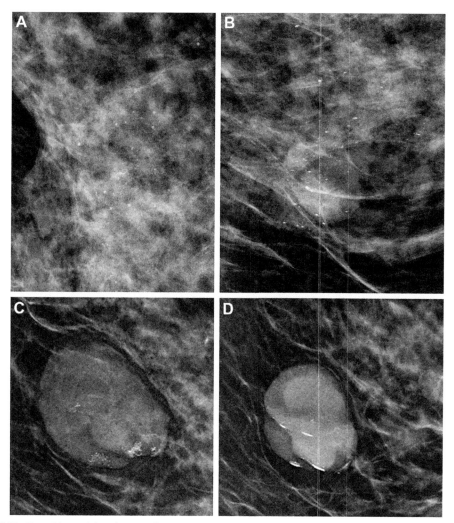

Fig. 4. CC (*A, C*) and lateral (*B, D*) magnification views in 2 patients recalled from screening for calcifications. In the first patient (*A, B*), amorphous calcifications on the CC view (*A*) change morphology and demonstrate teacup layering on the lateral view (*B*), consistent with benign milk of calcium in microcysts. In the second patient (*C, D*), a mass with associated calcifications on the CC view (*C*) is found to reflect milk of calcium sedimenting within macrocysts on the lateral view (*D*), also a benign finding.

for definitive diagnosis. Proliferative changes without atypia, specifically complex sclerosing lesions and radial scars, account for most of these distortions.[40] Cysts, apocrine metaplasia, and fibrosis are also found in benign biopsies of architectural distortion.[41,42] Rarely, proliferative changes with atypia (ADH and ALH) may also present with architectural distortion.[41]

Uncommonly, focal fibrocystic change may present as a developing asymmetry (**Fig. 6**A–F) or solid mass (**Fig. 7**A–C).[43,44] These masses may have suspicious imaging features, including posterior acoustic shadowing.[45] Biopsy is recommended for masses demonstrating any suspicious features.

Fibrocystic changes on MR imaging are typically seen as either nonmass enhancement (NME) or focal mass; as with mammography, these findings can be seen together.[46–48] MR imaging cannot distinguish between nonproliferative and proliferative changes.[49]

NME may be in any distribution (linear, segmental, or regional)[50,51] with typically benign enhancement kinetics.[50] Microcysts and apocrine metaplasia can present as an oval mass with a circumscribed margin that shows increased T2 signal and enhances.[52] Focal fibrocystic change and stromal fibrosis can present as a focus of enhancement, mass, or NME and are often associated with increased signal intensity on T2-weighted images and variable enhancement (**Fig. 8**A–C). There can be overlap with MR features of malignancy with rapid enhancement and

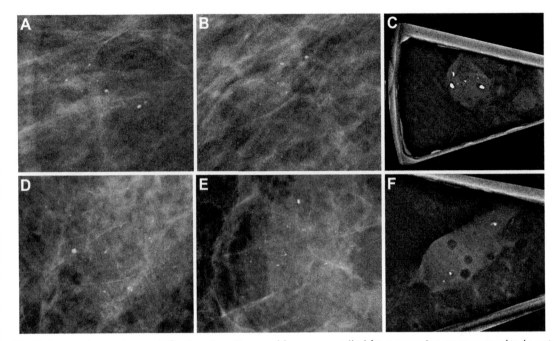

Fig. 5. Grouped amorphous calcifications in a 45-year-old woman recalled from screening mammography do not change shape between magnification CC (*A*) and ML (*B*) views. Stereotactic biopsy was recommended. Specimen radiograph (*C*) demonstrates appropriate sampling of the calcifications. Pathology showed microcalcifications associated with fibrocystic changes (stromal fibrosis, adenosis, and cyst formation). Pathology was considered benign and concordant. Similarly, grouped calcifications in a different 47-year-old woman recalled from screening mammography were thought to be suspicious based on fine pleomorphic morphology on both CC (*D*) and ML (*E*) views. Stereotactic biopsy (*F*) showed fibrocystic changes (apocrine metaplasia, cysts, stromal fibrosis, and columnar cell change) with associated calcifications. Pathologic condition was also considered benign and concordant.

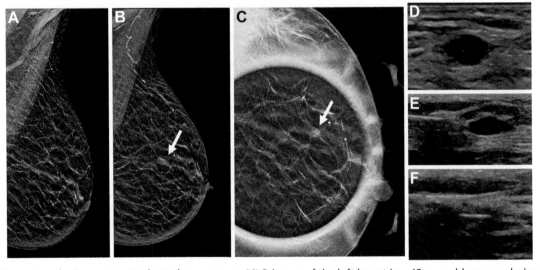

Fig. 6. Developing asymmetry (*arrow*) was seen on MLO image of the left breast in a 48-year-old woman during screening mammography (prior year, *A*; current year, *B*). Spot compression view (*C*) confirmed persistent asymmetry (*arrow*). Ultrasound demonstrated an oval mass with angular margins (*D*) and biopsy was performed (*E*). The mass disappeared after the first sample was taken. Clip was placed at site of biopsy (*F*). Pathology showed cyst wall with benign epithelial lining, associated mild acute inflammation and stromal fibrosis. Pathologic condition was considered benign and concordant.

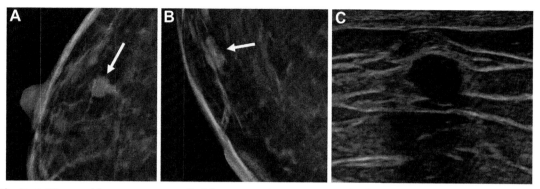

Fig. 7. A 53-year-old woman was recalled from screening mammography for the evaluation of a right breast mass. Spot compression CC (*A*) and ML (*B*) tomosynthesis images confirmed a round mass with indistinct margins (*arrows*). Ultrasound demonstrated a corresponding round, hypoechoic mass with indistinct margins (*C*). Ultrasound-guided biopsy showed benign proliferative changes, including usual ductal hyperplasia, columnar cell change, microcysts with focal apocrine metaplasia and stromal fibrosis. Pathologic condition was considered benign and concordant.

washout kinetics.[53,54] Biopsy is typically required for definitive diagnosis in these cases.

DIAGNOSTIC CRITERIA

A simple cyst must be anechoic, round or oval, circumscribed, and show posterior acoustic enhancement without internal vascularity (see **Fig. 2**A–E).[32,35] Simple cysts are benign.[35]

Complicated cysts have the same imaging features as those for a simple cyst but with low-level internal echoes (see **Fig. 2**A–E). The internal echoes within a complicated cyst may be mobile and may show a fluid level.[33] Complicated cysts in the setting of multiple other cysts may be considered benign. Isolated complicated cysts may be followed with short interval follow-up or aspiration.[35]

Clustered microcysts are masses that are entirely composed of individual 2 to 3 mm anechoic masses with thin septations between each mass (<0.5 mm; see **Fig. 2**A–E).[33,35]

Clustered microcysts do not have a solid component within any of the cysts. When clearly composed of simple cysts, clustered microcysts may be considered benign. If there is uncertainty, short interval follow-up may be appropriate.[35]

Diffuse, bilateral calcifications that are punctate, round, or amorphous may be considered benign (see **Fig. 1**A, B).[35] If grouped, calcifications that definitively layer on a lateral view may also be considered benign milk of calcium (see **Fig. 4**A–D). These typically demonstrate a change in shape between the craniocaudal (CC) view and lateral view.[35]

Biopsy should be recommended for imaging findings not meeting these diagnostic criteria (see **Fig. 5**A–F).

DIFFERENTIAL DIAGNOSIS

Fibrocystic change can have a similar imaging appearance to other benign entities and, in some cases, to malignancies. This is particularly true for focal fibrocystic change.[55]

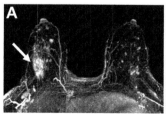
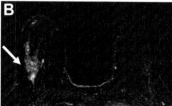
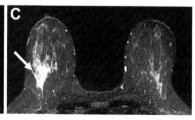

Fig. 8. Maximal intensity projection of T1-weighted, fat-saturated, subtracted postcontrast (*A*), T1-weighted, fat-saturated, subtracted postcontrast (*B*), and fluid-sensitive (STIR) (*C*) axial MR images of both breasts in a 42-year-old woman undergoing high-risk screening show segmental NME in the lateral right breast, new from the prior study (*arrows*). Small T2-bright masses are present throughout the area of NME. MR-guided biopsy was performed showing fibrocystic changes (apocrine metaplasia, usual ductal hyperplasia, fibrosis, cyst formation, columnar cell changes, and columnar cell hyperplasia). Pathologic condition was considered benign and concordant.

Cysts should be distinguished from complex masses, which are partially cystic and partially solid[32] with thick septations or thick wall (≥0.5 mm) or that contain solid masses.[33] Papillary lesions often present as complex masses.[32,56,57] High-grade invasive tumors with central necrosis may also present as complex masses with a thick wall.[58] It is important to confirm the lack of vascularity within an anechoic mass. High-grade malignancies such as triple-negative carcinomas and lymphoma can present as nearly anechoic masses with posterior acoustic enhancement but will demonstrate internal vascularity.[59]

Fat necrosis,[60,61] hematoma or postoperative fluid collection,[62] abscess,[58] and galactocele[63] can also present as cystic masses. These entities typically have unique imaging and clinical features.[64] Phyllodes tumors and some fibroadenomas may also present as masses with cystic spaces.[32,65,66]

Calcifications that are not classically benign may reflect DCIS and stereotactic biopsy is required to establish the diagnosis.[38] Biopsy is also required for architectural distortion, which may reflect invasive malignancy.[40]

The primary differential diagnosis for MR imaging findings includes DCIS for NME and invasive malignancy for masses.[51,67] Mucinous carcinoma should also be included on the differential for T2-bright masses on MR imaging given their internal mucin content. In contrast to benign cysts, mucinous carcinomas typically are irregular in shape and margins are not circumscribed.[68]

CLINICAL APPLICATIONS

Definitively benign imaging findings do not require further evaluation or biopsy.[69] For symptomatic patients, therapeutic cyst aspiration can be offered.

Cyst aspiration may be recommended for isolated complicated cysts or in cases with diagnostic uncertainty. If cyst aspiration is performed, cyst fluid that is yellow, straw-colored, milky, or green can be discarded.[17] If cyst fluid returns that is dark red/bloody, fluid should be sent for cytology. If purulent material is aspirated, the fluid should be sent for microbiology and culture.[70] If cyst aspiration does not result in complete collapse of the mass, core needle biopsy should be performed of the remaining component, including the cyst wall.

Any finding that does not meet diagnostic criteria described above should be biopsied. Biopsy markers should be placed to allow for surgical excision and localization if needed.[71] Clip placement is important because the initial imaging finding may no longer be present after the biopsy.

Special consideration should be given to post-menopausal patients not on hormone replacement therapy presenting with cystic masses because the incidence of fibrocystic change decreases considerably after menopause,[8,72] whereas the incidence of cancer increases. Although subclinical fibrocystic change is found pathologically in many postmenopausal women,[73] the threshold for recommending aspiration and/or biopsy should be lower in this group of women.

For all patients, no further management is required if a biopsy is performed and pathology is benign and concordant.[74] If pathology returns with atypia, the patient should be referred for surgical consultation. If results are discordant, either a repeat biopsy or surgical excision should be recommended.

Despite benign findings, patients who initially presented with breast pain may still inquire about the management of fibrocystic change. Reassurance is appropriate for these patients.[75] If pain is persistent, conservative nonpharmacological therapies should be attempted. Many patients treated with the use of sports bra during regular activities found pain relief.[76] Modifications to caffeine, iodine, alcohol, or fat intake have not been shown to significantly reduce breast pain.[77–79] There is no convincing data to support the routine use of vitamins E and B6 or evening primrose oil.[80–83]

For patients who experience severe or persistent pain that does not respond to conservative therapy, consultation to a clinical breast specialist should be considered. Topical nonsteroidal anti-inflammatory drugs,[84] danazol,[85,86] and tamoxifen[87–89] have shown utility in treating breast pain.

CASE STUDY PRESENTATION

A 46-year-old woman was recalled from screening mammography for architectural distortion seen on the mediolateral oblique (MLO) view of the left breast (Fig. 9A–E). This was persistent on spot compression view. Ultrasound demonstrated a questionable correlate for the distortion, with multiple simple and complicated cysts seen throughout the left breast. The patient reported that she had been previously evaluated several times in the past for palpable findings and found to have benign cysts. Although fibrocystic changes could account for architectural distortion, the finding was not classically benign, and biopsy was therefore recommended. This was performed with tomosynthesis guidance because the finding was better seen mammographically. Pathologic condition showed low-grade invasive ductal carcinoma.

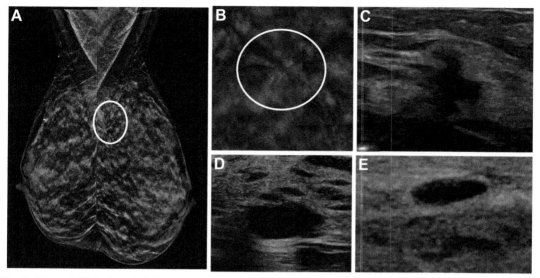

Fig. 9. Bilateral MLO views (*A*) from screening mammogram in a 46-year-old woman with history of fibrocystic change shows an area of architectural distortion in the upper left breast (*circle*). Distortion was persistent on spot compression tomosynthesis image (*B*) (*circle*). Ultrasound showed questionable correlate for the distortion (*C*), as well as multiple benign simple (*D*) and complicated (*E*) cysts throughout the breast. Biopsy was performed with stereotactic/tomosynthesis guidance. Biopsy showed invasive ductal carcinoma. Although architectural distortion can be caused by fibrocystic changes, biopsy is required for definitive diagnosis.

SUMMARY

Fibrocystic changes are commonly encountered in breast imaging practice, both from symptomatic patients and during imaging workup of screening-detected findings. Fibrocystic changes encompass a broad spectrum of benign pathologic entities. Recognition of classically benign findings of fibrocystic changes can prevent unnecessary follow-ups and biopsies. In cases of diagnostic uncertainty, however, core needle biopsy may be warranted.

CLINICS CARE POINTS

- Fibrocystic changes are common in both symptomatic and asymptomatic women.
- The imaging appearance of fibrocystic change is broad and varied. Simple cysts and complicated cysts in the setting of multiple other cysts may be considered benign (breast imaging reporting and data system [BI-RADS] 2) without the need for further intervention.
- Isolated complicated cysts may be appropriate for short-term follow-up (BI-RADS 3).
- Complex masses have both solid and cystic components or thick septations or walls (>0.5 mm) and should be biopsied (BI-RADS 4).

- Although fibrocystic change can account for imaging findings such as solid mass, developing asymmetry, architectural distortion, and mass and NME on MR imaging, biopsy is generally required for diagnosis in these cases.
- Aspiration should be offered for symptomatic benign cysts.
- Cysts in which aspiration is attempted but the mass does not aspirate to completion should be biopsied with tissue marker placement.

DISCLOSURE

The authors have nothing to disclose.

REFERENCES

1. Guray M, Sahin AA. Benign breast diseases: classification, diagnosis, and management. Oncol 2006; 11(5):435–49.
2. LiVolsi VA, Stadel BV, Kelsey JL, et al. Fibrocystic breast disease in oral-contraceptive users. A histopathological evaluation of epithelial atypia. N Engl J Med 1978;299(8):381–5.
3. Hughes LE, Mansel RE, Webster DJ. Aberrations of normal development and involution (ANDI): a new perspective on pathogenesis and nomenclature of benign breast disorders. Lancet 1987;2(8571):1316–9.
4. Dupont WD, Page DL. Risk factors for breast cancer in women with proliferative breast disease. N Engl J Med 1985;312(3):146–51.

5. Hartmann LC, Sellers TA, Frost MH, et al. Benign breast disease and the risk of breast cancer. N Engl J Med 2005;353(3):229–37.

6. Dyrstad SW, Yan Y, Fowler AM, et al. Breast cancer risk associated with benign breast disease: systematic review and meta-analysis. Breast Cancer Res Treat 2015;149(3):569–75.

7. Román M, Louro J, Posso M, et al. Breast density, benign breast disease, and risk of breast cancer over time. Eur Radiol 2021;31(7):4839–47.

8. Johansson A, Christakou AE, Iftimi A, et al. Characterization of benign breast diseases and association with age, hormonal factors, and family history of breast cancer among women in sweden. JAMA Netw Open 2021;4(6):e2114716.

9. Ghosh K, Vierkant RA, Frank RD, et al. Association between mammographic breast density and histologic features of benign breast disease. Breast Cancer Res 2017;19(1):134.

10. Ghosh K, Hartmann LC, Reynolds C, et al. Association between mammographic density and age-related lobular involution of the breast. J Clin Oncol 2010;28(13):2207–12.

11. Owen WA, Brazeal HA, Shaw HL, et al. Focal breast pain: imaging evaluation and outcomes. Clin Imag May-Jun 2019;55:148–55.

12. Ortman H, Abdo J, Tillman R, et al. Management of cystic conditions. Surg Clin North Am 2022;102(6):1089–102.

13. Egwuonwu OA, Anyanwu SN, GU Chianakwana, et al. Breast pain: clinical pattern and aetiology in a breast clinic in eastern nigeria. Niger J Surg Jan-Jun 2016;22(1):9–11.

14. Deschamps M, Band PR, Coldman AJ, et al. Clinical determinants of mammographic dysplasia patterns. Cancer Detect Prev 1996;20(6):610–9.

15. Guinebretière JM, Menet E, Tardivon A, et al. Normal and pathological breast, the histological basis. Eur J Radiol 2005;54(1):6–14.

16. Pitanguy I, Torres E, Salgado F, et al. Breast pathology and reduction mammaplasty. Plast Reconstr Surg 2005;115(3):729–34. ; discussion 735.

17. Mannello F, Tonti GA, Papa S. Human gross cyst breast disease and cystic fluid: bio-molecular, morphological, and clinical studies. Breast Cancer Res Treat 2006;97(2):115–29.

18. Quinn CM, D'Arcy C, Wells C. Apocrine lesions of the breast. Virchows Arch. Jan 2022;480(1):177–89.

19. Shin S, Ko ES, Han BK, et al. Stromal fibrosis of the breast: outcome analysis. Acta Radiol 2014;55(4):409–15.

20. Strickland S, Turashvili G. Are columnar cell lesions the earliest non-obligate precursor in the low-grade breast neoplasia pathway? Curr Oncol 2022;29(8):5664–81.

21. Visscher DW, Nassar A, Degnim AC, et al. Sclerosing adenosis and risk of breast cancer. Breast Cancer Res Treat 2014;144(1):205–12.

22. Bahl M. Management of High-Risk Breast Lesions. Radiol Clin North Am 2021;59(1):29–40.

23. Haagensen CD, Lane N, Lattes R, et al. Lobular neoplasia (so-called lobular carcinoma in situ) of the breast. Cancer 1978;42(2):737–69.

24. Morrow M, Schnitt SJ, Norton L. Current management of lesions associated with an increased risk of breast cancer. Nat Rev Clin Oncol 2015;12(4):227–38.

25. Pugh CM, Domont ZB, Salud LH, et al. A simulation-based assessment of clinical breast examination technique: do patient and clinician factors affect clinician approach? Am J Surg 2008;195(6):874–80.

26. Boyd NF, Sutherland HJ, Fish EB, et al. Prospective evaluation of physical examination of the breast. Am J Surg 1981;142(3):331–4.

27. Rosner D, Blaird D. What ultrasonography can tell in breast masses that mammography and physical examination cannot. J Surg Oncol 1985;28(4):308–13.

28. Klein KA, Kocher M, Lourenco AP, et al. ACR appropriateness criteria® palpable breast masses: 2022 update. J Am Coll Radiol 2023;20(5s):S146–s163.

29. Noroozian M, Hadjiiski L, Rahnama-Moghadam S, et al. Digital breast tomosynthesis is comparable to mammographic spot views for mass characterization. Radiology 2012;262(1):61–8.

30. Posso M, Alcántara R, Vázquez I, et al. Mammographic features of benign breast lesions and risk of subsequent breast cancer in women attending breast cancer screening. Eur Radiol 2022;32(1):621–9.

31. Sickles EA. Breast masses: mammographic evaluation. Radiology 1989;173(2):297–303.

32. Berg WA, Campassi CI, Ioffe OB. Cystic lesions of the breast: sonographic-pathologic correlation. Radiology 2003;227(1):183–91.

33. Mendelson EB, Berg WA, Merritt CR. Toward a standardized breast ultrasound lexicon, BI-RADS: ultrasound. Semin Roentgenol 2001;36(3):217–25.

34. Kushwaha AC, O'Toole M, Sneige N, et al. Mammographic-pathologic correlation of apocrine metaplasia diagnosed using vacuum-assisted stereotactic core-needle biopsy: our 4-year experience. AJR Am J Roentgenol 2003;180(3):795–8.

35. D'Orsi CJSE, Mendelson EB, Morris EA, et al. ACR BI-RADS® Atlas, breast imaging reporting and data system. American College of Radiology; 2013.

36. Iglesias A, Arias M, Santiago P, et al. Benign breast lesions that simulate malignancy: magnetic resonance imaging with radiologic-pathologic correlation. Curr Probl Diagn Radiol 2007;36(2):66–82.

37. Moy L, Slanetz PJ, Yeh ED, et al. The pendent view: an additional projection to confirm the diagnosis of milk of calcium. AJR Am J Roentgenol 2001;177(1):173–5.

38. Sanders MA, Roland L, Sahoo S. Clinical implications of subcategorizing BI-RADS 4 breast lesions

associated with microcalcification: a radiology-pathology correlation study. Breast J 2010;16(1):28–31.

39. Bent CK, Bassett LW, D'Orsi CJ, et al. The positive predictive value of BI-RADS microcalcification descriptors and final assessment categories. AJR Am J Roentgenol 2010;194(5):1378–83.

40. Bahl M, Baker JA, Kinsey EN, et al. Architectural Distortion on Mammography: Correlation With Pathologic Outcomes and Predictors of Malignancy. AJR Am J Roentgenol 2015;205(6):1339–45.

41. Ambinder EB, Plotkin A, Euhus D, et al. Tomosynthesis-guided vacuum-assisted breast biopsy of architectural distortion without a sonographic correlate: a retrospective review. AJR Am J Roentgenol 2021;217(4):845–54.

42. Vijapura C, Yang L, Xiong J, et al. Imaging features of nonmalignant and malignant architectural distortion detected by tomosynthesis. AJR Am J Roentgenol 2018;211(6):1397–404.

43. Liang A, Baraban E, Myers KS, et al. Developing asymmetries without sonographic correlate at digital breast tomosynthesis. Radiology 2022;302(3):525–32.

44. Shetty MK, Shah YP. Sonographic findings in focal fibrocystic changes of the breast. Ultrasound Q 2002;18(1):35–40.

45. Guirguis MS, Adrada B, Santiago L, et al. Mimickers of breast malignancy: imaging findings, pathologic concordance and clinical management. Insights Imaging 2021;12(1):53.

46. Chen JH, Liu H, Baek HM, et al. Magnetic resonance imaging features of fibrocystic change of the breast. Magn Reson Imaging 2008;26(9):1207–14.

47. Gao Y, Dialani V, DeBenedectis C, et al. Apocrine metaplasia found at mr biopsy: is there something to be learned? Breast J 2017;23(4):429–35.

48. Maglione KD, Lee AY, Ray KM, et al. Radiologic-pathologic correlation for benign results after MRI-guided breast biopsy. AJR Am J Roentgenol 2017;209(2):442–53.

49. Milosevic ZC, Nadrljanski MM, Milovanovic ZM, et al. Breast dynamic contrast enhanced mri: fibrocystic changes presenting as a non-mass enhancement mimicking malignancy. Radiol Oncol 2017;51(2):130–6.

50. van den Bosch MA, Daniel BL, Mariano MN, et al. Magnetic resonance imaging characteristics of fibrocystic change of the breast. Invest Radiol 2005;40(7):436–41.

51. Liberman L, Morris EA, Dershaw DD, et al. Ductal enhancement on MR imaging of the breast. AJR Am J Roentgenol 2003;181(2):519–25.

52. Choe AI, Kasales C, Mack J, et al. Fibrocystic changes of the breast: radiologic–pathologic correlation of MRI. Journal of Breast Imaging 2021;4(1):48–55.

53. Chen JH, Nalcioglu O, Su MY. Fibrocystic change of the breast presenting as a focal lesion mimicking breast cancer in MR imaging. J Magn Reson Imaging 2008;28(6):1499–505.

54. Lee SJ, Mahoney MC, Khan S. MRI features of stromal fibrosis of the breast with histopathologic correlation. AJR Am J Roentgenol. Sep 2011;197(3):755–62.

55. Lin X, He Y, Fu S, et al. The ultrasonographic characteristics of focal fibrocystic change of the breast and analysis of misdiagnosis. Clin Breast Cancer 2022;22(3):252–60.

56. Muttarak M, Lerttumnongtum P, Chaiwun B, et al. Spectrum of papillary lesions of the breast: clinical, imaging, and pathologic correlation. AJR Am J Roentgenol 2008;191(3):700–7.

57. Soo MS, Williford ME, Walsh R, et al. Papillary carcinoma of the breast: imaging findings. AJR Am J Roentgenol 1995;164(2):321–6.

58. Athanasiou A, Aubert E, Vincent Salomon A, et al. Complex cystic breast masses in ultrasound examination. Diagn Interv Imaging 2014;95(2):169–79.

59. Berg WA, Sechtin AG, Marques H, et al. Cystic breast masses and the ACRIN 6666 experience. Radiol Clin North Am 2010;48(5):931–87.

60. Soo MS, Kornguth PJ, Hertzberg BS. Fat necrosis in the breast: sonographic features. Radiology 1998;206(1):261–9.

61. Bilgen IG, Ustun EE, Memis A. Fat necrosis of the breast: clinical, mammographic and sonographic features. Eur J Radiol 2001;39(2):92–9.

62. Chansakul T, Lai KC, Slanetz PJ. The postconservation breast: part 1, expected imaging findings. AJR Am J Roentgenol 2012;198(2):321–30.

63. Gao Y, Slanetz PJ, Eisenberg RL. Echogenic breast masses at US: to biopsy or not to biopsy? Radiographics 2013;33(2):419–34.

64. Hines N, Slanetz PJ, Eisenberg RL. Cystic masses of the breast. AJR Am J Roentgenol 2010;194(2):W122–33.

65. Duman L, Gezer NS, Balcı P, et al. Differentiation between phyllodes tumors and fibroadenomas based on mammographic sonographic and MRI Features. Breast Care 2016;11(2):123–7.

66. Liberman L, Bonaccio E, Hamele-Bena D, et al. Benign and malignant phyllodes tumors: mammographic and sonographic findings. Radiology 1996;198(1):121–4.

67. Jansen SA, Shimauchi A, Zak L, et al. The diverse pathology and kinetics of mass, nonmass, and focus enhancement on MR imaging of the breast. J Magn Reson Imaging 2011;33(6):1382–9.

68. Chaudhry AR, El Khoury M, Gotra A, et al. Imaging features of pure and mixed forms of mucinous breast carcinoma with histopathological correlation. Br J Radiol 2019;92(1095):20180810.

69. Bevers TB, Niell BL, Baker JL, et al. NCCN guidelines® insights: breast cancer screening and diagnosis, version 1.2023. J Natl Compr Canc Netw 2023;21(9):900–9.

70. Daly CP, Bailey JE, Klein KA, et al. Complicated breast cysts on sonography: is aspiration necessary to exclude malignancy? Acad Radiol 2008;15(5): 610–7.

71. Phillips SW, Gabriel H, Comstock CE, et al. Sonographically guided metallic clip placement after core needle biopsy of the breast. AJR Am J Roentgenol 2000;175(5):1353–5.

72. Dang BQ, Miles B, Young P, et al. An interesting imaging presentation of a common benign entity: fibrocystic changes in a postmenopausal patient. Cureus 2023;15(3):e36292.

73. Sarnelli R, Squartini F. Fibrocystic condition and "at risk" lesions in asymptomatic breasts: a morphologic study of postmenopausal women. Clin Exp Obstet Gynecol 1991;18(4):271–9.

74. Lee SJ, Mahoney MC, Redus Z. The Management of benign concordant mri-guided brest biopsies: lessons learned. Breast J 2015;21(6):665–8.

75. Barros AC, Mottola J, Ruiz CA, et al. Reassurance in the treatment of mastalgia. Breast J 1999;5(3): 162–5.

76. Hadi MS. Sports brassiere: is it a solution for mastalgia? Breast J 2000;6(6):407–9.

77. Millet AV, Dirbas FM. Clinical management of breast pain: a review. Obstet Gynecol Surv 2002;57(7): 451–61.

78. Goodwin PJ, Miller A, Del Giudice ME, et al. Elevated high-density lipoprotein cholesterol and dietary fat intake in women with cyclic mastopathy. Am J Obstet Gynecol 1998;179(2):430–7.

79. Boyd NF, McGuire V, Shannon P, et al. Effect of a low-fat high-carbohydrate diet on symptoms of cyclical mastopathy. Lancet 1988;2(8603):128–32.

80. Ernster VL, Goodson WH 3rd, Hunt TK, et al. Vitamin E and benign breast "disease": a double-blind, randomized clinical trial. Surgery 1985;97(4):490–4.

81. Meyer EC, Sommers DK, Reitz CJ, et al. Vitamin E and benign breast disease. Surgery 1990;107(5): 549–51.

82. Pruthi S, Wahner-Roedler DL, Torkelson CJ, et al. Vitamin E and evening primrose oil for management of cyclical mastalgia: a randomized pilot study. Altern Med Rev 2010;15(1):59–67.

83. Blommers J, de Lange-De Klerk ES, Kuik DJ, et al. Evening primrose oil and fish oil for severe chronic mastalgia: a randomized, double-blind, controlled trial. Am J Obstet Gynecol 2002;187(5):1389–94.

84. Colak T, Ipek T, Kanik A, et al. Efficacy of topical nonsteroidal antiinflammatory drugs in mastalgia treatment. J Am Coll Surg 2003;196(4):525–30.

85. Pye JK, Mansel RE, Hughes LE. Clinical experience of drug treatments for mastalgia. Lancet 1985; 2(8451):373–7.

86. O'Brien PM, Abukhalil IE. Randomized controlled trial of the management of premenstrual syndrome and premenstrual mastalgia using luteal phase-only danazol. Am J Obstet Gynecol 1999;180(1 Pt 1):18–23.

87. Fentiman IS, Caleffi M, Hamed H, et al. Dosage and duration of tamoxifen treatment for mastalgia: a controlled trial. Br J Surg. Sep 1988;75(9):845–6.

88. Kontostolis E, Stefanidis K, Navrozoglou I, et al. Comparison of tamoxifen with danazol for treatment of cyclical mastalgia. Gynecol Endocrinol 1997; 11(6):393–7.

89. Srivastava A, Mansel RE, Arvind N, et al. Evidence-based management of Mastalgia: a meta-analysis of randomised trials. Breast 2007;16(5):503–12.

Understanding Risk

Breast Density
Where Are We Now?

Eric Kim, MD[a], Alana A. Lewin, MD[a,b,*]

KEYWORDS

• Breast density • Breast cancer risk • Dense breasts • Supplemental breast cancer screening

KEY POINTS

- Breast density is a heritable and dynamic trait associated with age, race/ethnicity, body mass index and hormonal factors.
- Increased breast density may have a masking effect on mammography and is an independent risk factor for breast cancer.
- The American College of Radiology has published appropriate use criteria for supplemental screening based on breast density due to the negative impact of breast density on mammographic sensitivity.

INTRODUCTION

Breast density refers to the amount of fibroglandular tissue relative to fat and is determined either visually or quantitatively on mammography. The assessment of breast density is important as it indicates the possibility that a lesion could be obscured by normal tissue. Fibroglandular tissue absorbs relatively more ionizing radiation compared with fatty tissue and projects as gradations of white on mammography. In an attempt to standardize the description of breast density, the Breast Imaging Reporting and Data System (BI-RADS) fifth edition described four categories of breast density: category A (almost entirely fatty), B (scattered fibroglandular tissue), C (heterogeneously dense), and D (extremely dense).[1] (Fig. 1, Table 1). Dense breasts are common as approximately 36% of women more than 40 year old have heterogeneously dense breasts and 7% have extremely dense breasts.[2] Previously, the breast density categories were defined by the total amount of fibroglandular tissue within the breast. However, in order to reflect the relationship between breast density and the risk of masking breast cancer, the BI-RADS fifth edition changed the definition of density to reflect the densest area[1] of fibroglandular tissue within the breast (Fig. 2).

As a result, breast density remains an important factor in the interpretation of screening mammography. Breast density not only has the potential to mask a malignancy but is an independent risk factor for breast cancer. Dense breast tissue also is associated with an increased risk of interval breast cancer[3] and an increased incidence of high-risk lesions and nonproliferative benign breast disease.[4] Owing to the ongoing attention toward personalized care in medicine and in particular breast cancer screening, there is increasing interest in breast density as a modifiable risk factor for breast cancer and a tool for risk stratification. In addition, there is enhanced focus on methods to optimize breast cancer screening and offer supplemental tools to improve cancer detection in women with dense breasts.

ASSESSMENT OF BREAST DENSITY
Visual Assessment

The most commonly used method to categorize breast density is subjective visual assessment. The fourth edition of BI-RADS which was released in 2003 used quartile ranges of the percentage of

[a] Department of Radiology, New York University Grossman School of Medicine, New York, NY, USA; [b] New York University Grossman School of Medicine, New York University Langone Health, Laura and Isaac Perlmutter Cancer Center, 160 East 34th Street 3rd Floor, New York, NY 10016, USA
* Corresponding author. 160 East 34th Street, 3rd Floor, New York, NY 10016.
E-mail address: Alana.Amarosa@nyulangone.org

Radiol Clin N Am 62 (2024) 593–605
https://doi.org/10.1016/j.rcl.2023.12.007

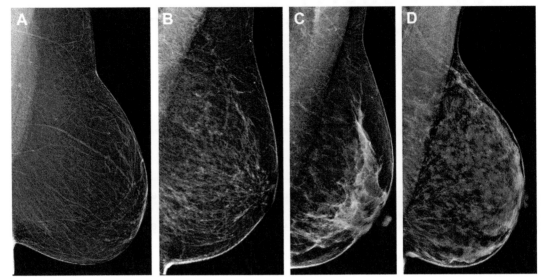

Fig. 1. Left mediolateral oblique (MLO) views demonstrate the BI-RADS fifth edition breast density categories: (*A*) Almost entirely fatty. (*B*) Scattered fibroglandular density. (*C*) Heterogeneously dense. (*D*) Extremely dense.

dense fibroglandular tissue (<25%, 25%–50%, 50%–75%, and >75%) for the four density categories. However, the fifth edition of BI-RADS which was released in 2013 has removed these percentage ranges. Instead, BI-RADS now emphasizes the text descriptions of breast density to focus on the masking effect of dense fibroglandular tissue to detect breast cancer.

According to BI-RADS, radiologists should make an overall assessment of breast density based on the relative possibility of normal fibroglandular tissue to obscure an underlying breast lesion. This should be based on the densest area of tissue within the breast; therefore, a breast may be categorized as dense even when only a focal area of dense tissue is present in an otherwise predominantly fatty breast (see **Fig. 2**). In breasts that have areas of primarily dense tissue with other areas that are primarily fatty, BI-RADS suggests that it may be helpful to the referring clinician to describe the location of the denser tissue. In breasts that are not of equal density, the denser breast should be used to categorize breast density.

A well-known limitation of visual assessment is that there is considerable intraobserver and interobserver variation in the categorization of breast density.[5–8] This may be due to multiple individual factors including reader fatigue, the predisposition to overestimate or underestimate density, and variable reading room conditions. A study which involved 30 radiology facilities in the United States from the Population-based Research Optimizing Screening through Personalized Regimens consortium demonstrated a wide range (6.3%–84.5%) of screening mammograms that were interpreted as dense by radiologists.[8] In a recent study, statistically significant interobserver variability also was seen at the international level when comparing breast imaging radiologists practicing in Indonesia, the Netherlands, South Africa, and the United States.[9] Because of this variability, quantitative and deep learning methods have emerged in an effort to standardize the assessment of breast density.

Quantitative Assessment

Fully automated quantitative methods have been developed which calculate either the volume or area-based density percentage on mammography. The two most well-known commercially available and Food and Drug Administration

Table 1
Breast density categories based on the breast imaging reporting and data system (BI-RADS) fifth edition

Category	Terms
A	The breasts are almost entirely fatty
B	There are scattered areas of fibroglandular density
C	The breasts are heterogeneously dense, which may obscure small masses
D	The breasts are extremely dense, which lowers the sensitivity of mammography

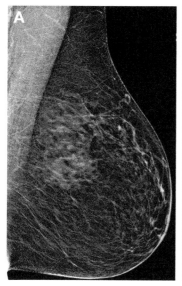
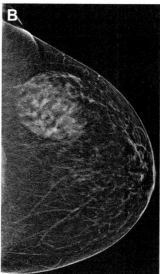

Fig. 2. Left mediolateral oblique (MLO) (*A*) and craniocaudal (CC) (*B*) views of a 46-year-old woman who presented for screening mammogram. Dense fibroglandular tissue is visualized in the upper breast. Even though the percentage density in the breast is less than 50%, the mammogram was classified as heterogeneously dense according to the BI-RADS fifth edition which states that density should be based on the ability of the densest area of tissue within the breast to mask a lesion.

(FDA)-approved methods are Volpara (Volpara Health, Wellington, New Zealand) (**Fig. 3**) and Quantra (Hologic, Danbury, Connecticut). Both calculate the volumetric breast density percentage by dividing the volume of fibroglandular tissue by the total breast volume and convert this into an appropriate BI-RADS breast density category. These automated methods have been shown to be both consistent and reproducible.[10,11] However, studies have shown mixed results in regard to correlation between different automated methods as well as between automated methods and radiologists.[12–15]

Previously, area-based density percentage methods also were used, primarily in the research setting. The most well-known is Cumulus (University of Toronto, Toronto, Ontario, Canada), which is a semiautomated method that requires human input including segmentation of the breast. These methods have limited clinical utility because they are time-consuming and less reliable than volume-based methods.[10,16] Fully automated area-based methods also were developed but never achieved widespread use.

Artificial Intelligence

Recently, deep learning-based methods have been developed to categorize breast density on mammograms with encouraging results.[17–19] Lehman and colleagues trained a deep convolutional neural network to assess breast density on more than 41,000 screening mammograms. They were one of the first to implement their model in the clinical

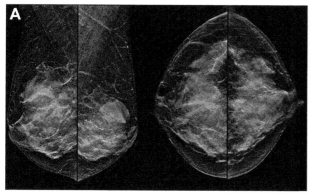
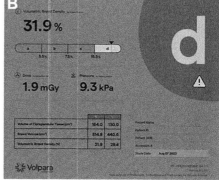

Fig. 3. Bilateral mediolateral oblique (MLO) and craniocaudal (CC) views from screening mammogram demonstrate dense breast tissue (*A*). The volumetric breast density percentage was calculated using fully-automated Volpara software and results in BI-RADS breast density category D or extremely dense breasts (*B*). (*Courtesy of* Dr. Stamatia DeStounis.)

setting and demonstrated very good (94%) agreement between their model and radiologists in the binary categorization of dense versus non-dense breasts.[17] In a more recent prospective study with more than 85,000 consecutive screening mammograms, Dontchos and colleagues evaluated clinical implementation of their deep learning model at three sites. Interestingly, they demonstrated a significant reduction in the radiologist classification of mammograms as dense after exposure to their deep learning model. They also reported reduced reader variability in density assessment at the sites exposed to the model.[20]

There are now multiple FDA-approved AI and machine learning tools to assess breast density including commercial options from Volpara and Quantra.[21] The limitations of deep learning models include the need to verify the models in diverse patient populations, across different mammographic vendors, and across multiple institutions. Further studies need to be performed to compare the results in breast density categorization between deep learning methods and quantitative volume-based methods.

FACTORS THAT INFLUENCE BREAST DENSITY

Breast density is a heritable and dynamic trait. Studies show that the heritability of breast density is high, with genetic factors accounting for 58% to 67% of breast density variation.[22–24] Breast density is associated with age, hormonal factors, race/ethnicity, and body mass index (BMI).[25]

Hormonal

Exogenous and endogenous hormonal factors impact breast density. Generally, mammographic density gradually decreases as age increases in the premenopausal period, with the exception of pregnancy and breastfeeding (**Fig. 4**). This inverse relationship with mammographic density and age continues postmenopausally and is most pronounced in the menopausal transition. These age-related density changes are seen across ethnic groups of women worldwide, suggesting a common intrinsic biological mechanism.[26] Parity is inversely associated with breast density.[27,28] In addition, two recent studies[27,28] found that older age at first birth and older age at menarche are associated with higher density. A retrospective study of BRCA1/2 mutation carriers who underwent bilateral oophorectomy showed that breast density significantly decreased after oophorectomy.[29] Younger patients demonstrated greater absolute decreases compared with older patients.[29]

Menopausal hormone therapy (MHT) is used to relieve the common symptoms of menopause, including hot flashes, sleep disturbances, mood alteration, muscle, and joint pain. Studies have shown an association between systemic MHT and increased density. Specifically, estrogen plus progestin MHT is associated with higher density than estrogen alone.[27] Mammographic density at least partially accounts for the association between MHT and breast cancer.[27,30]

Tamoxifen, a selective estrogen receptor modulator, can reduce breast density and breast cancer risk. High-risk women receiving tamoxifen chemoprevention who experienced ≥ 10% reduction in breast density had a 63% reduction in breast cancer risk compared with placebo group.[31] Women who had less than 10% reduction in breast density had no breast cancer risk reduction.[31] Further research has shown a large decrease in breast density over the first year of tamoxifen therapy with continued decline thereafter.[32] Studies on aromatase inhibitors and breast density reduction demonstrate mixed results.[33–35]

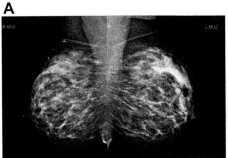 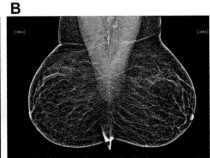

Fig. 4. Bilateral mediolateral oblique (MLO) views from a 35-year-old woman who presents for mammogram while breastfeeding demonstrate heterogeneously dense breasts (*A*). Bilateral mediolateral oblique views when the same patient presents for screening mammogram 5 years later demonstrate interval decreased breast density, now characterized as scattered areas of fibroglandular density (*B*).

Race/Ethnicity

Studies on breast density and its association with race and ethnicity have shown mixed results.[36] Breast density is well studied among Asian women who have a high prevalence of heterogeneously dense and extremely dense breasts.[14] According to the Breast Cancer Surveillance Consortium (BCSC), in the United States, Asian women have the highest proportion of dense breasts, followed in descending order by non-Hispanic White women, Hispanic/Latina women, and non-Hispanic Black/African American women.[25] However, the effect of race and ethnicity on breast density are often limited by confounding factors such as use of hormone replacement therapy, BMI, and reproductive factors.[37] When correcting for these factors, there is still variability in breast density by race/ethnicity.[38]

Nonetheless, higher breast density is associated with an increased risk of breast cancer within certain racial/ethnic groups,[38] Although a smaller proportion of Black/African American women have dense breasts, Black/African American women with dense breasts are at an increased risk of breast cancer compared with Black/African American women with nondense breasts.[39]

Lifestyle and Environmental Factors

There is growing interest in the impact of lifestyle and environmental factors on breast density. BMI is inversely related to breast density in adulthood.[40] Interestingly, high BMI increases the risk of developing postmenopausal breast cancer, but not premenopausal breast cancer.[38,41] Reduced breast cancer risk following weight loss or bariatric surgery may be due in part to reduction in total volume of dense breast tissue.[42,43] In light of this information, breast density must be corrected for BMI and age in the Tyrer-Cuzick (TC) model to add the independent contribution of breast density to breast cancer risk.[44]

The role of alcohol and tobacco use on breast density has also been explored. Studies show that there is a relationship between higher breast density and alcohol intake and lower breast density and tobacco use.[27,45]

CLINICAL IMPLICATIONS
Masking Effect on Mammography: Decreased Sensitivity

Mammographic performance and resultant screening outcomes are significantly impacted by breast density. Both increased false-positive findings[46,47] and reduced cancer detection rates are seen in women with dense breasts[48] (Fig. 5).

Although malignant calcifications remain well visualized, noncalcified cancers (approximately 45% of invasive cancers[49]) can be masked by dense tissue. The sensitivity of mammography to detect breast cancer diminishes with increasing breast density. The sensitivity range of mammography is 81% to 93% for fatty breasts, 84% to 90% for breasts with scattered fibroglandular density, 69% to 81% for heterogeneously dense breasts, and 57% to 71% for extremely dense breasts.[46] In addition, women with dense breasts have more interval cancers, which are cancers diagnosed in between successive screening mammograms, than women with nondense breasts.[50,51] Even with the use of tomosynthesis,[52] approximately 25% of breast cancers are missed on mammography in women with heterogeneously dense breasts and about 40% in women with extremely dense breasts[46,48,50]

Independent Risk Factor for Breast Cancer

Multiple studies have demonstrated that breast density is an independent risk factor for the development of breast cancer, although there is continued debate about the degree to which it increases lifetime risk. This was first described by Wolfe when he demonstrated an increased risk for developing breast cancer based solely on a classification system for the appearance of breast parenchyma on mammography.[53,54] Since then, numerous additional studies have been published confirming that dense breast tissue increases the risk of breast cancer.

In a meta-analysis which included 42 studies, McCormack and colleagues demonstrated a 4.64-fold (95% CI 3.65–5.91) increased risk of breast cancer in patients with the most dense breasts compared with those with the least dense breasts.[55] A more recent meta-analysis by Bodewes and colleagues published in 2022 analyzed studies which used the breast density classification system from the more recent BI-RADS fifth edition.[56] The analysis included nine studies which together demonstrated a 3.89-fold (95% CI 2.47–6.13) increased breast cancer risk in patients with extremely dense breast tissue in comparison with those with extremely fatty breast tissue. However, less than 10% of women have either extremely dense or extremely fatty breasts. Therefore, the investigators also investigated the relative risk of patients with dense breasts to those with scattered density, which they described as the average breast density. In this comparison, they found a 1.28-fold increase (95% CI 1.19–1.37) in women with heterogeneously dense breasts and a 2.11-fold (95% CI 1.84–2.42) in women with

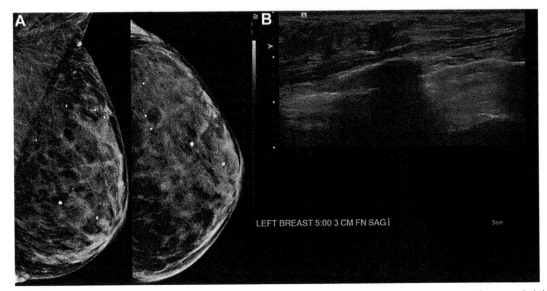

Fig. 5. A 67-year-old woman who presented for annual screening mammogram and screening ultrasound. (*A*) Left mediolateral oblique (MLO) and craniocaudal (CC) views demonstrate breast density category D: extremely dense. There is no mammographic evidence of malignancy. However, screening ultrasound (*B*) demonstrates a 0.6 cm irregular, hypoechoic mass at left 5:00, 3 cm from the nipple. This underwent ultrasound core biopsy yielding invasive ductal carcinoma, well-differentiated, estrogen receptor positive, progesterone receptor positive, HER2-neu receptor negative.

extremely dense breasts compared with those with scattered density.

In a literature review including 102 studies, increased breast density has been associated with increased tumor size, although there are conflicting data regarding lymph node status and no evidence to support an increased risk of distant metastasis.[57]

Increased mammographic density has also been shown to be associated with an increased rate of interval cancers.[58,59] This may be in part due to the masking effect of breast density, although some suggest that underlying biological changes may also play a role. The findings are important because interval cancers are known to be more aggressive and have a poorer prognosis than screen-detected cancers.[60] A pooled analysis which included six studies and 3492 invasive breast cancers demonstrated a positive correlation between percent mammographic density with an increased risk of breast cancer across all molecular subtypes of breast cancer.[61] Interestingly, a recently published longitudinal study found that the decrease in breast density over time was slower in patients who developed breast cancer, suggesting that breast density is a dynamic risk factor which can change over time.[62]

Overview of Risk Models

There are several models used to assess the risk for developing breast cancer, although there are multiple limitations in the use of current risk models. Most of the currently used risk models provide general risk estimates at the population level rather than at the individual level, and different models are known to underestimate breast cancer risk in different subgroups of patients.[63] A recently published study also showed that there is substantial variability between different models in estimating breast cancer risk.[64]

The most common risk models currently used are the Gail, TC, and BCSC models. Each model uses a different combination of factors to calculate individual risk (**Table 2**). For instance, the Gail model, also known as the Breast Cancer Risk Assessment Tool, includes criteria such as reproductive history, history of breast biopsies, and first-degree relatives with breast cancer. The TC model, also known as the International Breast Intervention Study model, is more comprehensive, including additional criteria such as greater family history (first- and second-degree relatives with history of breast cancer) and BMI.

Breast density is not included as a factor in many of the risk models, such as the widely used Gail model. However, at least three models, including the latest version of the TC model, the BSCS model, and the Breast and Ovarian Analysis of Disease Incidence and Carrier Estimation Algorithm model, include breast density information. Studies have shown that the addition of breast density improves the performance of the Gail

Table 2
Factors included in commonly used breast cancer risk models

Gail	Tyrer-Cuzick (Version 8)	Breast Cancer Surveillance Consortium
• Age	• Age	• Age
• Age at menarche	• Age at menarche	• Race/ethnicity
• Age at first live birth	• Age at first live birth	• Family history of breast cancer
• Race/ethnicity	• Age at menopause	○ First-degree relatives
• Family history of breast cancer	• Body mass index	• History of prior breast biopsies
○ First-degree relatives	• Breast density	• BI-RADS breast density
• History of prior breast biopsies	• Hormone replacement therapy use	
	• BRCA gene	
	• Family history of breast cancer	
	○ First-degree relatives	
	○ Second-degree relatives	
	• History of prior breast biopsies	
	• History of ovarian cancer	

and TC risk models.[65–67] In a systematic review with 11 studies including mammographic breast density improved risk prediction in all of the tested breast cancer risk models.[68] McCarthy and colleagues demonstrated that the BCSC model had higher accuracy than other models that they tested, including the Gail and TC models, in predicting breast cancer risk among women who had breast density information available in their cohort of more than 35,000 women.[69] Volume-based breast density percentage has been shown to be more strongly associated with breast cancer risk than area-based breast density percentage.[70]

Recently, deep learning models trained on mammographic images have been developed to estimate breast cancer risk. Early results demonstrate improvement over breast density-based scores and models,[71,72] suggesting that there is more image-based information than density alone which plays an important role in risk prediction. Newer risk models are being developed to include additional information such as genetics to further improve breast cancer risk prediction. Improving the performance of risk models is critical in identifying patients who may benefit from supplemental imaging or chemoprevention.

SUPPLEMENTAL SCREENING BASED ON BREAST DENSITY

Although mammography reduces breast cancer mortality,[73] the impact of breast density on mammographic performance underscores the need for more effective screening strategies.

Changes to Dense Breast Notification Laws

In 2009, Connecticut was the first state to enact dense breast notification laws, mandating that patients are notified about their breast density. In 2011, the FDA Mammography Quality Assurance Advisory Committee advised that the FDA should require breast density reporting both in mammography reports to health care providers and in lay language summaries to patients. On March 10, 2023, the FDA issued a rule (effective September 10, 2024) that will require the BI-RADS density category (using the 2013 BI-RADS language[1]) to be included in mammography reports sent to health care providers.[74] This also stipulates specific language in mammography letters sent to patients, which cannot be altered (**Fig. 6**).

In addition, facilities will have to comply with all applicable federal, state, and local reporting requirements. The FDA estimates that there will be reduced mortality and reduced breast cancer treatment costs as a result of density notification.[74] However, in order to observe these benefits, women and their providers must be educated about supplemental screening and have access to supplemental screening modalities.

Supplemental Screening Based on Breast Density

Research shows that there are socioeconomic, geographic, racial, and ethnic disparities in both the awareness of breast density and its implications for supplemental screening.[75] The modalities available to patients with dense breasts are impacted by practice type (academic vs private practice) and geography.[76] The most common supplemental modalities available are whole-breast ultrasound (WBUS), digital breast tomosynthesis (DBT), and breast MR imaging.

In 2021, the American College of Radiology (ACR) published appropriate use criteria for

> **Non-dense breast notification:** "Breast tissue can be either dense or not dense. Dense tissue makes it harder to find breast cancer on a mammogram and also raises the risk of developing breast cancer. Your breast tissue is not dense. Talk to your healthcare provider about breast density, risks for breast cancer, and your individual situation."
>
> **Dense breast notification:** "Breast tissue can be either dense or not dense. Dense tissue makes it harder to find breast cancer on a mammogram and also raises the risk of developing breast cancer. Your breast tissue is dense. In some people with dense tissue, other imaging tests in addition to a mammogram may help find cancers. Talk to your healthcare provider about breast density, risks for breast cancer, and your individual situation."

Fig. 6. Food and Drug Administration (FDA) language required in mammogram results letters to patients as of September 10, 2024. Breasts assessed by the radiologist as "not dense" include BI-RADS density category A (almost entirely fatty) and B (scattered areas of fibroglandular density). "Dense" breasts include those assessed as BI-RADS category C (heterogeneously dense, which may obscure small masses) and D (extremely dense, which lowers the sensitivity of mammography).

supplemental breast cancer screening based on breast density.[77] The document reviewed six clinical scenarios based on breast cancer risk and breast density and presented evidence for the appropriate use of various imaging studies in the specific contexts. In 2023, the ACR released updated breast cancer screening guidelines[78] (**Table 3**), some of which address scenarios of patients with varying risk factors and different breast density.

Multiple studies confirm the incremental cancer detection of WBUS. Whole-breast screening ultrasound (WBUS) increases the detection of early invasive node-negative breast cancers in women with mammographically dense breast tissue and varying patient risk factors[73,79,80] with an incremental cancer detection rate (CDR) of 2 to 2.7/1000.[81] However, as demonstrated in the multi-institutional ACRIN 6666 trial and other studies, the supplemental cancer detection with ultrasound is associated with high screening recall rates, high rate of short-term follow-up, and lower positive predictive value for biopsy compared with mammography, and MR imaging.[82–84] Therefore, the ACR recommends that women with elevated risk due to breast density may consider adjunctive screening with ultrasound after weighing the risks and benefits.[78]

Multiple prospective studies in women at higher-than-average risk of breast cancer demonstrate that breast MR imaging has higher sensitivity than mammography, ultrasound, and mammography plus ultrasound combined. The

Table 3
Comparison of the American College of Radiology recommendations for annual imaging (with consideration of breast density)

	ACR Recommendations 2018[76]	Updated ACR Recommendations 2023[77]
Lifetime risk ≥20% (regardless of breast density)	Annual DM ± DBT Annual MR imaging (starting at age 30 y)	Annual DM ± DBT Annual MR imaging (starting at age 30 y)
Personal history of breast cancer	Annual DM ± DBT (from the age of diagnosis) Annual MR imaging if dense breasts or if diagnosed before age 50	Annual DM ± DBT (from the age of diagnosis) Annual MR imaging if dense breasts or if diagnosed before age 50 y
Dense breast tissue	Annual DM ± DBT consider annual MR imaging or ultrasound (age 40 y or earlier if other risk factors)	Annual DM ± DBT annual MR imaging Consider CEM or ultrasound as alternative to MR imaging (age 40 y or earlier if other risk factors)

Abbreviations: DBT, digital breast tomosynthesis; DM, digital mammography; MR imaging, contrast-enhanced breast MR imaging.

Table adapted and modified from: Monticciolo DL et al. Breast Cancer Screening for Women at Higher-Than-Average Risk: Updated Recommendations From the ACR. J Am Coll Radiol 2023 May 5;S1546-1440(23)00334-4.

American Cancer Society advocates for screening with breast MR imaging in high-risk women regardless of breast density. In addition, the ACR recommends that women with genetics-based increased risk (including BRCA1 carriers), those with a calculated lifetime risk of $\geq$ 20%, and those exposed to chest radiation at a young age are recommended to have MR imaging surveillance starting at age 25 to 30 years, regardless of breast density.[78]

Breast MR imaging also is recommended for women with dense breasts who desire supplemental screening. For those who qualify for but cannot undergo breast MR imaging, contrast-enhanced mammography (CEM) or ultrasound may be considered.[78] A recent meta-analysis by Hussein and colleagues found that for women at average or intermediate risk for breast cancer with dense breasts, MR imaging was statistically superior to other supplemental modalities, with better cancer detection rate than ultrasound or DBT.[85] Given the recent evidence that women with dense breast tissue alone may benefit from supplemental screening with MR imaging,[86,87] the European Society of Breast Imaging has updated their recommendations to reflect this change.[88] In the DENSE (Breast Cancer Screening With MR imaging in Women Aged 50–75 Years With Extremely Dense Breast Tissue) randomized controlled trial in the Netherlands, the prevalence-round MR imaging screening in women with extremely dense breasts yielded 16.5/1000 cancers and a 50% reduction in interval cancer rate, suggesting a mortality benefit[89]; this was shown to be cost-effective in modeling.[90] In the second MR imaging screening round, the CDR was 5.8/1000 and the false-positive rate decreased from 79.8% to 26.3%.[91] It should be noted that women were invited for biennial screening and therefore that the impact of MR imaging on interval cancer rates might vary compared with a study evaluating annual screening.

Insurance Coverage

Issues with insurance coverage/denials and out-of-pocket costs remain a concern for patients recommended for supplemental screening. State insurance laws for supplemental screening are inconsistent. Currently, 21 states and the District of Columbia have enacted insurance laws for either supplemental US and/or MR imaging. Of note, for most of the state insurance laws, out-of-pocket costs such as copays and deductibles still apply. As of June 19, 2023, 14 states either have no-cost sharing legislation in effect or soon to be in effect (ie, no expense to the patient) for supplemental screening.[92] However, even when a state insurance law is in effect, some insurance plans are exempt from state laws, including national plans like Medicare and the Veterans Administration.

FUTURE DIRECTIONS
Textural Analysis and Radiomics

Breast density provides a global assessment of the relative amount of fibroglandular tissue in the breast. However, there is increasing interest in analyzing the more complex parenchymal pattern of the breast. These more granular textural features have been proposed as possible imaging biomarkers for breast cancer risk. The idea behind this is that medical images contain information reflecting underlying biological processes which can be analyzed quantitatively.[93] Radiomics refers to the practice of high-throughput extraction of mineable quantitative data from digital medical images. Advantages to this include reproducibility and scalability over subjective or qualitative methods. There is growing evidence that textural features have the ability to provide more information than breast density alone in breast cancer risk assessment.

One of the first studies to look at textural analysis was performed by Byng and colleagues.[94] The investigators conducted a nested case-control study using automated analysis of two textural mammographic features, one describing the distribution of breast density and the other characterizing texture. The study demonstrated a moderately increased relative risk of breast cancer with these two textural features after adjusting for the effect of other risk factors. Several additional studies since then have also demonstrated increased breast cancer risk after analyzing textural features from mammography.[95–97]

The investigators of a recent systematic review which included 28 articles published between 2016 and 2021 suggest that risk prediction model performance increases when textural features are added to breast density.[98] For example, Kontos and colleagues demonstrated a significant association of their radiomics-derived textural features from mammography with breast cancer. They also demonstrated improved performance of their model after including textural features compared with a baseline model which only included percentage density and BMI (area under the curve [AUC] of 0.84 vs 0.80).[99]

Most of the studies thus far have been retrospective case-control studies. As a result, additional and larger prospective studies are needed before textural features are included in breast cancer risk prediction models. Of note, it is also difficult to perform a meta-analysis or assess reproducibility in this area given the heterogeneity in the approach and number of features that are included. Despite academic interest, clinical application or evaluation of radiomic approaches are still lacking. However, radiomics remains a promising field with the potential to improve our knowledge of breast cancer risk, diagnosis, and treatment.

SUMMARY

Breast density is a heritable trait that is influenced by age, hormonal factors, race/ethnicity, and BMI. There are important clinical implications of having increased breast density including decreased mammographic sensitivity and increased risk of developing breast cancer. Standardized methods of density assessment that are reproducible and reliable are becoming increasingly important. This will allow for the addition of breast density information to improve the accuracy of risk assessment models and assess the need for supplemental screening on an individual basis. Breast density remains a significant and complex topic in breast imaging that will continue to evolve as we learn more about its associations and clinical implications.

CLINICS CARE POINTS

- Mammographic breast density is traditionally assessed visually, although there are now Food and Drug Administration-approved, fully automated quantitative, and artificial intelligence methods available.

- Reproducible and reliable breast density assessment is important to improve the accuracy of breast cancer risk assessment models and to optimize personalized breast cancer screening.

- Supplemental screening with whole-breast ultrasound, digital breast tomosynthesis, and breast MR imaging should be considered in patients with dense breasts.

DISCLOSURE

No relevant relationships.

REFERENCES

1. Acr. 2013 ACR BI-RADS Atlas: Breast Imaging Reporting and Data System. (2014). Available at: https://www.acr.org/Clinical-Resources/Reporting-and-Data-Systems/Bi-Rads.

2. Prevalence of mammographically dense breasts in the United States. J Natl Cancer Inst 2014;106.

3. Mandelson MT, Oestreicher N, White PL. Breast density as a predictor of mammographic detection: comparison of interval- and screen-detected cancers. J Natl Cancer Inst 2000;92:1081–7.

4. Boyd NF, Jensen HM, Cooke G, et al. Relationship between mammographic and histological risk factors for breast cancer. J Natl Cancer Inst 1992;84:1170–9.

5. Ciatto S, Houssami N, Apruzzese A, et al. Categorizing breast mammographic density: intra- and interobserver reproducibility of BI-RADS density categories. Breast 2005;14:269–75.

6. Ooms EA, Zonderland HM, Eijkemans MJ, et al. Mammography: interobserver variability in breast density assessment. Breast 2007;16:568–76.

7. Redondo A, Comas M, Macià F, et al. Inter- and intraradiologist variability in the BI-RADS assessment and breast density categories for screening mammograms. Br J Radiol 2012;85:1465–70.

8. Sprague BL, Conant EF, Onega T, et al. Variation in Mammographic Breast Density Assessments Among Radiologists in Clinical Practice: A Multicenter Observational Study. Ann Intern Med 2016;165:457–64.

9. Portnow LH, Malek L, Leung JWT, et al. International Interobserver Variability of Breast Density Assessment. J Am Coll Radiol 2023. https://doi.org/10.1016/j.jacr.2023.03.010.

10. Alonzo-Proulx O, Mawdsley GE, Patrie JT, et al. Reliability of automated breast density measurements. Radiology 2015;275:366–76.

11. Engelken F, Jasmin-Maya S, Eva-Maria F, et al. Volumetric breast composition analysis: reproducibility of breast percent density and fibroglandular tissue volume measurements in serial mammograms. Acta radiol 2014;55:32–8.

12. Lee HN, Sohn Y-M, Han KH. Comparison of mammographic density estimation by Volpara software with radiologists' visual assessment: analysis of clinical-radiologic factors affecting discrepancy between them. Acta radiol 2015;56:1061–8.

13. Morrish OWE, Tucker L, Black R, et al. Mammographic breast density: comparison of methods for quantitative evaluation. Radiology 2015;275:356–65.

14. Brandt KR, Scott CG, Ma L, et al. Comparison of Clinical and Automated Breast Density Measurements: Implications for Risk Prediction and Supplemental Screening. Radiology 2016;279:710–9.

15. Gweon HM, Youk JH, Kim J-A, et al. Radiologist assessment of breast density by BI-RADS categories versus fully automated volumetric assessment. AJR Am J Roentgenol 2013;201:692–7.

16. Yaffe MJ. Mammographic density. Measurement of mammographic density. Breast Cancer Res 2008;10:209.

17. Lehman CD, Yala A, Schuster T, et al. Mammographic Breast Density Assessment Using Deep Learning: Clinical Implementation. Radiology 2019;290:52–8.

18. Saffari N, Rashwan HA, Abdel-Nasser M, et al. Fully Automated Breast Density Segmentation and Classification Using Deep Learning. Diagnostics 2020;10.

19. Matthews TP, Singh S, Mombourquette B, et al. A Multisite Study of a Breast Density Deep Learning Model for Full-Field Digital Mammography and Synthetic Mammography. Radiol Artif Intell 2021;3: e200015.

20. Dontchos BN, Cavallo-Hom K, Lamb LR, et al. Impact of a Deep Learning Model for Predicting Mammographic Breast Density in Routine Clinical Practice. J Am Coll Radiol 2022;19:1021–30.

21. Center for Devices & Radiological Health. Artificial Intelligence and Machine Learning (AI/ML)- Enabled Medical Devices. U.S. Food and Drug Administration. 2022. Available at: https://www.fda.gov/medical-devices/software-medical-device-samd/artificial-intelligence-and-machine-learning-aiml-enabled-medical-devices. Accessed August 28, 2023.

22. Mavaddat N, Michailidou K, Dennis J, et al. Polygenic Risk Scores for Prediction of Breast Cancer and Breast Cancer Subtypes. Am J Hum Genet 2019;104:21–34.

23. Boyd NF, Dite GS, Stone J, et al. Heritability of mammographic density, a risk factor for breast cancer. N Engl J Med 2002;347:886–94.

24. Holowko N, Eriksson M, Kuja-Halkola R, et al. Heritability of Mammographic Breast Density, Density Change, Microcalcifications, and Masses. Cancer Res 2020;80:1590–600.

25. Chalfant JS, Hoyt AC. Breast Density: Current Knowledge, Assessment Methods, and Clinical Implications. J Breast Imaging 2022;4:357–70.

26. Burton A, Maskarinec G, Perez-Gomez B, et al. Mammographic density and ageing: A collaborative pooled analysis of cross- sectional data from 22 countries worldwide. PLoS Med 2017;14:e1002335.

27. Azam S, Sjölander A, Eriksson M, et al. Determinants of Mammographic Density Change. JNCI Cancer Spectr 2019;3:kz004.

28. Alexeeff SE, Odo NU, McBride R, et al. Reproductive Factors and Mammographic Density: Associations Among 24,840 Women and Comparison of Studies Using Digitized Film-Screen Mammography and Full-Field Digital Mammography. Am J Epidemiol 2019;188:1144–54.

29. Lecler A, Dunant A, Delaloge S, et al. Breast tissue density change after oophorectomy in BRCA mutation carrier patients using visual and volumetric analysis. Br J Radiol 2018;91(1083):20170163.

30. Rice MS, Bertrand KA, VanderWeele TJ, et al. Mammographic density and breast cancer risk: a mediation analysis. Breast Cancer Res 2016;18:94.

31. Cuzick J, Warwick J, Pinney E, et al. Tamoxifen-induced reduction in mammographic density and breast cancer risk reduction: a nested case-control study. J Natl Cancer Inst 2011;103:744–52.

32. Brentnall AR, Warren R, Harkness EF, et al. Mammographic density change in a cohort of premenopausal women receiving tamoxifen for breast cancer prevention over 5 years. Breast Cancer Res 2020;22:101.

33. Cigler T, Richardson H, Yaffe MJ, et al. A randomized, placebo-controlled trial (NCIC CTG MAP.2) examining the effects of exemestane on mammographic breast density, bone density, markers of bone metabolism and serum lipid levels in postmenopausal women. Breast Cancer Res Treat 2011;126:453–61.

34. Vachon CM, Suman VJ, Brandt KR, et al. Mammographic breast density response to aromatase inhibition. Clin Cancer Res 2013;19:2144–53.

35. Prowell TM, Blackford AL, Byrne C, et al. Changes in breast density and circulating estrogens in postmenopausal women receiving adjuvant anastrozole. Cancer Prev Res 2011;4:1993–2001.

36. McCarthy AM, Keller BM, Pantalone LM, et al. Racial Differences in Quantitative Measures of Area and Volumetric Breast Density. J Natl Cancer Inst 2016;108.

37. El-Bastawissi AY, White E, Mandelson MT, et al. Reproductive and hormonal factors associated with mammographic breast density by age (United States). Cancer Causes Control 2000;11:955–63.

38. Bissell MCS, Kerlikowske K, Sprague BL, et al. Breast Cancer Surveillance Consortium. Breast Cancer Population Attributable Risk Proportions Associated with Body Mass Index and Breast Density by Race/Ethnicity and Menopausal Status. Cancer Epidemiol Biomarkers Prev 2020;29(10):2048–56.

39. Friebel-Klingner TM, Ehsan S, Conant EF, et al. Risk factors for breast cancer subtypes among Black women undergoing screening mammography. Breast Cancer Res Treat 2021;189(3):827–35.

40. Lee KH, Chae SW, Yun JS, et al. Association between skeletal muscle mass and mammographic breast density. Sci Rep 2021;11:16785.

41. Premenopausal Breast Cancer Collaborative Group et al. Association of Body Mass Index and Age With Subsequent Breast Cancer Risk in Premenopausal Women. JAMA Oncol 4, e181771 (2018).

42. Hassinger TE, Mehaffey JH, Knisely AT, et al. The impact of bariatric surgery on qualitative and quantitative breast density. Breast J 2019;25:1198–205.

43. Williams AD, So A, Synnestvedt M, et al. Mammographic breast density decreases after bariatric surgery. Breast Cancer Res Treat 2017;165:565–72.

44. Brentnall AR, Cuzick J. Risk Models for Breast Cancer and Their Validation. Stat Sci 2020;35:14–30.

45. McBride RB, Fei K, Rothstein JH, et al. Alcohol and Tobacco Use in Relation to Mammographic Density

in 23,456 Women. Cancer Epidemiol Biomarkers Prev 2020;29:1039–48.

46. Kerlikowske K, Zhu W, Tosteson ANA, et al. Identifying women with dense breasts at high risk for interval cancer: a cohort study. Ann Intern Med 2015; 162:673–81.

47. Conant EF, Barlow WE, Herschorn SD, et al. Association of Digital Breast Tomosynthesis vs Digital Mammography With Cancer Detection and Recall Rates by Age and Breast Density. JAMA Oncol 2019;5:635–42.

48. Destounis S, Johnston L, Highnam R, et al. Using Volumetric Breast Density to Quantify the Potential Masking Risk of Mammographic Density. AJR Am J Roentgenol 2017;208:222–7.

49. Gajdos C, Tartter PI, Bleiweiss IJ, et al. Mammographic appearance of nonpalpable breast cancer reflects pathologic characteristics. Ann Surg 2002; 235:246–51.

50. Wanders JOP, Holland K, Karssemeijer N, et al. The effect of volumetric breast density on the risk of screen-detected and interval breast cancers: a cohort study. Breast Cancer Res 2017;19(1):67.

51. Holland K, van Gils CH, Mann RM, et al. Quantification of masking risk in screening mammography with volumetric breast density maps. Breast Cancer Res Treat 2017;162:541–8.

52. Berg WA, Rafferty EA, Friedewald SM, et al. Screening Algorithms in Dense Breasts: Expert Panel Narrative Review. AJR Am J Roentgenol 2021;216: 275–94.

53. Wolfe JN. Risk for breast cancer development determined by mammographic parenchymal pattern. Cancer 1976;37:2486–92.

54. Wolfe JN. Breast patterns as an index of risk for developing breast cancer. AJR Am J Roentgenol 1976;126:1130–7.

55. McCormack VA, dos Santos Silva I. Breast density and parenchymal patterns as markers of breast cancer risk: a meta-analysis. Cancer Epidemiol Biomarkers Prev 2006;15:1159–69.

56. Bodewes FTH, van Asselt AA, Dorrius MD, et al. Mammographic breast density and the risk of breast cancer: A systematic review and meta- analysis. Breast 2022;66:62–8.

57. Shawky MS, Huo CW, Henderson MA, et al. A review of the influence of mammographic density on breast cancer clinical and pathological phenotype. Breast Cancer Res Treat 2019;177:251–76.

58. Boyd NF, Guo H, Martin LJ, et al. Mammographic density and the risk and detection of breast cancer. N Engl J Med 2007;356:227–36.

59. Pollán M, Ascunce N, Ederra M, et al. Mammographic density and risk of breast cancer according to tumor characteristics and mode of detection: a Spanish population-based case-control study. Breast Cancer Res 2013;15:R9.

60. Mook S, Van 't Veer LJ, Rutgers EJ, et al. Independent prognostic value of screen detection in invasive breast cancer. J Natl Cancer Inst 2011;103:585–97.

61. Kleinstern G, Scott CG, Tamimi RM, et al. Association of mammographic density measures and breast cancer "intrinsic" molecular subtypes. Breast Cancer Res Treat 2021;187(1):215–24.

62. Jiang S, Bennett DL, Rosner BA, et al. Longitudinal Analysis of Change in Mammographic Density in Each Breast and Its Association With Breast Cancer Risk. JAMA Oncol 2023;9:808–14.

63. Amir E, Freedman OC, Seruga B, et al. Assessing women at high risk of breast cancer: a review of risk assessment models. J Natl Cancer Inst 2010; 102:680–91.

64. Paige JS, Lee CI, Pin-Chieh W, et al. Variability Among Breast Cancer Risk Classification Models When Applied at the Level of the Individual Woman. J Gen Intern Med 2023. https://doi.org/10.1007/s11606-023-08043-4.

65. Brentnall AR, Harkness EF, Astley SM, et al. Mammographic density adds accuracy to both the Tyrer-Cuzick and Gail breast cancer risk models in a prospective UK screening cohort. Breast Cancer Res 2015;17:147.

66. Brentnall AR, et al. A Case-Control Study to Add Volumetric or Clinical Mammographic Density into the Tyrer-Cuzick Breast Cancer Risk Model. J Breast Imaging 2019;1:99–106.

67. Tice JA, Cummings SR, Ziv E, et al. Mammographic breast density and the Gail model for breast cancer risk prediction in a screening population. Breast Cancer Res Treat 2005;94:115–22.

68. Vilmun BM, Vejborg I, Lynge E, et al. Impact of adding breast density to breast cancer risk models: A systematic review. Eur J Radiol 2020;127:109019.

69. McCarthy AM, Guan Z, Welch M, et al. Performance of Breast Cancer Risk-Assessment Models in a Large Mammography Cohort. J Natl Cancer Inst 2020;112(5):489–97.

70. Gastounioti A, Pantalone L, Scott CG, et al. Fully Automated Volumetric Breast Density Estimation from Digital Breast Tomosynthesis. Radiology 2021; 301(3):561–8.

71. Yala A, Lehman C, Schuster T, et al. A Deep Learning Mammography- based Model for Improved Breast Cancer Risk Prediction. Radiology 2019;292:60–6.

72. Dembrower K, Liu Y, Azizpour H, et al. Comparison of a Deep Learning Risk Score and Standard Mammographic Density Score for Breast Cancer Risk Prediction. Radiology 2020;294(2):265–72.

73. Smith RA, Duffy SW, Gabe R, et al. The randomized trials of breast cancer screening: what have we learned? Radiol Clin North Am 2004;42:793–806, v.

74. Website. Department of Health and Human Services. Food and Drug Administration Mammography

Quality Standards Act final rule. Available at: https://public-inspection.federalregister.gov/2023-04550.pdf.

75. Huang S, Houssami N, Brennan M, et al. The impact of mandatory mammographic breast density notification on supplemental screening practice in the United States: a systematic review. Breast Cancer Res Treat 2021;187:11–30.

76. Choudhery S, Patel BK, Johnson M, et al. Trends of Supplemental Screening in Women With Dense Breasts. J Am Coll Radiol 2020;17:990–8.

77. Expert Panel on Breast Imaging et al. ACR Appropriateness Criteria® Supplemental Breast Cancer Screening Based on Breast Density. J. Am. Coll. Radiol. 18, S456–S473 (2021).

78. Monticciolo DL, Newell MS, Moy L, et al. Breast Cancer Screening for Women at Higher-Than-Average Risk: Updated Recommendations From the ACR. J Am Coll Radiol 2023. https://doi.org/10.1016/j.jacr.2023.04.002.

79. Kolb TM, Lichy J, Newhouse JH. Comparison of the performance of screening mammography, physical examination, and breast US and evaluation of factors that influence them: an analysis of 27,825 patient evaluations. Radiology 2002;225:165–75.

80. Kim WH, Chang JM, Lee J, et al. Diagnostic performance of tomosynthesis and breast ultrasonography in women with dense breasts: a prospective comparison study. Breast Cancer Res Treat 2017;162:85–94.

81. Berg WA, Vourtsis A. Screening Breast Ultrasound Using Handheld or Automated Technique in Women with Dense Breasts. J Breast Imaging 2019;1:283–96.

82. Corsetti V, Houssami N, Ferrari A, et al. Breast screening with ultrasound in women with mammography-negative dense breasts: evidence on incremental cancer detection and false positives, and associated cost. Eur J Cancer 2008;44:539–44.

83. Berg WA, Zhang Z, Lehrer D, et al. Detection of breast cancer with addition of annual screening ultrasound or a single screening MRI to mammography in women with elevated breast cancer risk. JAMA 2012;307:1394–404.

84. Brem RF, Tabár L, Duffy SW, et al. Assessing improvement in detection of breast cancer with three-dimensional automated breast US in women with dense breast tissue: the SomoInsight Study. Radiology 2015;274:663–73.

85. Hussein H, Abbas E, Keshavarzi S, et al. Supplemental Breast Cancer Screening in Women with Dense Breasts and Negative Mammography: A Systematic Review and Meta-Analysis. Radiology 2023;306:e221785.

86. Chen S-Q, Huang M, Shen Y-Y, et al. Application of Abbreviated Protocol of Magnetic Resonance Imaging for Breast Cancer Screening in Dense Breast Tissue. Acad Radiol 2017;24:316–20.

87. Chen S-Q, Huang M, Shen Y-Y, et al. Abbreviated MRI Protocols for Detecting Breast Cancer in Women with Dense Breasts. Korean J Radiol 2017;18:470–5.

88. Mann RM, Athanasiou A, Baltzer PA, et al. Breast cancer screening in women with extremely dense breasts recommendations of the European Society of Breast Imaging (EUSOBI). Eur Radiol 2022;32:4036–45.

89. Bakker MF, de Lange SV, Pijnappel RM, et al. Supplemental MRI Screening for Women with Extremely Dense Breast Tissue. N Engl J Med 2019;381:2091–102.

90. Geuzinge HA, Bakker MF, Heijnsdijk EAM, et al. Cost-Effectiveness of Magnetic Resonance Imaging Screening for Women With Extremely Dense Breast Tissue. J Natl Cancer Inst 2021;113:1476–83.

91. Veenhuizen SGA, de Lange SV, Bakker MF, et al. Supplemental Breast MRI for Women with Extremely Dense Breasts: Results of the Second Screening Round of the DENSE Trial. Radiology 2021;299:278–86.

92. Berg WA, Seitzman RL, Pushkin J. Implementing the National Dense Breast Reporting Standard, Expanding Supplemental Screening Using Current Guidelines, and the Proposed Find It Early Act. J Breast Imaging 2023;wbad034.

93. Gillies RJ, Kinahan PE, Hricak H. Radiomics: Images Are More than Pictures, They Are Data. Radiology 2016;278:563–77.

94. Byng JW, Yaffe MJ, Lockwood GA, et al. Automated analysis of mammographic densities and breast carcinoma risk. Cancer 1997;80:66–74.

95. Manduca A, Carston MJ, Heine JJ, et al. Texture features from mammographic images and risk of breast cancer. Cancer Epidemiol Biomarkers Prev 2009;18:837–45.

96. Wei J, Ping Chan H, Yi-Ta W, et al. Association of computerized mammographic parenchymal pattern measure with breast cancer risk: a pilot case-control study. Radiology 2011;260:42–9.

97. Zheng Y, Keller BM, Ray S, et al. Parenchymal texture analysis in digital mammography: A fully automated pipeline for breast cancer risk assessment. Med Phys 2015;42:4149–60.

98. Anandarajah A, Chen Y, Colditz GA, et al. Studies of parenchymal texture added to mammographic breast density and risk of breast cancer: a systematic review of the methods used in the literature. Breast Cancer Res 2022;24:101.

99. Kontos D, Winham SJ, Oustimov A, et al. Radiomic Phenotypes of Mammographic Parenchymal Complexity: Toward Augmenting Breast Density in Breast Cancer Risk Assessment. Radiology 2019;290:41–9.

Background Parenchymal Enhancement
A Comprehensive Update

Sona A. Chikarmane, MD[a],*, Sharon Smith, MD[b]

KEYWORDS

- Breast MR imaging • Background parenchymal enhancement • Breast cancer

KEY POINTS

- Background parenchymal enhancement is the normal enhancement of breast tissue on MR imaging after administration of intravenous contrast.
- Background parenchymal enhancement (BPE) is influenced by a variety of factors including age, menopausal status, exogenous hormones, and breast cancer treatment.
- Breast cancer risk and treatment outcomes have been linked to the degree of BPE.
- Artificial intelligence may standardize the evaluation of BPE, which is currently based on visual inspection and therefore limited by interobserver variability.

INTRODUCTION

Breast cancer is the most common cause of cancer in the United States and the second leading cause of cancer death in women. There has been a 30% to 40% reduction in breast cancer mortality due to mammographic screening.[1] Despite the improved outcomes with screening mammography, high-risk patients may develop breast cancers[2,3] not detected mammographically. Breast MR imaging is a complementary screening tool for patients at high risk for breast cancer[4] and is also frequently used in the diagnostic setting. Normal enhancement of the breast tissue on MR imaging is called background parenchymal enhancement (BPE), which occurs after administration of an intravenous contrast agent.[5] Initially thought to be an incidental finding, BPE varies widely based on factors such as age, menstrual cycle phase, use of hormonal contraceptives, and menopausal status.[6] In addition, BPE has been shown to increase breast cancer risk and may predict treatment outcomes. The authors provide a comprehensive review of BPE describing its physiologic causes and hormonal influences. The authors also discuss quantitative and qualitative assessment of BPE, the impact of contrast and examination timing on BPE and BPE as a biomarker for predicting breast cancer risk and treatment outcomes. Finally, the authors describe how artificial intelligence (AI) has potential for BPE assessment.

PHYSIOLOGY OF BREAST PARENCHYMAL ENHANCEMENT

The typical breast is made up of fatty tissue, fibro-glandular tissue, minor ducts, and connective tissue.[7] There are limited data directly analyzing the pathophysiology of BPE, and the precise biological mechanism underlying the enhancement of breast parenchyma is not entirely understood. Histopathologic examinations have shed light on some of the contributing elements. Sung and colleagues examined the contralateral breasts of 80 patients with breast cancer who underwent prophylactic mastectomy before receiving any other form of treatment for their disease other than surgery.[8] The investigators found significant

[a] Breast Imaging Division, Department of Radiology, Brigham and Women's Hospital, 75 Francis Street, Boston, MA 02115, USA; [b] Department of Radiology, Brigham and Women's Hospital, 75 Francis Street, Boston, MA 02115, USA
* Corresponding author.
E-mail address: schikarmane@bwh.harvard.edu

Radiol Clin N Am 62 (2024) 607–617
https://doi.org/10.1016/j.rcl.2023.12.013
0033-8389/24/© 2024 Elsevier Inc. All rights reserved.

relationships between premenopausal women's qualitative baseline parenchymal enhancement and CD34 (marker of microvascular density), micro-vessel density, glandular concentration, and vascular endothelial growth factor (VEGF). These findings support the hypothesis that the expression of VEGF, density of blood vessels in the breast tissue, and amount of glandular tissue concentrations may impact BPE.

HORMONAL AND METABOLIC IMPACT ON BREAST PARENCHYMAL ENHANCEMENT

Research has shown BPE is highly dependent on the effects of endogenous and exogenous hormones. In premenopausal and younger women, the impact of estrogen explains the cyclical changes in BPE that occur during the menstrual cycle. Estrogen promotes the epithelial proliferation and differentiation of the acini throughout the first part of the menstrual cycle.[7] In the second half of the menstrual cycle, estrogen stimulates secretions to widen acini luminal size. BPE fluctuates with the menstrual cycle, peaking in weeks 3 and 4 and declining in week 2.[5,6,9] In postmenopausal women, increased BPE may be seen in women getting exogenous hormone replacement therapy and elevated BPE has been associated with increased levels of serum estrone and estradiol. Reciprocally, tamoxifen, an estrogen receptor blocker used to decrease breast cancer risk, is thought to decrease parenchymal enhancement.[10] The effect is reversed after discontinuation of tamoxifen with rebound effects of endogenous hormones on the fibroglandular tissue[6,9] resulting in increased BPE. BPE variations following risk-reducing salpingo-oophorectomies (RRSO) and menopause provide further indirect evidence of hormonal influence on BPE. After RRSO, BRCA 1 and 2 mutation carriers showed a significant decrease in BPE and fibroglandular tissue, indicating that the amount of endogenous estrogens can alter BPE.[11]

BPE may also reflect metabolic activity within normal parenchymal tissue. A study of 298 consecutive patients who underwent both breast MR imaging and F18-FDG PET/CT was performed, and the level of BPE was correlated with metabolic activity of normal glandular tissue by menstrual cycle. The study found that the metabolic activity of breast tissue is highest in the third week and lowest in the second week, moderately correlating with BPE.[12] Another study of 73 patients with breast MR imaging in newly diagnosed breast cancer and F18-FDG PET/CT within 1 week found significant association between BPE and metabolic uptake, when measured both qualitatively and quantitatively.[13]

QUALITATIVE AND QUANTITATIVE MEASUREMENT

The qualitative assessment of BPE involves visually evaluating the degree and extent of enhancement in normal fibroglandular tissue after contrast delivery. The assessment of BPE using a subjective method of four grades (minimal, mild, moderate, and marked) by radiologists may exhibit limited reliability due to significant inter-reader variability.[14] For example, in a 2012 preliminary study conducted by Scaranelo and colleagues,[15] a cohort of 147 women who underwent preoperative breast MR imaging was examined to assess the level of agreement between two independent readers for BPE. The results revealed a fair level of agreement between the two readers, with a weighted agreement coefficient of 0.37. Preibsch and colleagues[16] conducted a 2016 study examining inter-reader agreement in the assessment of BPE in relation to neoadjuvant chemotherapy. The researchers found that the level of agreement among readers was determined to be "substantial" ($\kappa = 0.73$–0.77) before therapy, and "moderate" ($\kappa = 0.43$–0.60) after therapy. However, with training among breast radiologists, there is potential for improved inter-reader agreement.[14]

Although not described fully in the literature, the use of the MIP image has been used as a method of BPE assessment[17] and has been described as a time-saving step when evaluating breast MR imagings. A study by Bignotti and colleagues in 2019 demonstrated similar reliability with MIP alone image and shorter reading time (4 seconds with MIP only vs 38 seconds), suggesting MIP can be used as a tool in BPE assessment.[18]

Quantitative evaluation, on the other hand, focuses on a more objective and measurable assessment. Computer algorithms and mathematical models are used to quantify the volume and intensity of breast enhancement with interest-based and segmentation-based enhancement being the most common reported approaches in the literature. For instance, studies have used qualitative methodologies such as signal enhancement ratios,[19–21] percentage enhancement,[15,22,23] and automaticity.[24–26] It is important to acknowledge there is limited standardization both among and within the various methodologies used in quantitative analyses; therefore, quantitative assessment is not yet in widespread clinical use.

INFLUENCE OF CONTRAST TIMING ON PARENCHYMAL ENHANCEMENT

The timing of contrast delivery is a crucial factor in the diagnosis and staging of breast cancer.

According to a study by Melsaether and colleagues in 2017,[27] BPE increases between the first (100 seconds) and second (210 seconds) post-contrast scans before stabilizing (approximately 320 seconds post-contrast). Typically, the radiologist responsible for image interpretation conducts a qualitative analysis of the background parenchymal enhancement (BPE) on the early post-contrast imaging categorizing the BPE. According to the guidelines set forth by the ACR,[28] the early post-contrast sequence should be used for BPE evaluation (90 seconds) as tumors exhibit the most pronounced level of enhancement within this specific temporal window. Interestingly, Tomida and colleagues[29] observed that normal breast tissue exhibits lower enhancement during the super early phase. These findings suggest that shorter MR imaging protocols known as ultrafast-dynamic contrast-enhanced (UF-DCE) MR imaging can potentially facilitate the identification of malignant tumors using kinetic and morphologic information from breast lesions in the extremely early post-contrast phase when BPE is not yet visualized. When compared with conventional DCE MR imaging, BPE has been shown to be lower on UF-DCE MR imaging than on conventional DCE MR while lesion detectability is improved on UF-DCE MR imaging versus DCE-MR imaging in patients with a greater degree of BPE.[30]

TIMING OF SCREENING BREAST MR IMAGING AND BREAST PARENCHYMAL ENHANCEMENT

Historically, breast MR imaging screening examinations were thought to be optimally scheduled between days 7 and 14 of the menstrual cycle when BPE is at its lowest levels in order to reduce any potential masking of small cancers by BPE. However, the "masking" effect of moderate or marked BPE to obscure possible malignancies has not been consistently demonstrated in the literature. In addition, some studies have shown no difference in BPE by week of menstrual cycle.[31] Dontchos and colleagues reported on 320 examinations in 224 premenopausal women and found that menstrual cycle timing did not affect performance benchmarks including abnormal interpretation rates (AIRs), cancer detection rates, or specificity. However, some larger retrospective studies have shown increased AIRs with increasing BPE. DeMartini and colleagues[32] retrospectively reviewed the prospectively reported BPE assessments in 736 women and found a significantly higher AIR with high BPE compared with low (30.5% vs 23.3%). Similarly, studies by Hambly and colleagues[33] and Ray and colleagues[34] demonstrated increased AIR with non-minimal BPE compared with minimal BPE. These mixed results suggest that the timing of screening breast MR imaging warrants further investigation.

TYPICAL AND ATYPICAL APPEARANCES OF BREAST PARENCHYMAL ENHANCEMENT ON BREAST MR IMAGING

Standard MR imaging protocols include pre-contrast T1 with fat suppression sequences with varying numbers of post-contrast T1 with dynamic sequences. BPE can present with different levels of enhancement on dynamic sequences and is characterized as minimal, mild, moderate, or marked based on theACRs Breast Imaging Reporting and Data System (BI-RADS) Atlas for Breast MR imaging [28] (Fig. 1A–D). Per the ACR, BPE should be assessed on the first post-contrast subtraction image. Otherwise, there is no standardization in BPE assessment, and inter-observer variability exists from institution to institution and radiologist to radiologist. BPE does not correlate with dense breast tissue on mammography or with dense fibroglandular tissue on breast MR imaging. For example, patients with dense fibroglandular tissue on mammography and breast MR imaging may have mild to minimal background parenchymal enhancement.[35]

The common appearance of BPE has been described as "picture-framing" when the enhancement occurs in the periphery of the parenchymal tissue and then fills centrally; this is thought to be secondary to a medial inflow pattern from the internal mammary artery, a lateral inflow from the lateral thoracic and thoracoacromial arteries, and the lateral cutaneous branches of the intercostal arteries. The enhancement gradually enters the central cone of the tissue, and the retroareolar region is the last to enhance.[6,9]

The most common pattern of BPE is bilateral and symmetric with persistent kinetics.[6] Other more typical patterns of BPE include scattered bilateral innumerable foci, larger areas of regional enhancement, and multiple bilateral focal areas of enhancement. Bilateral symmetric areas of enhancement are most likely to be BPE even if marked or nodular in appearance.[6] Comparison with prior breast MR imagings and correlation with patient factors such as menopausal status, exogenous hormones, and endocrine therapies are important to differentiate non-mass enhancement (NME) from BPE.

Although BPE may present in typical patterns, BPE can also present as an asymmetric or atypical enhancement pattern. Breast conservation therapy (radiation and lumpectomy) can cause decreased BPE in the treated breast which

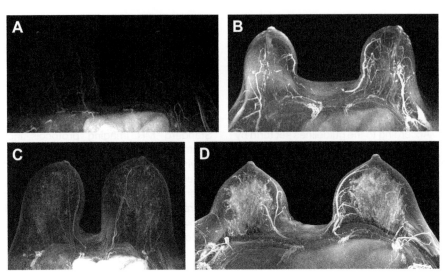

Fig. 1. Axial contrast-enhanced T1-weighted fat-suppressed subtraction maximal intensity projection (MIP) MR imaging demonstrating qualitative background enhancement assessments of minimal (*A*), mild (*B*), moderate (*C*), and marked (*D*).

appears asymmetric from the normal enhancement contralateral breast.[36] In addition, patients who received systemic treatment of endocrine therapy or chemotherapy may have decreased BPE in the unaffected breast.[6] Asymmetry can also be secondary to increased BPE secondary to rebound after tamoxifen cessation (**Fig. 2**A, B).

Other appearances of BPE may be diffuse, regional, or nodular, which may cause diagnostic challenges. Per Giess and colleagues in a 2014[6] review article: "in the setting of moderate or marked BPE, a focus or focal area that is dominant or enlarging or that has isolated suspicious kinetic features should raise more concern than numerous similar findings." If enhancement in the breast is difficult to differentiate from NME due to its distribution, the patient may be scheduled between days 7 to 10 of their menstrual cycle for an MR imaging-guided breast biopsy. If the finding persists, then biopsy can be performed; if the finding is no longer present, it is likely BPE and short interval follow-up may be recommended.[37,38] However, marked BPE which is bilateral and symmetric, even if in a pattern of multiple focal areas or foci, does not necessitate short interval follow-up and can be deemed benign (**Fig. 3**A–C).[39]

Marked background enhancement can be seen in lactating patients, as lactational breast tissue exhibits increased vascularity[40] (**Fig. 4**A, B). The marked BPE in lactation can theoretically be challenging in differentiating normal physiologic breast tissue from abnormal findings. However, a recent study by Nissan and colleagues, of 198 lactating

patients and 132 controls, found high sensitivity (93%) and negative predictive value (96.2%) for breast cancer detection for MR imaging in lactating patients.[41] The investigators demonstrated reduction in BPE among lactating breast cancer patients compared with lactating controls and attributed this reduction in BPE as a vascular steal phenomenon, which allowed for sufficient conspicuity of breast cancers on the first subtracted image. The vascular steal phenomenon was identified when comparing BPE of the normal contralateral breast in breast cancer cohort compared with healthy lactating controls. Other studies have also reported the high sensitivity of breast MR imaging in lactating patients and its use in screening lactating high-risk patients.[42–44]

ASSOCIATION OF BREAST PARENCHYMAL ENHANCEMENT WITH BREAST CANCER RISK

Studies have documented correlation between mammographic density and breast cancer risk. There is new and evolving evidence regarding the association between BPE and the elevated risk of developing breast cancer.[10,27,45–47] Studies have shown that women with dense breast tissue and mild or minimal BPE are not at higher risk of breast cancer, suggesting that BPE is an independent risk factor.[46] The first study exploring BPE and cancer risk was performed by King and colleagues.[10] The investigators found increased BPE correlated with higher rates of cancer in their cohort of 39 cancers in 1275 women who underwent breast MR imaging screening between

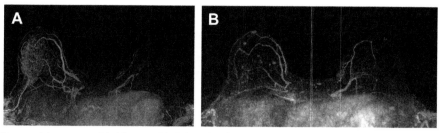

Fig. 2. A 57-year-old woman with history of left invasive breast cancer treated with breast conservation therapy (radiation and surgery), 6 years prior. Axial contrast-enhanced T1-weighted fat-suppressed subtraction maximal intensity projection (MIP) demonstrates new marked BPE in the right breast (*A*), after cessation of tamoxifen, when compared with 1 year prior (*B*). This is termed "tamoxifen rebound." In addition, there is persistently no/minimal BPE in the left breast, secondary to radiation treatment.

December 2002 and February 2008. In a retrospective study conducted by Melsaether and colleagues,[27] the researchers examined the correlation between BPE and patients diagnosed with breast cancer, comparing this group to a cohort without breast cancer. The study concluded that there was no statistically significant difference in BPE between the two groups. In contrast, a more recent study conducted by Watt and colleagues[48] included patients from the imaging and epidemiology (IMAGINE) multi-institutional study who enrolled any patients receiving diagnostic, screening or follow-up breast MR imaging between 2010 and 2017. The investigators examined the BPE in patients who were diagnosed with unilateral breast cancer compared with a control group of patients who had no previous or ongoing history of breast cancer. They found that premenopausal women with moderate to marked BPE had a higher likelihood of developing breast cancer compared with those with minimal to mild BPE. Sippo and colleagues[49] examined the association between BPE and the risk of developing breast cancer in high-risk populations undergoing screening MR imaging. The study included 4686 screening MR imaging examinations in 2446 women, grouping patients by minimal or mild BPE (3975/4686; 85%) versus moderate/marked BPE (711/4686; 15%) and by screening indication as BRCA carrier or history of thoracic radiation, breast cancer personal history, high-risk lesion, and breast cancer family history.

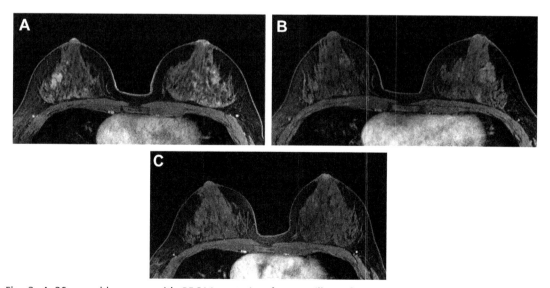

Fig. 3. A 36-year-old woman with BRCA1 mutation for surveillance breast MR imaging. On axial contrast-enhanced T1-weighted fat-suppressed dynamic sequences, there is moderate background enhancement in a focal pattern which appears symmetric to the contralateral side (*A*). The patient was placed in short interval follow-up for bilateral BPE. There is decreased bilateral BPE at 6-month (*B*) and 12-month (*C*) follow-up, after which she was placed in routine surveillance.

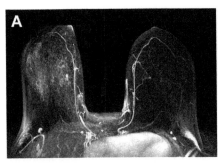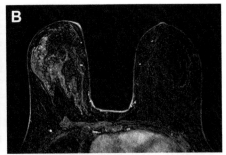

Fig. 4. A 39-year-old lactating woman with prior history of left breast cancer. There is asymmetry in the breast tissue with moderate BPE on the left, secondary to lactational changes, when compared with no/minimal BPE on the right, secondary to radiation treatment (*A*, MIP; *B*, Axial contrast-enhanced T1-weighted fat-suppressed subtraction).

The investigators determined that higher BPE was a significant and independent indicator of breast cancer in women who were undergoing screening MR imaging for these various high-risk indications. Since King's[10] initial article, there have been more than 25 studies on breast cancer risk and BPE.[50]

Finally, a comprehensive meta-analysis[51] was conducted on a total of 18 studies, which included a sample size of 1910 women diagnosed with breast cancer and 2541 control participants. After excluding studies with unmatched data from their analysis, the investigators found that women with a high-risk profile had a 2.1 increased odds of developing breast cancer when presenting with either moderate or mild BPE. The study did not confirm a significant association between a higher level of BPE and breast cancer presence in patients at average risk. However, more studies will be needed focused on patients at average and intermediate risk and may be particularly warranted given the heterogeneity of prior studies and the potential expansion of the MR imaging screening population with the increasing availability of abbreviated MR imaging protocols.

For patients with a prior history of breast cancer, studies have shown that higher BPE increases the likelihood of subsequent and interval breast cancers. Lee and colleagues reviewed 6489 consecutive breast MR imagings in 2860 women with 109 cancers (4%). The investigators found that greater than minimal BPE is associated with a doubled risk of developing second breast cancers[52] and the difference remained in subgroup analysis by age (> or < 45 years), hormonal receptor positive or negative tumor subtype, dense breast tissue on mammography, and in patients without a family history. Greater than minimal BPE was associated with both ipsilateral and contralateral breast cancers. Patients with breast cancer with higher BPE have been shown to have a higher risk not only of breast cancers but also of interval cancers. In

a study of 2809 women who underwent breast conservation therapy, Kim and colleagues found interval cancer rates of 1.5 per thousand. The interval cancers were significantly associated with moderate or marked BPE versus mild or minimal BPE (OR 10.8, $P < .001$).[53]

BREAST PARENCHYMAL ENHANCEMENT AS A PREDICTOR OF TREATMENT OUTCOMES

Breast MR imaging is used to evaluate extent of disease in newly diagnosed patients with breast cancer as well as to monitor treatment response in patients undergoing neoadjuvant treatment. More recently, BPE has been shown as a predictor and prognostic marker for women diagnosed with breast cancer and has been associated with tumor subtypes, response to neoadjuvant chemotherapy, and finally, recurrence-free survival (RFS).

Extent of disease is important in planning appropriate treatment and surgery, and there are limited data on the relationship of BPE on MR imaging and extent of disease accuracy. One of the first studies describing the effect of BPE and extent of disease examined 70 patients with single-site, multifocal and multicentric invasive and ductal carcinoma in situ (DCIS) breast cancers on breast MR imaging. The authors found that tumor measurement accuracy was higher in patients with minimal/mild BPE when compared with moderate/marked BPE. Four patients with single-site disease were mistakenly thought to have multifocal disease because of confounding moderate BPE. There was also one false-negative case of contralateral, synchronous DCIS obscured by diffuse moderate BPE. Subsequently, Baek and colleagues [54] examined 56 patients with DCIS and found that those with minimal or mild BPE had more accurate tumor measurements than those with moderate or marked background. In addition, Uematsu and colleagues[55] studied 131 biopsy-proven cases (104 malignant and 27 benign) and found that tumor extent accuracy is significantly higher in patients with minimal/mild BPE when compared with moderate/marked BPE. Other studies, however, have shown no association between degree of BPE and subsequent surgical margin status.[56,57]

Studies on BPE in patients on neoadjuvant treatment (NAT) and pathologic complete response (pCR) are evolving as well. Multiple studies have shown that pretreatment BPE may not be a predictor of treatment response.[58,59] However, post-NAT BPE on MR imaging may be a predictor of treatment response (Fig. 5A, B). In 2018, Oh and colleagues[60] studied 372 MR imagings in 186 women and found that post-NAT BPE was significantly lower in patients with a complete pathologic response when compared with patients with a non-complete pathologic response. The authors wrote that pathologic tumor response after NAT is important, as it can predict long-term outcomes in patients and is a marker for survival. In contrast, pretreatment MR imaging BPE was not a predictor of treatment response. A larger study by Onishi and colleagues[61] examined 3528 MR imaging examinations from 882 patients enrolled in the Investigation of Serial Studies to Predict Your Therapeutic Response with Imaging and Molecular Analysis 2 (I-SPY 2) TRIAL using automated BPE assessment. Patients in the trial underwent four MR imagings including baseline, early treatment, mid-regimen, and presurgery timepoints. The study found that in patients with hormone receptor positive cancer, the lack of BPE suppression in the contralateral breast indicated inferior treatment response. Similar results were found in patients with hormone receptor (HR)-negative tumors, but the data were not statistically significant. Similarly, in a study of 71 patients with unilateral human epidermal growth factor receptor-2 (HER2)-positive breast cancer treated with trastuzumab before surgery, decreased BPE after the second treatment cycle was significantly associated with complete pathologic response.[62] The cause for decreased BPE is uncertain and may be secondary to estrogen decreases due to ovarian suppression and/or breast parenchymal vascularity and proliferation. Because menopausal status was not a significant factor in the I-SPY study results, it suggests that there are more factors in play beyond ovarian suppression.

The data surrounding BPE associated with overall and risk free survival (RFS) are evolving with mixed results based on heterogeneous studies. In 2015, van der Valden and colleagues[63] studied 531 women with extent of disease MR imagings for ipsilateral invasive breast cancer and found that increased BPE was independently associated with improved overall survival. Other studies have shown that increased BPE is associated with decreased RFS or that there is no association between BPE and RFS.[64] A large recent study[65] in 2023 of 1432 women in 10 centers from the SELECT group (Stromal Enhancement on Breast MR imaging as a Biomarker for Survival with Endocrine Therapy) included patients with unilateral hormone positive, HER2-negative breast cancers in 10 Dutch hospitals who underwent preoperative breast MR imaging. BPE was quantified in the contralateral breast, as endocrine therapies have been shown to decrease BPE. The investigators found that increased contralateral BPE was associated with decreased overall survival, albeit marginally. In addition, the investigators reported no association with RFS or distant RFS.

As therapies are not without morbidity, it is important to explore noninvasive markers of treatment response, overall survival, and RFS. More studies are needed to evaluate the role of BPE in breast cancer outcomes as treatment moves to a more tailored approach.

ARTIFICIAL INTELLIGENCE AND BREAST PARENCHYMAL ENHANCEMENT

AI is poised to revolutionize radiology, including automating BPE assessment. As stated earlier, there is much variability in BPE assessment which limits its use in risk assessment, and this variability can be decreased with use of automation. Saha and colleagues[66] conducted a case control study of 133 women at high risk for developing cancer. They compared automatic features of BPE extracted by computer algorithm with subjective BPE scores from five breast radiologists and reported that quantitative BPE features exhibited superior predictive ability of detecting breast cancer in the future compared with the subjective BPE evaluations conducted by human readers.

A study from Memorial Sloan Kettering investigated two deep learning models (Slab AI; maximum intensity projection) to characterize BPE and compare it to radiology reports.[67] The investigators evaluated 5224 breast MR imaging with 3998 training, 444 validations, and 782 testing examinations, using three-reader consensus as the reference standard. They found that automated BPE models could outperform BPE assessments by radiologists. Similarly, a prospective case-control study of 536 cases of breast cancer compared with 940 noncancer controls was performed at the same institution.[68] The sample population is a subset of the IMAGINE study, a multisite cancer study, with multiple MR imaging magnets and protocols. The investigators

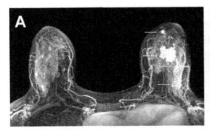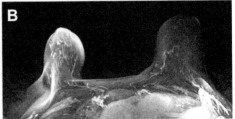

Fig. 5. A 47-year-old woman with newly diagnosed left-sided ER/PR+, HER2+ breast cancer. (*A*) Pretreatment axial contrast-enhanced T1-weighted fat-suppressed subtraction (MIP) demonstrates marked background enhancement in the bilateral breasts, with multiple enhancing masses on the left (biopsy-proven disease) (*arrows*). (*B*) Posttreatment MIP demonstrates complete imaging response with resolution of left-sided masses, along with now mild BPE. The patient also had a complete pathologic response. ER/PR+, estrogen and progesterone receptor positive

matched the contralateral or unaffected breast BPE with the same side in matched controls. An automated computer algorithm was used to segment fibroglandular tissue (FGT), fatty tissue, and quantify BPE (extent and intensity). They concluded that the quantitative algorithm correlated with BI-RADS BPE and was associated with increased odds of breast cancer. Other smaller case-control studies have shown similar results, including a study by Niell and colleagues of 19 cases of breast cancer and 76 controls who found that quantitative BPE extent models better identified patients who developed breast cancer when compared with subjective BPE assessment.[69] Further studies are needed to optimize quantification of BPE using AI to help tailor risk profiles in patients.

FUTURE DIRECTIONS AND SUMMARY

Initially thought to be an incidental finding on breast MR imaging, background parenchymal enhancement has now been shown to play a critical role in breast cancer risk and possibly treatment outcomes. BPE is quantified by radiologists as minimal, mild, moderate, and marked using ACR BI-RADS terminology, complicated by known interobserver variability. BPE is influenced by endogenous and exogenous hormones, as well as treatments including radiation, endocrine therapies, and chemotherapy. Although not shown to affect cancer detection, higher AIRs have been reported in patients with marked and moderate BPE compared with mild and minimal. Multiple studies have shown that BPE is associated with breast cancer risk in high-risk women. Data are limited in intermediate and average risk women, as breast MR imaging is used most exclusively in a higher risk patient population. However, there is potential use in the general screening population with newer breast MR imaging protocols, and therefore further research is needed in cancer risk with

elevated BPE in normal risk patients. Finally, AI is poised to help standardize BPE quantification, allowing for more accurate BPE assessments to tailor a patient's breast cancer risk profile.

CLINICS CARE POINTS

- Background parenchymal enhancement (BPE) refers to the normal enhancement of the breast tissue and can be influenced by a variety of factors.

- BPE is visually assessed as minimal, mild, moderate, and marked, with artificial intelligence tools on the horizon to standardize the inherent variability with visual assessment.

- BPE is associated with increased breast cancer risk in high-risk patients and response to therapy in those patients' undergoing neoadjuvant chemotherapy for breast cancer.

- Further research is necessary to evaluate the role of BPE in breast cancer risk, given the heterogeneity in studies to date.

DISCLOSURE

The authors have no commercial or financial conflicts of interest to disclose.

REFERENCES

1. Nicosia L, Gnocchi G, Gorini I, et al. History of mammography: analysis of breast imaging diagnostic achievements over the last century. Healthcare (Basel) 2023;11(11). https://doi.org/10.3390/healthcare11111596.

2. Santen RJ, Boyd NF, Chlebowski RT, et al. Critical assessment of new risk factors for breast cancer: considerations for development of an improved

risk prediction model. Endocr Relat Cancer 2007; 14(2):169–87.

3. Boyd NF, Guo H, Martin LJ, et al. Mammographic density and the risk and detection of breast cancer. N Engl J Med 2007;356(3):227–36.

4. Kuhl CK. Current status of breast MR imaging. Part 2. Clinical applications. Radiology 2007;244(3): 672–91.

5. Morris EA. Diagnostic breast MR imaging: current status and future directions. Magn Reson Imag Clin N Am 2010;18(1):57–74.

6. Giess CS, Yeh ED, Raza S, et al. Background parenchymal enhancement at breast MR imaging: normal patterns, diagnostic challenges, and potential for false-positive and false-negative interpretation. Radiographics 2014;34(1):234–47.

7. Lester SC, Hicks DG. Diagnostic pathology: breast, e-book: diagnostic pathology: breast, E-Book. Amsterdam: Elsevier Health Sciences; 2021.

8. Sung JS, Corben AD, Brooks JD, et al. Histopathologic characteristics of background parenchymal enhancement (BPE) on breast MRI. Breast Cancer Res Treat 2018;172(2):487–96.

9. Giess CS, Raza S, Birdwell RL. Patterns of nonmasslike enhancement at screening breast MR imaging of high-risk premenopausal women. Radiographics 2013;33(5):1343–60.

10. King V, Brooks JD, Bernstein JL, et al. Background parenchymal enhancement at breast MR imaging and breast cancer risk. Radiology 2011;260(1): 50–60.

11. Price ER, Brooks JD, Watson EJ, et al. The impact of bilateral salpingo-oophorectomy on breast MRI background parenchymal enhancement and fibroglandular tissue. Eur Radiol 2014;24(1):162–8.

12. An Y-S, Jung Y, Kim JY, et al. Metabolic activity of normal glandular tissue on 18F-fluorodeoxyglucose positron emission tomography/computed tomography: correlation with menstrual cycles and parenchymal enhancements. J Breast Cancer 2017; 20(4):386–92.

13. Mema E, Mango VL, Guo X, et al. Does breast MRI background parenchymal enhancement indicate metabolic activity? Qualitative and 3D quantitative computer imaging analysis. J Magn Reson Imag 2018;47(3):753–9.

14. Melsaether A, McDermott M, Gupta D, et al. Inter- and intrareader agreement for categorization of background parenchymal enhancement at baseline and after training. AJR Am J Roentgenol 2014; 203(1):209–15.

15. Scaranelo A. Breast screening with magnetic resonance imaging. CMAJ (Can Med Assoc J) 2012; 184(16):E877.

16. Preibsch H, Wanner L, Bahrs SD, et al. Background parenchymal enhancement in breast MRI before and after neoadjuvant chemotherapy: correlation with tumour response. Eur Radiol 2016;26(6): 1590–6.

17. Chalfant JS, Mortazavi S, Lee-Felker SA. Background parenchymal enhancement on breast MRI: assessment and clinical implications. Current Radiology Reports 2021;9(10):10.

18. Bignotti B, Calabrese M, Signori A, et al. Background parenchymal enhancement assessment: Inter- and intra-rater reliability across breast MRI sequences. Eur J Radiol 2019;114:57–61.

19. Kim S-A, Cho N, Ryu EB, et al. Background parenchymal signal enhancement ratio at preoperative MR imaging: association with subsequent local recurrence in patients with ductal carcinoma in situ after breast conservation surgery. Radiology 2014; 270(3):699–707.

20. Kim MY, Cho N, Koo HR, et al. Predicting local recurrence following breast-conserving treatment: parenchymal signal enhancement ratio (SER) around the tumor on preoperative MRI. Acta Radiol 2013; 54(7):731–8.

21. Hattangadi J, Park C, Rembert J, et al. Breast stromal enhancement on MRI is associated with response to neoadjuvant chemotherapy. AJR Am J Roentgenol 2008;190(6):1630–6.

22. Kim JY, Kim SH, Kim YJ, et al. Enhancement parameters on dynamic contrast enhanced breast MRI: do they correlate with prognostic factors and subtypes of breast cancers? Magn Reson Imaging 2015; 33(1):72–80.

23. Kajihara M, Goto M, Hirayama Y, et al. Effect of the menstrual cycle on background parenchymal enhancement in breast MR imaging. Magn Reson Med Sci 2013;12(1):39–45.

24. Mazurowski MA, Zhang J, Grimm LJ, et al. Radiogenomic analysis of breast cancer: luminal B molecular subtype is associated with enhancement dynamics at MR imaging. Radiology 2014;273(2):365–72.

25. Tagliafico A, Bignotti B, Tagliafico G, et al. Quantitative evaluation of background parenchymal enhancement (BPE) on breast MRI. A feasibility study with a semi-automatic and automatic software compared to observer-based scores. Br J Radiol 2015;88(1056):20150417.

26. Wu S, Weinstein SP, DeLeo MJ 3rd, et al. Quantitative assessment of background parenchymal enhancement in breast MRI predicts response to risk-reducing salpingo-oophorectomy: preliminary evaluation in a cohort of BRCA1/2 mutation carriers. Breast Cancer Res 2015;17:67.

27. Melsaether A, Pujara AC, Elias K, et al. Background parenchymal enhancement over exam time in patients with and without breast cancer. J Magn Reson Imag 2017;45(1):74–83.

28. American College of Radiology. ACR BI-RADS atlas: breast imaging reporting and data system ; mammography, ultrasound, magnetic resonance

imaging, follow-up and outcome monitoring, Data Dictionary. ACR. Reston, VA: American College of Radiology; 2013.

29. Tomida T, Urikura A, Uematsu T, et al. Contrast enhancement in breast cancer and background mammary-gland tissue during the super-early phase of dynamic breast magnetic resonance imaging. Acad Radiol 2017;24(11):1380–6.

30. Honda M, Kataoka M, Iima M, et al. Background parenchymal enhancement and its effect on lesion detectability in ultrafast dynamic contrast-enhanced MRI. Eur J Radiol 2020;129:108984.

31. Lee CH, Bryce Y, Zheng J, et al. Outcome of screening MRI in premenopausal women as a function of the week of the menstrual cycle. AJR Am J Roentgenol 2020;214(5):1175–81.

32. DeMartini WB, Liu F, Peacock S, et al. Background parenchymal enhancement on breast MRI: impact on diagnostic performance. AJR Am J Roentgenol 2012;198(4):W373–80.

33. Hambly NM, Liberman L, Dershaw DD, et al. Background parenchymal enhancement on baseline screening breast MRI: impact on biopsy rate and short-interval follow-up. AJR Am J Roentgenol 2011;196(1):218–24.

34. Ray KM, Kerlikowske K, Lobach IV, et al. Effect of background parenchymal enhancement on breast MR imaging interpretive performance in community-based practices. Radiology 2018;286(3):822–9.

35. Liao GJ, Henze Bancroft LC, Strigel RM, et al. Background parenchymal enhancement on breast MRI: A comprehensive review. J Magn Reson Imag 2020; 51(1):43–61.

36. Li J, Dershaw DD, Lee CH, et al. Breast MRI after conservation therapy: usual findings in routine follow-up examinations. AJR Am J Roentgenol 2010;195(3):799–807.

37. Pinnamaneni N, Moy L, Gao Y, et al. Canceled MRI-guided breast biopsies due to nonvisualization: follow-up and outcomes. Acad Radiol 2018;25(9): 1101–10.

38. Pinkney DM, Chikarmane SA, Giess CS. Do benign-concordant breast MRI biopsy results require short interval follow-up imaging? Report of longitudinal study and review of the literature. Clin Imag 2019; 57:50–5.

39. Chikarmane SA, Birdwell RL, Poole PS, et al. Characteristics, malignancy rate, and follow-up of BI-RADS category 3 lesions identified at breast MR Imaging: implications for MR image interpretation and management. Radiology 2016;280(3):707–15.

40. Geddes DT, Aljazaf KM, Kent JC, et al. Blood flow characteristics of the human lactating breast. J Hum Lact 2012;28(2):145–52.

41. Nissan N, Massasa EEM, Bauer E, et al. MRI can accurately diagnose breast cancer during lactation. Eur Radiol 2023;33(4):2935–44.

42. Taron J, Fleischer S, Preibsch H, et al. Background parenchymal enhancement in pregnancy-associated breast cancer: a hindrance to diagnosis? Eur Radiol 2019;29(3):1187–93.

43. Oh SW, Lim HS, Moon SM, et al. MR imaging characteristics of breast cancer diagnosed during lactation. Br J Radiol 2017;90(1078):20170203.

44. Peterson MS, Gegios AR, Elezaby MA, et al. Breast imaging and intervention during pregnancy and lactation. Radiographics 2023;43(10):e230014.

45. Dontchos BN, Rahbar H, Partridge SC, et al. Are qualitative assessments of background parenchymal enhancement, amount of fibroglandular tissue on MR images, and mammographic density associated with breast cancer risk? Radiology 2015;276(2):371–80.

46. Arasu VA, Miglioretti DL, Sprague BL, et al. Population-based assessment of the association between magnetic resonance imaging background parenchymal enhancement and future primary breast cancer risk. J Clin Oncol 2019;37(12):954–63.

47. Grimm LJ, Saha A, Ghate SV, et al. Relationship between background parenchymal enhancement on high-risk screening MRI and future breast cancer risk. Acad Radiol 2019;26(1):69–75.

48. Watt GP, Sung J, Morris EA, et al. Association of breast cancer with MRI background parenchymal enhancement: the IMAGINE case-control study. Breast Cancer Res 2020;22(1):138.

49. Sippo DA, Rutledge GM, Mercaldo SF, et al. Impact of background parenchymal enhancement on diagnostic performance in screening breast MRI. Acad Radiol 2020;27(5):663–71.

50. Acciavatti RJ, Lee SH, Reig B, et al. Beyond breast density: risk measures for breast cancer in multiple imaging modalities. Radiology 2023;306(3):e222575.

51. Thompson CM, Mallawaarachchi I, Dwivedi DK, et al. The association of background parenchymal enhancement at breast MRI with breast cancer: a systematic review and meta-analysis. Radiology 2019;292(3):552–61.

52. Lee SH, Jang M-J, Yoen H, et al. Background Parenchymal Enhancement at Postoperative Surveillance Breast MRI: Association with Future Second Breast Cancer Risk. Radiology 2023;306(1):90–9.

53. Kim GR, Cho N, Kim S-Y, et al. Interval cancers after negative supplemental screening breast MRI results in women with a personal history of breast cancer. Radiology 2021;300(2):314–23.

54. Baek JE, Kim SH, Lee AW. Background parenchymal enhancement in breast MRIs of breast cancer patients: impact on tumor size estimation. Eur J Radiol 2014;83(8):1356–62.

55. Uematsu T, Kasami M, Watanabe J. Does the degree of background enhancement in breast MRI affect the detection and staging of breast cancer? Eur Radiol 2011;21(11):2261–7.

56. Yoon J, Kim EK, Kim MJ, et al. Preoperative magnetic resonance imaging features associated with positive resection margins in patients with invasive lobular carcinoma. Korean J Radiol 2020;21(8):946–54.

57. Preibsch H, Richter V, Bahrs SD, et al. Repeated surgeries in invasive lobular breast cancer with preoperative MRI: Role of additional carcinoma in situ and background parenchymal enhancement. Eur J Radiol 2017;90:181–7.

58. You C, Gu Y, Peng W, et al. Decreased background parenchymal enhancement of the contralateral breast after two cycles of neoadjuvant chemotherapy is associated with tumor response in HER2-positive breast cancer. Acta Radiol 2018;59(7):806–12.

59. Dong J-M, Wang H-X, Zhong X-F, et al. Changes in background parenchymal enhancement in HER2-positive breast cancer before and after neoadjuvant chemotherapy: Association with pathologic complete response. Medicine 2018;97(43):e12965.

60. Oh SJ, Chae EY, Cha JH, et al. Relationship between background parenchymal enhancement on breast MRI and pathological tumor response in breast cancer patients receiving neoadjuvant chemotherapy. Br J Radiol 2018;91(1088):20170550.

61. Onishi N, Li W, Newitt DC, et al. Breast MRI during neoadjuvant chemotherapy: lack of background parenchymal enhancement suppression and inferior treatment response. Radiology 2021;301(2):295–308.

62. You C, Kaiser AK, Baltzer P, et al. The assessment of background parenchymal enhancement (BPE) in a high-risk population: what causes BPE? Transl Oncol 2018;11(2):243–9.

63. van der Velden BHM, Dmitriev I, Loo CE, et al. Association between parenchymal enhancement of the contralateral breast in dynamic contrast-enhanced MR imaging and outcome of patients with unilateral invasive breast cancer. Radiology 2015;276(3):675–85.

64. Shin GW, Zhang Y, Kim MJ, et al. Role of dynamic contrast-enhanced MRI in evaluating the association between contralateral parenchymal enhancement and survival outcome in ER-positive, HER2-negative, node-negative invasive breast cancer. J Magn Reson Imag 2018;48(6):1678–89.

65. Ragusi MAA, van der Velden BHM, Meeuwis C, et al. Long-term survival in breast cancer patients is associated with contralateral parenchymal enhancement at MRI: outcomes of the select study. Radiology 2023;307(4):e221922.

66. Saha A, Grimm LJ, Ghate SV, et al. Machine learning-based prediction of future breast cancer using algorithmically measured background parenchymal enhancement on high-risk screening MRI. J Magn Reson Imag 2019;50(2):456–64.

67. Eskreis-Winkler S, Sutton EJ, D'Alessio D, et al. Breast MRI background parenchymal enhancement categorization using deep learning: outperforming the radiologist. J Magn Reson Imag 2022;56(4):1068–76.

68. Watt GP, Thakran S, Sung JS, et al. Association of breast cancer odds with background parenchymal enhancement quantified using a fully automated method at MRI: the imagine study. Radiology 2023;308(3):e230367.

69. Niell BL, Abdalah M, Stringfield O, et al. Quantitative measures of background parenchymal enhancement predict breast cancer risk. AJR Am J Roentgenol 2021;217(1):64–75.

Artificial Intelligence for Breast Cancer Risk Assessment

Kathryn P. Lowry, MD[a,b,*], Case C. Zuiderveld, BS[c]

KEYWORDS

• Artificial intelligence • Deep learning • Breast cancer • Mammography

KEY POINTS

- Existing clinical risk models have limitations in predicting individual breast cancer risk, particularly for underrepresented race and ethnicity groups.
- Artificial intelligence (AI) algorithms using mammography images can outperform clinical risk prediction models, with 5 year area under the receiver operating curves ranging from 0.63 to 0.79.
- AI models have the potential to improve equity of performance and reduce misclassification of risk of women in underrepresented race and ethnicity groups.
- Future studies are needed to validate the accuracy of AI risk models, characterize cancer outcomes for high versus average risk individuals, and inform guidelines for the use of these new technologies in clinical practice.

INTRODUCTION

It is well known that on average, female persons (hereafter referred to as "women") born in the United States have a "1 in 8" risk of being diagnosed with breast cancer during their lifetime.[1] As medicine has shifted away from a "one-size-fits-all" approach to a more individualized approach in the era of precision medicine, there is growing demand for more refined breast cancer risk profiling. Women known to be at elevated risk for breast cancer can benefit from more intensive screening beyond routine mammography, with current guidelines supporting the use of MR imaging in women with lifetime risk exceeding 20%.[2,3] However, to maximize the impact of high-risk screening, reliable tools for individual breast cancer risk assessment are necessary to ensure that supplemental screening is offered to women most likely to benefit.

Ideally, a risk prediction model used in the clinical setting would demonstrate adequate *discrimination* and *calibration*.[4] Model discrimination refers to the distribution of risk scores and the ability to distinguish between individual women who do and do not develop breast cancer. It is typically assessed using the area under the receiver operating curve (AUC) which is expressed as a continuous measure ranging from 0 to 1, with 0.5 indicating complete overlap of risk scores between cases and controls (equivalent to "random guessing").[4,5] Model calibration refers to the ability to accurately predict absolute risk in groups of women with similar scores, typically measured as the ratio of expected-to-observed (E/O) cases. Ratios less than 1 indicate the model underpredicts risk, while ratios greater than 1 indicate the model overpredicts risk.

In the clinical setting, breast cancer risk has traditionally been assessed using the prediction models that incorporate hereditary and nonhereditary factors known to increase breast cancer risk. Some of the most commonly used models include the Breast Cancer Risk Assessment Tool (BCRAT; formerly known as the Gail model),[6] BRCAPRO,[7] BODICEA,[8] the Breast Cancer Surveillance

a Department of Radiology, University of Washington School of Medicine, Seattle, WA, USA; b Fred Hutchinson Cancer Center, Seattle, WA, USA; c University of Washington School of Medicine, Seattle, WA, USA
* Corresponding author. 1144 Eastlake Avenue East, LG-215, Seattle, WA 98109.
E-mail address: kplowry@uw.edu

Radiol Clin N Am 62 (2024) 619–625
https://doi.org/10.1016/j.rcl.2024.02.004
0033-8389/24/© 2024 Elsevier Inc. All rights reserved.

Consortium (BCSC),[9] and Tyrer-Cuzick models.[10] The specific inputs and complexity vary by model, but most current versions of these models incorporate age, family history, prior biopsy results, and breast density. Despite the evolution and adaptation of these models over time, in general, they have demonstrated only modest accuracy in predicting individual-level breast cancer risk, with AUCs typically ranging between 0.61 and 0.64 in external validation studies.[11] Importantly, models perform even less well in underrepresented minority groups, including Black women and Hispanic women in whom these models perform only slightly better than random chance, with AUCs of 0.56 and 0.51, respectively.[12]

In the last decade, there has been a surge in interest in the application of artificial intelligence (AI), particularly deep learning (DL), for prediction of clinical outcomes. A growing body of work suggests that AI algorithms have the potential to advance the field of risk prediction, performing as well or superior to traditional clinical risk models.[13] In this review, we summarize the current evidence on the utility of AI for breast cancer risk prediction. We also note current knowledge gaps and future opportunities to leverage AI to improve our ability to identify women most at risk for breast cancer.

Overview of Artificial Intelligence and Deep Learning

AI is broadly defined as the use of computer systems to interpret data in novel situations and produce output. Machine learning (ML) is a subset of AI that "learns" or extracts patterns from raw data without explicit human programming. DL is a type of ML that uses neural networks (similar to the structure of the human brain) to train for complex tasks.[14] One of the most common types of DL models is called a convolutional neural network (CNN). A CNN contains numerous layers of interconnected nodes, which send and receive signals and collectively produce the model output.[14] CNNs are trained using an iterative process performed on a large amount of input data with known outcomes. For each iteration, the model makes a prediction based on the input data and compares the predicted output to the known output, and the weights are adjusted. This process is repeated numerous times, each time adjusting the weights until the model output consistently matches the known (human-provided) outcome.[14] After completing model training, the model is then validated on a test data set (often a subset of the original data set reserved for testing) and the accuracy of model performance is assessed.

Applications of AI—and particularly DL—for imaging applications have grown exponentially in recent years due to advances in computer processing power and the increasing accessibility of large imaging data sets with known outcomes. Drawing on prior work demonstrating that some mammography features are associated with breast cancer risk, such as density and texture,[15,16] the DL algorithms have been developed for breast cancer risk prediction using mammography images as inputs. The task of breast cancer risk prediction lends itself particularly well to DL, as there are large-scale data with standardized inputs (ie, 4 view screening mammogram) with a single binary outcome (cancer or no cancer). As a result, the development of mammography-based AI breast cancer risk prediction models has progressed rapidly within the past 5 years.[13] While most algorithms have only been utilized in the research setting to date, multiple AI breast cancer risk prediction tools are currently undergoing review for FDA approval[17] and may soon disseminate into clinical practice.

Current Evidence

Table 1 provides an overview of the largest published studies to date of performance of mammography-based AI breast cancer risk prediction algorithms.[18–27] In general, most studies have reported on the performance of risk models using mammography-based AI risk scores alone and in combination with basic clinical risk factor information. Most studies have focused on model discrimination, with AUC as the primary outcome, and many performed a head-to-head comparison with currently used traditional risk factor-based models.

Two systematic reviews of AI-based breast cancer risk prediction model performance have been performed (see studies conducted by Gao and colleagues[23] and Schopf and colleagues[13]), reporting pooled and median AUCs of 0.73[23] and 0.72,[13] respectively. In both reviews, performance of AI-based risk models was generally superior to traditional risk factor-based models across studies. Importantly, there was significant heterogeneity across studies as well as concerns with study quality, including the need for performance data on model calibration as well as large-scale, diverse validation studies which are needed to demonstrate generalizability.[13,23]

Current evidence: Artificial intelligence risk model discrimination

In one of the earliest landmark studies of AI for breast cancer risk prediction, a DL risk model was trained using screening mammograms from a large US screening population.[18] This was the first to

Table 1
Studies evaluating image-based artificial intelligence breast cancer risk prediction model performance

Study	Data Set Population	Risk Timeframe	Clinical Risk Model Comparison	Model Type	AUC
Yala et al,[18] 2019	39,558 Massachusetts General Hospital	5 y	TC8	Image only Hybrid	0.68 0.70
Dembrower et al,[19] 2020	14,034 Cohort of Screen-aged Women	Lifetime	None	Hybrid	0.66
Yala et al,[20] 2021	70,811 Massachusetts General Hospital, 7353 Karolinska Mammography Project for Risk Prediction of Breast Cancer, 13,356 Chang Gung Memorial Hospital	5 y	TC8	Hybrid	0.78–0.79
Lehman et al,[22] 2022	57,493 Mass General Brigham	5 y	TC8, BCRAT	Hybrid	0.68
Dadsetan et al,[21] 2022	200 University of Pittsburgh Medical Center	Lifetime	None	Image only	0.67
Gastounioti et al,[28] 2022	5139 Hospital of the University of Pennsylvania	2 y	Gail	Image + age	0.68
Arasu et al,[29] 2023	324,009 Kaiser Permanente Northern California	0–5 y	BCSC	Mirai GMIC MammoScreen ProFound AI Mia	0.67 0.64 0.65 0.65 0.63
Li et al,[25] 2023	99 MD Anderson Cancer Center and University of Chicago Medical Center	Lifetime	None	Image-only	0.65
Michel et al,[27] 2023	23,467 Columbia Institute Irvine Medical Center	Lifetime	BCSC	Hybrid	0.65
Eriksson et al,[24] 2023	10,426 Karolinska Mammography Project for Risk Prediction of Breast Cancer	1–10 y	TC8	Image-only	0.69 5 y 0.65 10 y
Vachon et al,[33] 2023	6841 San Francisco Mammography Registry, 3239 Mayo Clinic Rochester	Lifetime	None	Image + age, BMI, density	0.63

Abbreviations: BCRAT, Breast Cancer Risk Assessment Tool; BCSC, Breast Cancer Surveillance Consortium; GMIC, Globally-Aware Multiple Instance Classifier; TC8, Tyrer-Cuzick version 8.

demonstrate the superior performance of an image-based AI risk model to a clinical risk prediction model in a large US screening population[18] The authors developed 3 models to predict 5 year risk of breast cancer: a logistic regression model using traditional clinical risk factors, a DL model using mammography images alone, and a hybrid DL model using both mammography images and risk factors. In their test set of 3937 mammograms with known cancer outcomes, the hybrid DL and image-only DL models achieved AUCs of 0.70 and 0.68, respectively, with the hybrid DL model significantly outperforming a traditional clinical model (Tyrer-Cuzick version 8 [TC8]). The image-only DL algorithm has since been adapted to enable risk prediction at multiple time points, incorporate clinical risk factor information when available, predict missing risk factor information, and produce consistent estimates across mammography vendors.[20,26] The updated algorithm (called Mirai) was trained using approximately 200,000 mammograms from Massachusetts General Hospital, of which 81% of controls and 86% of cases were performed in White women, 4.7% of controls and 3.9% of cases in Black women, 4.5% of controls and 3.0% of cases in Asian/Pacific Islander women, and 1.1% of controls and 1.2% of cases in Hispanic women. Mirai was subsequently validated on screening mammograms Massachusetts General Hospital as well as data sets from Karolinska University (Sweden) and Chang Gung Memorial Hospital (Taiwan).[20] In this validation, Mirai achieved 5 year AUCs ranging from 0.76 to 0.81 across cohorts, again outperforming TC8 (AUC of 0.64 in the MGH subset of data). In the largest validation study of Mirai performed using mammography data from 7 international sites, Mirai achieved AUCs of 0.75 to 0.84.[26] The updated Mirai has also continued to demonstrate superior performance to clinical risk factor-based models, including the TC8 and BCRAT in a recent study using screening mammograms performed at Mass General Brigham facilities.[22]

Gastounioti and colleagues[28] developed a short-term (2 year) breast cancer risk prediction model trained on mammograms from a Swedish population which produces risk estimates based on extracted imaging features, including density, masses, calcifications, and asymmetries. In a case-control validation study using screening mammograms from US women, the AI risk model significantly outperformed the BCRAT (AUC of 0.68 vs 0.55).[28] In a separate case-cohort study using mammograms from the Swedish KARMA cohort, the model's short- and long-term performance was examined for breast cancer risk prediction over a 10 year time horizon.[24] The model demonstrated better discrimination than TC8 during all years of the study, with AUCs of 0.69 and 0.65 for 5 and 10 year risk, respectively (vs 0.60 at 5 and 10 years for the TC8).[24] The AI model also produced similar results for estrogen receptor (ER)-negative breast cancers and ER-positive cancers, invasive cancers versus in ductal carcinoma in situ, and screen-detected versus symptomatic cancers.

The promising performance of mammography-based AI risk prediction was reinforced in a multimodel case-cohort US validation study which compared 2 open source models and 3 commercial models to the BCSC clinical risk model for 5 year risk prediction.[29] All 5 AI risk models performed significantly better than the BCSC model, with time-dependent AUCs ranging from 0.63 to 0.67 (vs 0.61 for the BCSC model). Performance was significantly better for both invasive cancer and ductal carcinoma in situ, as well as in the subset of women with negative screening mammograms.[29]

Current evidence: Artificial intelligence risk model calibration and risk classification

While there is growing evidence across multiple studies that AI-based breast cancer risk models can demonstrate discriminatory accuracy comparable to or better than traditional risk factor-based models, there are few reports of AI risk model calibration. In the multimodel case-cohort validation study,[29] calibration of Mirai and the BCSC risk models was compared using E/O ratios. While the BCSC model was well calibrated (E/O 1.02), Mirai considerably underestimated 5 year risk (E/O 0.60). This finding is noteworthy given that calibration is particularly important for tools such as breast cancer risk models which guide management based on absolute risk thresholds.

Other studies have compared risk classification using AI-based models versus clinical risk factor-based models. In their comparison of the Mirai versus TC8 and BCRAT models, Lehman and colleagues[22] compared the percentage of women with cancers identified as high risk by different models. Using the 50th percentile of risk or higher, the AI model identified 75% of women with cancers as high risk versus 35% and 39% of women with cancers identified based on risk scores produced by the BCRAT and TC8, respectively. Similarly, the 2 year AI-based risk model evaluated by Eriksson and colleagues identified 20% of women with cancers as high risk using a 2 year cutoff of 2.33% versus 7% of those identified as high risk based on 10 year risk estimates using TC8.[24]

Current evidence: Artificial intelligence risk model performance in subpopulations

Importantly, studies to date of AI-based breast cancer risk prediction suggest that AI models based on mammography images have the potential to improve the equity of breast cancer risk prediction. Multiple studies of traditional clinical risk factor-based models have demonstrated poorer performance in underrepresented minority groups compared to White women, including Black, Hispanic, Asian and Pacific Islander women.[30–32] In contrast, not only do mammography-based AI models demonstrate better performance than risk factor-based models in non-White women but also studies to date have demonstrated similar performance of AI risk models across race and ethnicity groups[18,20,22,27,28] and across international settings[26] without additional model training.

Studies have shown mixed results when comparing performance across other subpopulations. Some studies have found that AI risk models perform similarly across women when grouped by breast density[27] and menopausal status.[18,24] Others have found differential performance in some groups, including women younger than age 60 years[33] and women with a family history of breast cancer.[24] The reasons for these discrepancies have not been fully elucidated, and further investigation is needed with large screening populations to enable examination in these groups of women.

Current evidence: Mammography-only artificial intelligence models versus hybrid artificial intelligence and risk factor models

One of the appeals of mammography-based AI risk models is their efficiency, since they can produce risk estimates using images alone versus traditional risk models which require collecting a detailed history (Table 2). However, one consideration is whether a hybrid approach combining AI model output with clinical risk factors can improve risk prediction versus mammography-based AI risk model output alone. In general, this approach has had mixed results. In a recent systematic review,[13] 6 of 7 studies that compared performance of hybrid AI and risk factor models versus mammography-based AI models alone showed no difference in AUC, with the remaining study demonstrating a small improvement in AUC (0.06) with the addition of risk factors. In a multimodel comparison of 5 AI risk models,[29] AUCs for each model when combined with the BCSC 5 year risk model were significantly higher than for the AI models alone (AUCs for hybrid models ranging from 0.66–0.68 versus 0.63–0.67 for image-only models).[29] In a nested case-control study examining the Transpara AI model, when AI risk scores were added to density measures AUCs improved by 0.059-0.064 versus models with density measures alone.[33] However, it is not yet clear whether these small differences in discriminatory accuracy justify the additional time and complexity of collection and entry of risk factor information for model inputs. Implementation studies in the clinical setting are needed to further evaluate the impact and trade-offs of mammography-only AI models versus hybrid models combining AI scores and clinical risk factors.

Future Directions

There are important knowledge gaps that must be addressed prior to large scale implementation of these models in clinical practice. First, most studies thus far have relied on small convenience samples, and studies of performance in real-world screening settings are needed.[13] Additionally, while there are numerous studies that have compared discriminatory accuracy of AI risk models versus currently used models, only one has compared model calibration.[29] In this study, the clinical risk factor-based model was considerably better calibrated than the AI risk model. Model calibration is particularly important when risk models are used to determine eligibility based on an absolute risk threshold,[4] and therefore, calibration has important clinical implications and

Table 2
Risk factors and data leveraged by traditional and artificial intelligence breast cancer risk assessment models

Factors	Traditional Models				AI Models			
	TC8	BCRAT	BCSC	Mirai	Transpara	ProFound	Mia	GMIC
Age	X	X	X	X[b]		X[a]		
Height/weight	X		X	X[b]				
Breast density	X		X	X[b]				
History of biopsy	X	X	X	X[b]				
Family history of breast or ovarian cancer	X	X	X	X[b]				
Hormone therapy status	X		X	X[b]				
Race/ethnicity	X	X	X	X[b]				
Age at menarche	X	X	X	X[b]				
Age at first birth	X	X	X	X[b]				
Age at menopause	X		X	X[b]				
Screening Mammogram				X	X	X	X	X

Abbreviations: BCRAT, Breast Cancer Risk Assessment Tool; BCSC, Breast Cancer Surveillance Consortium; GMIC, Globally-Aware Multiple Instance Classifier; TC8, Tyrer-Cuzick version 8.
[a] Age is extracted from mammography images.
[b] Risk factors can be directly provided or generated based on imaging alone if unavailable.

warrants further study. Finally, more work is needed to determine how the risk estimates produced by these models should guide clinical care in terms of recommendations for both primary and secondary prevention.

SUMMARY

In summary, there is a compelling body of literature demonstrating similar if not superior performance of mammography-based AI models for breast cancer risk prediction compared to traditional models currently used in clinical practice. These models may address a critical shortcoming of risk factor-based models by improving equity of risk prediction across race and ethnicity groups. Many AI risk models perform well using mammographic images alone, suggesting these models may also improve efficiency by obviating the need for collection and manual entry of clinical risk factor information. Future studies are needed to validate these findings in diverse, real-world screening populations, examine model calibration, and guide recommendations for primary and secondary prevention.

CLINICS CARE POINTS

- AI breast cancer risk prediction models using mammography images have demonstrated similar or better accuracy than traditional clinical risk factor-based models used in clinical practice.

- Mammography-based AI risk models may especially improve risk prediction in women in underrepresented race and ethnicity groups.

- Further research is needed to validate AI risk model performance in real-world screening settings and inform clinical guidelines regarding their use.

DISCLOSURE

The authors have nothing to disclose.

FUNDING

Dr Lowry is funded by a research grant from the American Cancer Society (21-078-01-CPSH).

REFERENCES

1. Breast Cancer Statistics | How Common Is Breast Cancer? | American Cancer Society. Available at: https://www.cancer.org/cancer/types/breast-cancer/about/how-common-is-breast-cancer.html. [Accessed 22 August 2023].

2. Monticciolo DL, Newell MS, Moy L, et al. Breast Cancer Screening in Women at Higher-Than-Average Risk: Recommendations From the ACR. J Am Coll Radiol 2018;15(3 Pt A):408–14.

3. Saslow D, Boetes C, Burke W, et al. American Cancer Society guidelines for breast screening with MRI as an adjunct to mammography. CA Cancer J Clin 2007;57(2):75–89.

4. Steyerberg EW, Vickers AJ, Cook NR, et al. Assessing the Performance of Prediction Models. Epidemiology 2010;21(1):128–38.

5. Mandrekar JN. Receiver Operating Characteristic Curve in Diagnostic Test Assessment. J Thorac Oncol 2010;5(9):1315–6.

6. Gail MH, Brinton LA, Byar DP, et al. Projecting Individualized Probabilities of Developing Breast Cancer for White Females Who Are Being Examined Annually. JNCI Journal of the National Cancer Institute 1989;81(24):1879–86.

7. Parmigiani G, Berry DA, Aguilar O. Determining Carrier Probabilities for Breast Cancer–Susceptibility Genes BRCA1 and BRCA2. Am J Hum Genet 1998;62(1):145–58.

8. Lee A, Mavaddat N, Wilcox AN, et al. BOADICEA: a comprehensive breast cancer risk prediction model incorporating genetic and nongenetic risk factors. Genet Med 2019;21(8):1708–18.

9. Tice JA, Cummings SR, Smith-Bindman R, et al. Using Clinical Factors and Mammographic Breast Density to Estimate Breast Cancer Risk: Development and Validation of a New Predictive Model. Ann Intern Med 2008;148(5):337.

10. Tyrer J, Duffy SW, Cuzick J. A breast cancer prediction model incorporating familial and personal risk factors. Stat Med 2004;23(7):1111–30.

11. McCarthy AM, Guan Z, Welch M, et al. Performance of Breast Cancer Risk-Assessment Models in a Large Mammography Cohort. J Natl Cancer Inst 2020;112(5):489–97.

12. Allman R, Dite GS, Hopper JL, et al. SNPs and breast cancer risk prediction for African American and Hispanic women. Breast Cancer Res Treat 2015;154(3):583–9.

13. Schopf CM, Ramwala OA, Lowry KP, et al. Artificial Intelligence-Driven Mammography-Based Future Breast Cancer Risk Prediction: A Systematic Review. J Am Coll Radiol 2023. https://doi.org/10.1016/j.jacr.2023.10.018.

14. Hosny A, Parmar C, Quackenbush J, et al. Artificial intelligence in radiology. Nat Rev Cancer 2018;18(8):500–10.

15. Anandarajah A, Chen Y, Colditz GA, et al. Studies of parenchymal texture added to mammographic breast density and risk of breast cancer: a systematic

review of the methods used in the literature. Breast Cancer Res 2022;24(1).

16. Bodewes FTH, van Asselt AA, Dorrius MD, et al. Mammographic breast density and the risk of breast cancer: A systematic review and meta-analysis. Breast 2022;66:62–8.

17. Available at: https://www.fda.gov/medical-devices/software-medical-device-samd/artificial-intelligence-and-machine-learning-aiml-enabled-medical-devices. Accessed November 1, 2023.

18. Yala A, Lehman C, Schuster T, et al. A deep learning mammography-based model for improved breast cancer risk prediction. Radiology 2019;292(1):60–6.

19. Dembrower K, Liu Y, Azizpour H, et al. Comparison of a deep learning risk score and standard mammographic density score for breast cancer risk prediction. Radiology 2020;294(2):265–72.

20. Yala A, Mikhael PG, Strand F, et al. Toward robust mammography-based models for breast cancer risk. Sci Transl Med 2021;13(578). https://doi.org/10.1126/scitranslmed.aba4373.

21. Dadsetan S, Arefan D, Berg WA, et al. Deep learning of longitudinal mammogram examinations for breast cancer risk prediction. Pattern Recognit 2022;132. https://doi.org/10.1016/j.patcog.2022.108919.

22. Lehman CD, Mercaldo S, Lamb LR, et al. Deep Learning vs Traditional Breast Cancer Risk Models to Support Risk-Based Mammography Screening. J Natl Cancer Inst 2022;114(10):1355–63.

23. Gao Y, Li S, Jin Y, et al. An Assessment of the Predictive Performance of Current Machine Learning–Based Breast Cancer Risk Prediction Models: Systematic Review. JMIR Public Health Surveill 2022; 8(12). https://doi.org/10.2196/35750.

24. Eriksson M, Czene K, Vachon C, et al. A Clinical Risk Model for Personalized Screening and Prevention of Breast Cancer. Cancers 2023;15(12):3246.

25. Li H, Robinson K, Lan L, et al. Temporal Machine Learning Analysis of Prior Mammograms for Breast Cancer Risk Prediction. Cancers 2023;15(7). https://doi.org/10.3390/CANCERS15072141.

26. Yala A, Mikhael PG, Strand F, et al. Multi-Institutional Validation of a Mammography-Based Breast Cancer Risk Model. J Clin Oncol 2022;40(16):1732–40.

27. Michel A, Ro V, McGuinness JE, et al. Breast cancer risk prediction combining a convolutional neural network-based mammographic evaluation with clinical factors. Breast Cancer Res Treat 2023;200(2): 237–45.

28. Gastounioti A, Eriksson M, Cohen EA, et al. External Validation of a Mammography-Derived AI-Based Risk Model in a U.S. Breast Cancer Screening Cohort of White and Black Women. Cancers 2022; 14(19):4803.

29. Arasu VA, Habel LA, Achacoso NS, et al. Comparison of Mammography AI Algorithms with a Clinical Risk Model for 5-year Breast Cancer Risk Prediction: An Observational Study. Radiology 2023;307(5). https://doi.org/10.1148/RADIOL.222733/ASSET/IMAGES/LARGE/RADIOL.222733.VA.JPEG.

30. Banegas MP, John EM, Slattery ML, et al. Projecting Individualized Absolute Invasive Breast Cancer Risk in US Hispanic Women. J Natl Cancer Inst 2016; 109(2). https://doi.org/10.1093/JNCI/DJW215.

31. Gail MH, Costantino JP, Pee D, et al. Projecting individualized absolute invasive breast cancer risk in African American women. J Natl Cancer Inst 2007; 99(23):1782–92.

32. Matsuno RK, Costantino JP, Ziegler RG, et al. Projecting individualized absolute invasive breast cancer risk in Asian and pacific islander American women. J Natl Cancer Inst 2011;103(12):951–61.

33. Vachon CM, Scott CG, Norman AD, et al. Impact of Artificial Intelligence System and Volumetric Density on Risk Prediction of Interval, Screen-Detected, and Advanced Breast Cancer. J Clin Oncol 2023;41(17): 3172–83.

Hereditary Breast Cancer
BRCA Mutations and Beyond

Miral M. Patel, MD*, Beatriz Elena Adrada, MD, FSBI

KEYWORDS

- Breast cancer • Genetic mutation • Hereditary breast cancer • Screening

KEY POINTS

- Genetic testing should be available to all patients with newly diagnosed breast cancer or a personal history of breast cancer.
- Patients who have previously undergone genetic testing may benefit from updated testing, specifically, patients with prior negative BRCA1/2. If the genetic testing was performed before 2014, relevant mutations may not have been included.
- Certain high and moderate penetrance genes have specific breast cancer associations including triple negative, luminal, HER2+, lobular cancers and contralateral breast malignancy.
- Breast MR imaging remains the current adjunct screening modality of choice, in addition to annual mammography (in most higher risk patients). Abbreviated MR imaging is a promising imaging modality for high-risk screening, with cancer detection rate (CDR) comparable to standard breast MR imaging.
- In patients in whom breast MR imaging is contraindicated, contrast-enhanced mammography or bilateral ultrasound is a reasonable alternative to supplement mammography.

OVERVIEW

Breast cancer is the most common cancer worldwide and is the second leading cause of cancer-related death among women in the United States after lung cancer.[1] Approximately 5% to 10% of breast cancers have been attributed to germline mutations.[2] Of these, up to 30% of hereditary breast and ovarian cancer syndromes are associated with mutations in the BRCA1/2 genes located on chromosomes 13 and 17, respectively.[3] However, many individuals with a family history of breast cancer do not carry these genetic mutations, suggesting the existence of other genetic risk factors. Previously, only single gene testing was available. With the development of next-generation sequencing (NGS) technology, multiple genes can be simultaneously analyzed, altering the landscape of inherited breast cancer. Multigene panels have the potential effect of increasing the likelihood of detecting a breast cancer-associated variant and identifying at-risk family members. In fact, multiple genes with varying degrees of penetrance and breast cancer risk have now been identified. Consequently, genetic counseling and genetic testing have become an integral part of the management of women with newly diagnosed breast and ovarian cancer and for women with a personal or family history suggestive of an inherited syndrome.[4]

GENETIC TESTING

Hereditary cancers are frequently manifested by pathogenic and likely pathogenic (P/LP) variants with an increased risk for certain malignancies inherited from either parent. They typically develop at a young age and exhibit an autosomal dominant inheritance pattern. A person suspected of being at risk for inherited cancer should receive genetic

Funded by: NIHHYB. Grant number(s): P30 CA016672.
Department of Breast Imaging, The University of Texas MD Anderson Cancer Center, 1515 Holcombe, CPB5. 3208, Houston, TX 77030, USA
* Corresponding author.
E-mail address: MPatel6@mdanderson.org

counseling.[5] Until 2013, national guidelines were implemented only to identify patients with an increased risk of a breast cancer gene (BRCA) genetic mutation, as genetic testing was costly and only the presence of BRCA mutations could be identified.[3] NGS has since made it possible to identify additional genetic mutations with high and moderate penetrance. Gene penetrance is defined as the probability that a specific genetic mutation will manifest clinically.[6] The penetrance expresses the breast cancer risk that is genetically determined. A high penetrance gene is associated with a lifetime risk greater than 50% or a relative risk greater than 5 (ie, >5 times that of average risk population); an intermediate penetrance gene has a lifetime risk of 20% to 50% or a relative cancer risk of 1.5 to 5; and a low penetrance gene has a lifetime risk of less than 20% or a relative cancer risk less than 1.5[7] (**Fig. 1**). For many of these genetic pathologic variants (PVs), the degree of breast cancer risk is still unclear. In addition to the high and intermediate penetrance genetic mutations, genome-wide association studies have identified low penetrance single nucleotide pleomorphism (SNP). An individual SNP carries a low breast cancer risk but the combined effect of multiple SNPs might contribute up to 14% of hereditable breast cancer.[8]

There is still substantial controversy regarding the selection of patients with breast cancer who should undergo genetic testing and which genes should be included. The National Comprehensive Cancer Network (NCCN) has established criteria for identifying women with breast cancer, ovarian cancer, or both who should undergo genetic testing according to their personal and familial histories.[9] Conversely, the American Society of Surgeons proposes all women with breast cancer should undergo genetic testing[10] (**Table 1**).

The NCCN guidelines outline appropriate clinical scenarios for hereditary cancer testing. Patients with a personal history of breast cancer of 50 years or lesser as well as those diagnosed at any age with specific histories, including triple-negative breast cancers, multiple primary breast cancers (synchronous or metachronous), lobular breast cancer with personal or family history of gastric cancer, male patients, or patients of Ashkenazi Jewish ancestry warrant testing for high penetrance genes (including BRCA1, BRCA2, CDH1, PALB2, phosphatase and tensin homolog [PTEN], and TP53). Patients with breast cancer and with a family history of at least one close relative with either breast cancer under the age of 50 years, male breast cancer, ovarian cancer, pancreatic cancer, prostate cancer with metastatic disease, or in a high/very high-risk group should also be tested. Testing is also recommended for patients with a personal history of breast cancer and at least 3 total diagnoses of breast cancer in the patient/close blood relative or at least 2 close blood relatives with either breast or prostate cancer. In addition, more specific guidelines for testing for Li-Fraumeni syndrome and Cowden syndrome/PTEN Hamartoma Tumor syndrome are also outlined.[9]

Genetic testing in a patient with a newly diagnosed breast cancer has implications for surgical planning (eg, in determining the appropriateness of bilateral mastectomy), radiation treatment (radiation avoidance in TP53), and in the selection of systemic therapy (use of poly [ADP-ribose] polymerase inhibitors in PVs of PALB2 and BRCA).[6] With the identification of new genetic mutations, patients who previously tested negative for BRCA1/2 mutations or underwent genetic testing before 2014, should undergo repeat genetic testing.[10] Individuals who test positive for these genetic mutations should be counseled regarding various risk management strategies including chemoprevention, enhanced imaging screening, and risk-reducing surgery.[10]

PENETRANCE OF GENE MUTATIONS
High Penetrance Genes (TP53, PTEN, CDH1, STK11, PALB2)

Combined with BRCA1, BRCA2, pathogenic mutations in these high penetrance genes increase breast cancer risk by more than 4 times and are responsible for 25% of all hereditary breast cancers.[11]

TP53

TP53 is a tumor suppressor gene encoding transcription factor protein p53, which is involved in the preservation of an intact genome by regulating cell cycle, DNA repair, apoptosis, cellular senescence, and metabolism.[12] Breast cancer is the

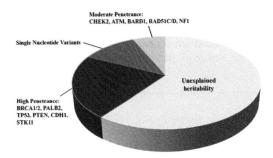

Fig. 1. Penetrance of genes conferring increased risk of breast cancer.

Table 1
Recommendations for genetic testing in patients without and with a personal history of breast cancer

NCCN Guidelines (Version 3.2023)	ASbrS Guidelines (February 2019)
Indications for Patients Without a Personal History of Breast Cancer	
• Blood relative with a known pathogenic/likely pathogenic variant in a cancer susceptibility gene • Meet above criteria and previously tested negative with limited (single gene testing) who are interested in multigene testing • Meet Li-Fraumeni, Cowden or Lynch syndrome testing criteria • A first or second-degree blood relative with a personal history of breast cancer meeting the criteria below (exception is for systemic therapy decision-making) • Probability of >5% of a BRCA1/2 pathogenic variant based on probability models (eg, Tyrer-Cuzick, BRCAPro, and CanRisk) • Testing *may* be considered for an individual of Ashkenazi Jewish ancestry without additional risk factors or with a personal history of serous endometrial cancer	• Test per NCCN guidelines • Testing an affected relative first is more informative than an unaffected individual undergoing testing • If this is not feasible, unaffected family member can undergo testing with pretest counseling • Reasonable to order a multigene panel if family history is incomplete or other cancers are found in the family history
Indications for patients with a personal history of breast cancer	

• Age≤50 y old
• At any age:
  *To assist in treatment decisions
  *If pathology/histology is triple-negative breast cancer, multiple primary breast cancers (synchronous or metachronous), lobular breast cancer with personal or family history of diffuse gastric cancer
  *Male breast cancer
  *Ashkenazi Jewish ancestry
  *Family history:
  ○ 1 or more close blood relative with breast cancer≤50, male breast cancer, ovarian cancer, pancreatic cancer, prostate cancer with metastasis or high/very high-risk group
  ○ 3 or more total diagnoses of breast cancer in patient and/or close blood relatives
  ○ 2 or more close blood relatives with either breast or prostate cancer
	• Genetic testing should be made available to all patients with a personal history of breast cancer

Data from Refs.[9,10]

most frequent malignancy for female TP53 carriers and 1% of women diagnosed with breast cancer before the age of 50 years have a TP53 mutation **(Fig. 2)**.[12–14]

Li-Fraumeni syndrome is characterized by germline TP53 mutations inherited in an autosomal dominant pattern exhibiting early onset multiple primary cancers involving the breast, brain, and adrenal gland.[12,15,16] Breast cancer is the most common cancer diagnosed in women with Li-Fraumeni syndrome with an estimated lifetime risk of 85% by the age of 60 years.[4,11] Most DCIS and invasive ductal carcinomas in patients

with Li Fraumeni syndrome are hormone receptor positive and/or HER-2 positive.[17]

NCCN guidelines recommend breast awareness starting at the age of 18 years and clinical breast examination every 6 to 12 months starting at the age of 20 years for these patients. Annual breast MR imaging is recommended between ages 20 to 29 years with the addition of annual mammogram beginning at the age of 30 years. Discussion of risk-reducing mastectomy is also recommended. Radiation therapy is avoided when possible due to increased risk of radiation-induced secondary malignancies. In addition,

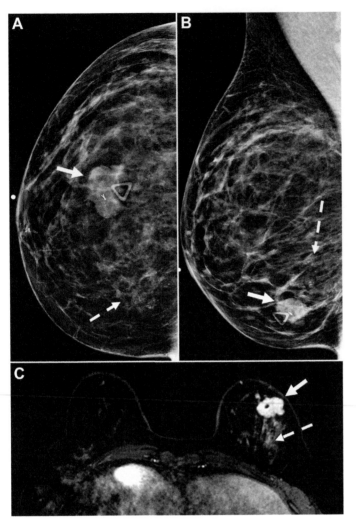

Fig. 2. A 29-year-old woman with TP53 germline pathogenic variant and history of osteosarcoma and pituitary microadenoma with newly diagnosed palpable invasive ductal carcinoma, ER+, PR+, HER2+ and ductal carcinoma in situ, grade 3, Patient's genetic mutation was discovered after referral to genetic counseling based on presentation of early-onset breast cancer. (A, B) Right CC and MLO mammographic views demonstrate a high density, irregular mass with associated marker clip (white arrows). Pleomorphic calcifications are noted in the lower inner quadrant of the right breast (dashed arrow). (C) Axial T1W contrast-enhanced breast MR image shows the enhancing irregular mass (arrow) with the associated nonmass enhancement in the right breast (dashed arrow). Patient underwent bilateral mastectomies.

diagnostic radiation should be minimized without sacrificing accuracy.[9]

PTEN

Phosphatase tensin homolog on chromosome 10q23.3 has a tumor suppressor role. When abnormal, cell cycle arrest and apoptosis cannot be activated leading to uncontrolled cell survival.[12,18] A mutation in PTEN is present in disorders such as Cowden syndrome or PTEN hamartoma tumor syndrome. Breast cancer is the most common malignancy in Cowden syndrome. Although Cowden syndrome is responsible for less than 1% of all breast cancers, those with this syndrome have a 25% to 50% lifetime risk of breast cancer with one study reporting up to 85% increased lifetime risk.[19,20] Patients with Cowden syndrome are more likely to have early onset breast cancer.[12,20,21]

Breast cancers are more frequently multifocal and bilateral in Cowden syndrome.[12,22,23] In addition, patients may also have breast hamartomas that can be multiple and bilateral.[12,24]

The NCCN guidelines recommend educating these patients on breast awareness starting at the age of 18 years and advise reporting any breast changes. Additionally, clinical breast examination is recommended every 6 to 12 months starting at the age of 25 or 5 to 10 years before the earliest known breast cancer in the family (whichever comes first). Annual mammography and breast are recommended starting at the age of 35 or 10 years before the earliest known breast cancer in the family (whichever comes first). Risk reduction mastectomy can be discussed in the appropriate clinical setting.[9]

CDH1

The CDH1 gene codes for epithelial cadherin (e-cadherin), located in the membrane surrounding epithelial cells and involved in cell adhesion, tumor suppression, cell maturation and movement, and gene regulation.[4] PV in CDH1 is found in hereditary diffuse gastric cancer, conferring an 80% lifetime risk of diffuse gastric cancer.[4] Female carriers of this gene have a 52% cumulative risk of breast cancer development by the age of 75 years with lobular carcinoma being a frequent breast tumor in CDH1 mutation carriers.[11,25,26]

NCCN screening guidelines recommend annual mammography and consideration for breast MR imaging starting at the age of 30 years. The option of risk-reducing mastectomy can also be discussed.[9]

STK11

Genetic mutations in STK11/LKB1, a serine/threonine kinase gene functioning as a tumor suppressor, are identified in Peutz-Jeghers syndrome. The highest cumulative cancer risks are for cancers of the gastrointestinal (GI) tract; however, for women, the major extraintestinal cancer risk is for breast cancer.[27] There is an associated 45% increased risk of ductal cancer by the age of 70 years compared with 7% in the general population.[11,27]

NCCN guidelines recommend annual mammogram and breast MR imaging starting at the age of 30 years with discussion of risk-reducing mastectomy.[9]

PALB2

The PALB2 gene codes for a protein scaffolding the BRCA2 protein during the DNA repair process.[11,28] When only 1 of the 2 gene copies (alleles) carries a variant, it is termed monoallelic and when both gene copies carry a variant it is termed biallelic.[29] Monoallelic versus biallelic states can have different effects on a disease.[29] Biallelic pathogenic variants in PALB2 cause Fanconi Anemia Type-N, a recessively inherited subtype with an elevated risk of solid tumors and leukemia in early infancy. Monoallelic PALB2 mutation carriers have an increased risk of breast and pancreatic cancer with a recent study demonstrating the cumulative risk of breast cancer to be 35% by the age of 70 years.[11,28] Absolute breast cancer risk is noted to increase in carriers with 2 or more first-degree relatives with breast cancer at the age of 50 years.[28] PALB2 breast cancers may more commonly be triple negative and at higher risk for a subsequent contralateral breast cancer.[4,30,31] A summary of risk associations and breast cancer histologic characteristics and biological marker subtypes is provided in **Table 2**.

NCCN guidelines recommend annual mammogram and breast MR imaging starting at the age of 30 years with discussion of the option of risk-reducing mastectomy.[9]

Moderate Penetrance Genes (CHEK2, ATM, BARD1, RAD51C/D, NF1)

Genes with intermediate penetrance are less prevalent in the population than high penetrance genes.[32] The lifetime risk from these genes ranges from 20% to 50%. These genes frequently interact with the BRCA1, BRCA2 pathways to repair DNA damage.[4]

Checkpoint kinase 2

The cell-cycle-checkpoint kinase 2 gene (CHEK2) is a serine/threonine kinase found on chromosome 22. It is a component of the ATM-CHK2-p53 pathway, which is activated in response to DNA double-stranded breaks.[33] Loss of kinase activity has been associated with an increased risk of developing breast, prostate, kidney, thyroid, and colon malignancies. Although CHEK2 is a gene mutation with moderate penetrance, this germline mutation is common in the population. The prevalence of the germline CHEK2 mutation varies by geography and ethnicity, with the mutation being more prevalent in Caucasian people of Eastern and Northern European descent.[34] A specific CHEK2 pathogenic variant (CHEK2*1100delC) is often observed in those with Northern and Eastern European descent; increasing the breast cancer risk by 3-fold to 5-fold, with a 37% cumulative risk of breast cancer by the age of 70 years.[35] If the CHEK2 carrier has first-degree and second-degree relatives with breast cancer, the breast cancer risk increases from 20% to 44%.[36,37]

Breast cancers in CHEK2 carriers exhibit similar characteristics. Protein truncating variants of CHEK2 have been associated with breast cancer of luminal subtype and with a higher incidence of bilateral breast cancers (**Fig. 3**).[31] Additionally,

Table 2
Risk associations and breast cancer histologic characteristics and biological marker subtypes

Breast Cancer Subtype	Gene Mutations
HER2+	TP53, NF1
ER+	ATM-CHEK2, CDH1
ER−	BRCA1, BRCA2, BARD1, PALB2, RAD51C
Triple-negative breast cancer	BRCA1, BRCA2, BARD1, PALB2, RAD51C
Invasive lobular carcinoma	CDH1, CHEK2
Asynchronous contralateral breast cancer	BRCA1, BRCA2, CHEK2, PALB2, PTEN

Data from Refs.[11,12,31]

CHEK2 mutations have been reported to predispose patients to lobular breast cancer. Men with CHEK2 mutations have been shown to have a higher risk of breast cancer.[38]

NCCN guidelines recommend annual mammography starting at the age of 40 years and consideration of breast MR imaging starting at the age of 30 to 35 years. Currently, there is insufficient evidence for risk-reducing mastectomy, and this may be considered based on family history.[9]

Ataxia-telangiectasia-mutated gene

The ataxia-telangiectasia-mutated (ATM) gene encodes a kinase implicated in the DNA double-strand breast repair mechanism. Ataxia-telangiectasia is a neurodegenerative disorder associated with the ATM gene. Although this recessive disease is uncommon, the frequency of heterozygous variants is not. Approximately 3% of Caucasians in the United States are estimated to be ATM heterozygotes.[6] Similar to CHEK2 mutations, ATM mutations bear a moderate breast cancer risk but they are detected more frequently than other mutations. A meta-analysis showed that ATM PV carriers have a 38% risk for developing cancer (**Fig. 4**).[39] The ATM gene predisposes to develop estrogen (ER) + breast cancers.[40] Carriers of ATM mutations also have an elevated risk of pancreatic, prostate, and ovarian malignancies.

The evidence for radiotoxicity in the setting of an ATM mutation is controversial. According to the WECARE study, exposure to radiation may be associated with an increased risk for asynchronous contralateral breast cancer in women who carry extremely uncommon ATM missense variants. However, these variants are not P/LP, and a meta-analysis of 5 studies revealed that exposure to ionizing radiation for diagnostic purposes or radiation therapy (with conventional doses) is not contraindicated for patients with a heterozygous ATM P/LP variant.[39]

NCCN guidelines recommend annual mammography starting at the age of 40 years and consideration of breast MR imaging starting at the age of 30 to 35 years. Currently, there is insufficient evidence for risk-reducing mastectomy, and this may be considered based on family history.[9]

BRCA1-associated ring domain

BRCA1-associated ring domain (BARD1) is a gene that interacts closely with BRCA1 to repair double-stranded breaks in DNA. Evidence regarding the function of the BRAD1 gene in breast and ovarian malignancies is limited and sometimes contradictory.[41,42] Weber-Lasalle and colleagues reported an association between the BARD1 mutation and early breast cancer onset.[43] Other studies have

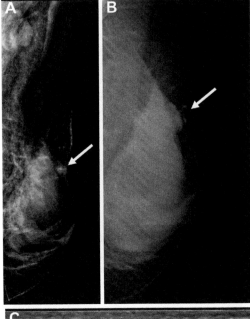

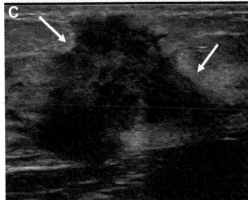

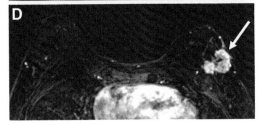

Fig. 3. A 43-year-old woman with palpable mass and skin changes in the left breast. She has a family history of breast cancer and a father with prostate cancer. Genetic testing was performed showing a CHEK2 c.1100 del pathogenic variant. (*A, B*) Left MLO DM and large paddle spot compression DBT views show a 2 cm oval mass with partially obscured margins associated with focal skin retraction at the area of palpable abnormality (*arrows*). (*C*) Longitudinal US shows an irregular hypoechoic mass extending to the overlying skin (*arrows*). Ultrasound-guided biopsy yielded IDC, ER+, PR+, and HER2−. Metastatic axillary level I to III lymph nodes were seen (not shown). (*D*) Axial T1W contrast-enhanced breast MR image shows multiple enhancing masses in the left breast. The index mass (*arrow*) is irregular in shape with noncircumscribed margins (*arrow*).

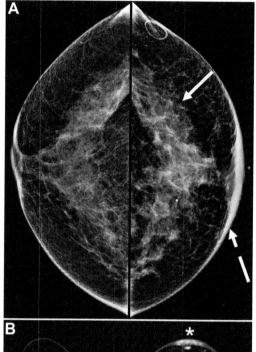

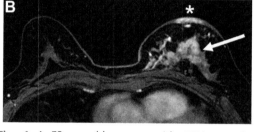

Fig. 4. A 52-year-old woman with ATM mutation and screening mammography-detected left TNBC. She had only been undergoing annual mammography screening. (A) Bilateral CC mammogram images demonstrate a global asymmetry (*white arrow*) in the left breast with associated skin thickening (*dashed arrow*) more prominent in the anterior region of the left breast. (B) Axial T1W contrast-enhanced breast MR image shows the malignancy presenting as nonmass enhancement (*white arrow*) involving the entire left breast with involvement of the nipple-areolar complex (*asterisk*). Core biopsy yielded IDC, ER−, PR−, and HER2−.

shown that BARD1 carriers are susceptible to developing ER-negative breast cancers, specifically triple-negative breast cancer (TNBC).[30,40]

NCCN guidelines recommend annual mammography and consideration for annual breast MR imaging starting at the age of 40 years. Currently, there is insufficient evidence of risk-reducing mastectomy, and this may be considered based on family history.[9]

RAD51C and RAD51D

RAD51C is a gene implicated in DNA repair via homologous recombination. Fanconi anemia is associated with the homozygous mutation of RAD51C.

RAD51D gene is also involved in the homologous recombination of the DNA repair. It increases the risk of ovarian cancer primarily.

Despite conflicting data, it has been reported that heterozygous carriers of RAD51C and RAD1D have an increased risk of breast and ovarian cancer. If a woman has a first-degree relative with ovarian or breast cancer, her breast cancer risk increases.[44] The estimated cumulative risk for developing breast cancer by the age of 80 years is 21% (95% CI = 15% to 29%) for RAD51C and 20% (95% CI = 14% to 28%) for RAD51D PV carriers.[44] RAD51C and RAD51D have also been linked to ER-negative breast cancer and TNBC. RAD51C has been related with bilateral TNBC.[45]

NCCN guidelines for both genetic mutations recommend annual mammography and consideration for breast MR imaging beginning at the age of 40 years.[9]

NF1 (Neurofibromatosis type 1)

NF1 (also known as von Recklinghausen's disease) is an autosomal dominant disorder characterized by mutations in the neurofibromin-coding NF1 gene. Loss of neurofibromin leads to uncontrolled cell proliferation and a susceptibility for the development of multiple malignancies. The estimated incidence of NF1 is 1 in 3000 individuals.[46] Individuals with NF1 have a 5% to 15% higher risk of developing malignancies than the general population, with a younger age of onset and a poorer prognosis. Optic gliomas, malignant peripheral nerve sheath tumors, rhabdomyosarcoma, GI stromal tumors, and breast cancer are common among those with NF1.[47,48] Women with -NF1 have a 3-fold to 5-fold increased incidence of breast cancer.[49] Seminog and colleagues found that women aged 30 to 39 years have a 6.5-fold increased breast risk compared with women aged 40 to 49 years (4.4) and 50 to 59 years (2.6).[50] The median age of women with NF1 who develop breast cancer is 46 years.

Breast malignancies are typically more aggressive and are larger at detection, higher grade, hormone receptor negative, and HER2-positive, resulting in worse overall survival.[48] Furthermore, Yap and colleagues reported resistance of breast cancer in NF1 women to standard cytotoxic and HER2-targeted therapies.[48]

NCCN guidelines recommend annual screening mammography beginning at the age of 30 years and consideration for breast MR imaging from ages 30 to 50 years. Currently, there is insufficient evidence for risk-reducing mastectomy, and this may be considered based on family history.[9]

IMAGING IN HEREDITARY BREAST CANCER
Imaging Modalities

Women with genetic mutations should undergo more intensive screening with mammography and breast MR imaging to detect small cancers with negative lymph nodes and reduce the incidence of interval cancers. As BRCA1/2 are the most well-known genetic mutations, most of the evidence to support this imaging recommendation is based on studies in BRCA1/2 mutation carriers.

Digital mammography and digital breast tomosynthesis

Mammography has repeatedly proven to be the most effective screening test for reducing breast cancer mortality. However, mammography underperforms in genetically predisposed women with lower sensitivity ranging from 25% to 59%.[51,52] Numerous variables have been attributed to the low mammographic performance in this population including dense breast tissue, early breast cancer onset, and accelerated tumor growth. The interval cancer rate in high-risk women only monitored with mammography is high, ranging from 35% to 50% with half presenting with nodal involvement at the time of presentation.[53–55]

Digital breast tomosynthesis (DBT), approved in 2011, has been gradually incorporated in the screening setting. DBT provides pseudo tridimensional images of the breast generated by multiple low-dose projections acquired across an arc-like movement (15°–60°) of the x-ray tube, using reconstruction algorithms. Overall cancer detection and interval cancer rates are equivalent between digital mammography (DM) and DBT alone.[56,57] Other prospective studies have revealed DBT plus DM has a higher cancer detection than DM alone.[58,59] Screen detected cancer biologic profile between DBT and DM is similar, mostly luminal tumors.[60] The addition of DBT to mammography seems to lead to higher specificity and fewer false positives without an increase in incremental cancer detection rate in high-risk patients (those with a personal history of breast cancer).[61,62] Data from the currently ongoing Tomosynthesis Mammographic Imaging screening trial will provide more accurate information in the performance of DBT in high-risk populations.

Given the limitations of mammography in women with inherited breast cancer and concerns about radiation exposure for BRCA and other high-risk mutation carriers causing patients to be more sensitive to the DNA-damaging effect of ionizing radiation, the added value of mammography in this population has been questioned with a suggestion to obviate mammography and follow these patients only with MR imaging.[51,63–65] Although Chiarelly and colleagues showed no significant increase in mammographic sensitivity when mammography was added to MR imaging in mutation carriers aged 30 to 39 years (100.0% vs 96.8%), a significant increase in sensitivity was observed when mammography was added to breast MR imaging in mutation carriers aged 50 to 69 years (92.7%, vs 83.5%).[66] Similarly, Obdeijn and colleagues showed the value of mammography in BRCA2 patients was significant in carriers aged 50 years and older.[67] A recent update of the American College of Radiology (ACR) guidelines advises starting mammography at the age of 40 years for patients with lifetime risk greater than 20%.[68]

Breast MR imaging

Breast MR imaging is highly beneficial for women with inherited breast cancer as a supplemental screening examination when added to annual mammography (Fig. 5). Cancers detected by MR imaging are generally an early stage with negative lymph node involvement (Fig. 6).[69–71] Most studies evaluating breast MR imaging screening in patients with germline mutations have been conducted on BRCA1/2 carriers. A meta-analysis revealed that mammography has a sensitivity of 55% compared with 89% for breast MR imaging, with specificities of 94% for mammography and 83% for breast MR imaging.[72] However, breast MR imaging specificity increases in subsequent screening rounds as demonstrated in multiple studies.[69,70,73] A combined protocol (mammography and breast MR imaging) increases sensitivity to 98%; however, specificity decreases to 79%. A prospective study by Leach and colleagues demonstrated that breast MR imaging outperforms mammography, and this effect is more pronounced in BRCA1 carriers.[73] This is likely due to the low sensitivity of mammography in BRCA1 carriers. In addition, breast MR imaging has a high negative predictive value (99.6%),[51] with a cancer detection rate of 21.8 per 1000 examinations compared with 7.2 per 1000 examinations for mammography.[74]

One study has evaluated the efficacy of intensive surveillance in women with PTEN Hamartoma Tumor syndrome.[75] A retrospective evaluation of 65 women using MR imaging and mammography revealed a high CDR of 45 per 1000 rounds for these patients.[75] As reported in previous studies, mammography underperforms when compared with MR imaging. The cancers detected on this study were small and node negative.[75]

Although evidence-based specific guidelines for non-BRCA genetic mutation carriers have yet to be established, Lowry and colleagues performed a comparative simulation modeling analysis using

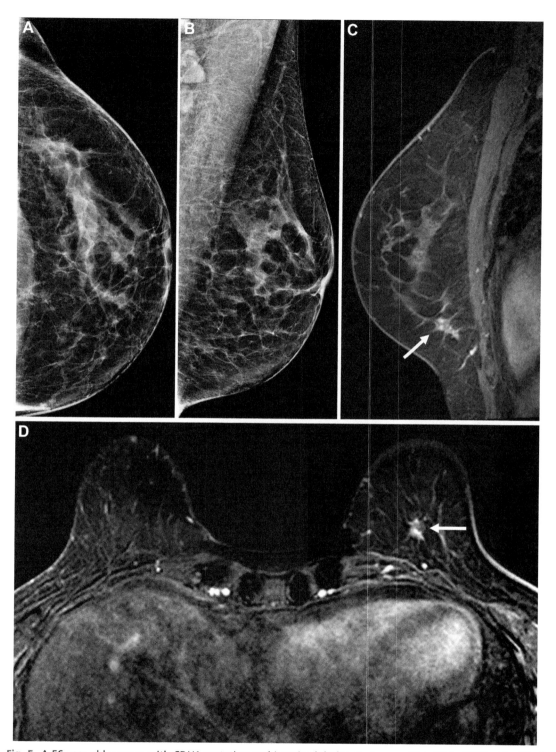

Fig. 5. A 56-year-old woman with CDH1 mutation and invasive lobular carcinoma, ER+, PR+, HER2– identified on screening breast MR imaging. She was treated with mastectomy with negative nodal basins. (A, B) Left CC and MLO mammographic views demonstrate no suspicious mass, calcifications, or distortion. (C, D) Sagittal post-contrast delayed and axial subtraction MR images from screening breast MR imaging performed 6 months later show focal nonmass enhancement in the inferior left breast (arrow). MR imaging-guided biopsy yielded ILC, ER+, PR+, HER2–. ILC, invasive lobular carcinoma.

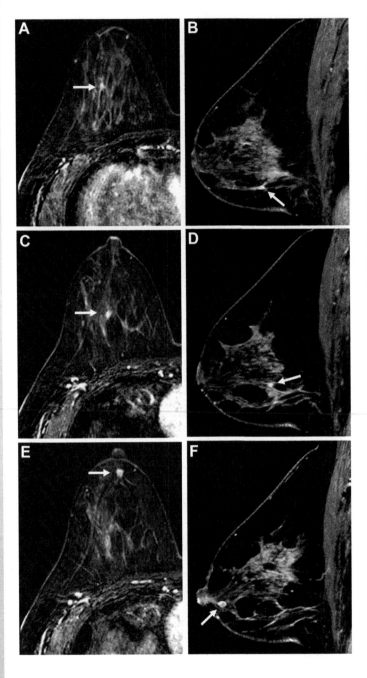

Fig. 6. A 48-year-old woman with Li-Fraumeni syndrome and multifocal DCIS, ER+, PR + identified on screening breast MR imaging. (A, B) Axial subtraction and sagittal postcontrast delayed breast MR images show an enhancing mass (arrows) in the right breast 6 o'clock position. MR imaging-guided biopsy yielded DCIS, high nuclear grade. ER+, PR+. (C, D) Axial subtraction and sagittal postcontrast delayed breast MR images show an enhancing mass (arrows) in the central breast. MR imaging-guided biopsy yielded DCIS, high nuclear grade. ER+, PR+. (E, F) Axial subtraction and sagittal postcontrast delayed breast MR images show an enhancing mass (arrows) in the retroareolar region. Second look US demonstrated a sonographic correlate (not shown) for which core biopsy yielded DCIS, intermediate nuclear grade, ER+, PR+.

models from the Cancer Intervention and Surveillance Modeling Network and using risk estimates from the Cancer Risk Estimates Related to Susceptibility Consortium to investigate the screening strategies with mammography and breast MR imaging at different start ages for women with ATM, -CHEK2, and PALPB2 pathogenic variants.[76] They determined that annual MR imaging screening beginning between 30 and 35 years of age, followed by combined annual MR imaging and mammography at 40 years of age, provides the optimal balance between screening benefits and harms. An estimate of a 52% to 60% reduction in breast cancer mortality in women screened with breast MR imaging and PVs in ATM, CHEK2, or PALB2, indicates that MR imaging is beneficial in the population with moderate genetic susceptibility.[76] In agreement with previous studies, mammography screening before the age of 40 years may be of little benefit for women undergoing annual MR imaging screening in this subset of genetic mutations.

Abbreviated breast MR imaging

With increasing use of breast MR imaging in the screening setting, abbreviated breast MR (AB-MR) imaging has been developed as an effort to reduce costs and increase accessibility. AB-MR imaging, a shortened MR imaging protocol with only 1 or 2 postcontrast sequences, seems to be a viable option to screen high-risk patients. The rationale of an abbreviated protocol is that cancer often enhances in the first sequence without the need for additional postcontrast sequences.[77] AB-MR imaging can enhance workflow efficiency while saving significant resources in the screening setting because it is less costly, requires less time to acquire the images, allows for faster interpretation, and is better tolerated by patients.[78] Harvey and colleagues retrospectively reviewed 568 high-risk screening MR imaging cases using the abbreviated and standard protocols. There was no difference in the number of malignancies detected but the AB-MR imaging required significantly less time to interpret (1.5 minutes) than the standard protocol (6.4 minutes). The scan time for standard breast MR imaging was 23.2 versus 4.4 minutes for the AB-MR imaging.[78] The CDR for AB-MR imaging ranged from 13.3 to 18.2 per 1000 examinations equivalent to standard breast MR imaging.[78,79]

Studies have demonstrated AB-MR imaging demonstrates similar performance metrics to standard breast MR imaging protocols in average-risk and high-risk patients. A retrospective study comparing standard MR imaging to AB-MR imaging with or without T2 images in 292 BRCA1/2 carriers yielded a pooled sensitivity for AB-MR imaging with T2 images comparable to that of standard MR imaging (90% vs 94%), with positive predictive value (PPV) (20% vs 19%), negative predictive value (NPV) (99% vs 100%), and area under the curve (AUC) (0.90, vs 0.92), respectively. The pooled specificity was significantly higher in the AB-MR imaging group (83% vs 80%).[80] Additional studies performed in high-risk patients have observed the performance metrics in the high-risk population are comparable with standard breast MR imaging.[81,82] Plaza and colleagues have suggested performing a baseline standard breast MR imaging followed by AB-MR imaging on subsequent rounds of screening.[82] To our knowledge, studies evaluating AB-MR imaging in specific mutation carriers other than BRCA1/2 have not been performed. Currently, there are no standardized protocols for AB-MR imaging.

Contrast-enhanced mammography

Contrast-enhanced digital mammography (CEM) using iodinated contrast is a promising technique for detecting tumor angiogenesis. In 2011, the United States Food and Drug Administration approved CEM for clinical use as an adjunct to mammography. The CEM technique obtains a precontrast image followed by multiple postcontrast images during the course of 5 to 7 minutes in the same imaging views performed for mammography. CEM begins image acquisition 2 to 2.5 minutes after contrast injection, whereas breast MR imaging begins earlier image acquisition with one before and one approximately 90 seconds after contrast administration. Subtracting the precontrast image from the postcontrast image highlights the contrast uptake.[83]

A small number of clinical studies evaluating CEM in high-risk settings have demonstrated performance comparable to breast MR imaging, with slightly less sensitivity and more specificity.[83,84] Sung and colleagues retrospectively reviewed 904 high-risk women, 27.3% of whom had a family history of breast cancer in a first-degree relative aged younger than 50 years. CEM had a CDR of 15.5 per 1000 examinations, sensitivity of 87.5%, specificity of 93.7%, and NPV of 99.7%.[84] Therefore, the ACR has suggested CEM can be considered as an alternative when breast MR imaging is contraindicated.[68] A currently ongoing trial entitled Screening-Contrast Enhanced Mammography as an Alternative to MR imaging will provide more information regarding CEM recommendations in the screening setting.[85]

It is important to note, contrast reaction risk, a smaller field of view compared with breast MR imaging, and the lack of widespread biopsy capability are disadvantages of CEM.

Ultrasound

In the population of high-risk women who undergo intensified surveillance with mammography and breast MR imaging, breast ultrasound provides no additional benefit despite being a low-cost, radiation-free, and widely accessible imaging technique. In a multicenter study comparing mammography, ultrasound, and breast MR imaging, ultrasound had a substantially lower sensitivity than breast MR imaging (52% vs 91%).[51] Van Zelst and colleagues conducted a prospective multicenter study on women with BRCA1/BRCA2 mutations evaluating multimodal high-risk surveillance with DM, breast MR imaging, and biannual automated ultrasound (ABUS).[86] The combination of breast MR imaging and DM showed the highest sensitivity of 76.3% with a specificity of 93.6%. ABUS did not reveal any malignancies beyond those identified by breast MR imaging or DM. ABUS had a lower sensitivity than MR imaging (32.1% vs 68.1%) and similar specificity (95% vs

95%).[86] For patients in whom breast MR imaging is contraindicated, ultrasound can serve as a supplemental screening imaging modality.

Molecular breast imaging

According to the ACR, molecular breast imaging is not recommended for supplemental screening in higher-than-average risk women.[68] Whole body radiation exposure remains an issue of concern.

CURRENT SCREENING GUIDELINES

Breast cancer imaging surveillance in the setting of hereditary cancer gene mutations varies among organizations (Table 3). The NCCN has imaging recommendations outlined in its annual report, which vary based on the specific genetic mutations as discussed above.[9] Within the field of radiology, specific guidelines are also outlined by the ACR with the most recent update simplifying the

Table 3
Screening recommendations for high-risk patients

Gene Mutation	Lifetime Risk for Breast Cancer (%)	NCCN Version 3.2023 Imaging Guidelines	ACR 2023 Guidelines
BRCA1/2	>60	Breast MR imaging: age 25–29 y[a] Annual mammogram and breast MR imaging: age 30–75 y	Risk assessment for all women by age 25 y, especially Black women and women of Ashkenazi Jewish heritage Women with genetic mutations (and untested first-degree relatives): • Annual mammogram ± DBT age 30 y (or age 40 y if annual MR imaging is performed) • Annual MR imaging age 25–30 y
TP53 (Li-Fraumeni syndrome)	>60	Annual MR imaging: age 20–29 y Annual mammogram and breast MR imaging: age 30–75 y	
PTEN (Cowden/PTEN hamartoma syndrome)	40–60	Annual mammography and breast MR imaging: age 35 or 10 y before the earliest known breast cancer in the family	
CDH1 (Hereditary diffuse gastric cancer)	41–60	Annual mammogram and consider breast MR imaging: age 30 y	
PALB2	41–60	Annual mammography and breast MR imaging: age 35 y	
STK11 (Peutz-Jeghers syndrome)	32–54	Annual mammogram and breast MR imaging: age 30 y	
CHEK2	20–40	Annual mammogram: age 40 y Consider breast MR imaging: age 30–35 y	
ATM	20–40	Annual mammogram: age 40 y Consider breast MR imaging: age 30–35 y	
BARD1	20–40	Annual mammogram: age 40 y Consider breast MR imaging: age 40 y	
NF1	20–40	Annual mammogram: age 30 y Consider breast MR imaging: age 30–50 y	
RAD51 C	20–40	Annual mammogram: age 40 y Consider breast MR imaging: age 40 y	
RAD51D	20–40	Annual mammogram and consider breast MR imaging: age 40 y	

Abbreviations: DBT, digital breast tomosynthesis; DM, digital mammography; MR, magnetic resonance.
[a] Individualized screening is considered if there is a family history of breast cancer diagnosed before the age of 30 y.
Data from Refs.[9,68]

recommendation for all patients with hereditary cancer gene mutations to annual DM with or without tomosynthesis beginning at the age of 40 years if annual breast MR imaging is also performed or age 30 if annual breast MR imaging is not performed. Annual breast MR imaging is recommended to begin at ages 25 to 30 years.[68]

SUMMARY

In addition to BRCA1/2, multiple genes conferring increased risk for breast cancer have now been identified. These include high penetrance genes, which increase the risk by more than 4 times as well as moderate penetrance genes, which increase the lifetime risk of breast cancer from 20% to 50%. The NCCN guidelines outline appropriate clinical scenarios for genetic testing with the goal to ensure those who are at an increased risk undergo appropriate supplemental screening for the early detection of breast cancer. Currently the most studied adjunct screening modality is breast MR imaging with most research conducted in the BRCA1/2 mutation carriers. Future research specific to additional supplemental breast cancer screening of patients with other high and moderate penetrance genes would be beneficial.

CLINICS CARE POINTS

- All women by the age of 25 years, especially Black women and women of Ashkenazi Jewish heritage should have an evaluation for calculation of breast risk assessment.

- Radiologists can play a crucial role in identifying patients who may benefit from genetic counseling and providing screening recommendations guidance for this high-risk population.

- Patients with high and moderate penetrance genetic mutations should follow specific screening strategies designed to detect cancer at an earlier stage. The age of starting this screening depends on the genetic mutation.

- Women with genetic mutations often develop breast cancer at a younger age. The sensitivity of mammography is lower in younger women. Therefore, breast MR imaging remains the current adjunct screening modality of choice.

ACKNOWLEDGMENTS

The authors acknowledge the National Institutes of Health, United States/National Cancer Institute Cancer Center Support Grant P30 CA016672 and the Department of Breast Imaging, The University of Texas MD Anderson Cancer Center. The authors also acknowledge the contributions of many others that could not be discussed due to space limitations.

DISCLOSURE

None.

REFERENCES

1. American Cancer Society. Breast Cancer Facts and Figures. 2023. Available at: https://www.cancer.org/research/cancer-facts-statistics/breast-cancer-facts-figures.html. Accessed August 8, 2023.
2. Lacroix M, Leclercq G. The "portrait" of hereditary breast cancer. Breast Cancer Res Treat 2005; 89(3):297–304.
3. Valencia OM, Samuel SE, Viscusi RK, et al. The Role of Genetic Testing in Patients With Breast Cancer: A Review. JAMA Surg 2017;152(6):589–94.
4. Piccinin C, Panchal S, Watkins N, et al. An update on genetic risk assessment and prevention: the role of genetic testing panels in breast cancer. Expert Rev Anticancer Ther 2019;19(9):787–801.
5. Daly MB, Pal T, Berry MP, et al. Genetic/Familial High-Risk Assessment: Breast, Ovarian, and Pancreatic, Version 2.2021, NCCN Clinical Practice Guidelines in Oncology. J Natl Compr Canc Netw 2021;19(1):77–102.
6. Graffeo R, Rana HQ, Conforti F, et al. Moderate penetrance genes complicate genetic testing for breast cancer diagnosis: ATM, CHEK2, BARD1 and RAD51D. Breast 2022;65:32–40.
7. Economopoulou P, Dimitriadis G, Psyrri A. Beyond BRCA: new hereditary breast cancer susceptibility genes. Cancer Treat Rev 2015;41(1):1–8.
8. Eccles D, Tapper W. The influence of common polymorphisms on breast cancer. Cancer Treat Res 2010;155:15–32.
9. National Comprehensive Cancer Network. NCCN clinical practice guidelines in oncology: genetic/familial high-risk assessment: breast and ovarian, and pancreatic V3.2023. Published February 13, 2023. Accessed August 8, 2023.
10. Manahan ER, Kuerer HM, Sebastian M, et al. Consensus Guidelines on Genetic' Testing for Hereditary Breast Cancer from the American Society of Breast Surgeons. Ann Surg Oncol 2019;26(10): 3025–31.
11. Kleibl Z, Kristensen VN. Women at high risk of breast cancer: Molecular characteristics, clinical presentation and management. Breast 2016;28:136–44.
12. Kwong A, Chen JW, Shin VY. A new paradigm of genetic testing for hereditary breast/ovarian cancers. Hong Kong Med J 2016;22(2):171–7.

13. Birch JM, Blair V, Kelsey AM, et al. Cancer phenotype correlates with constitutional TP53 genotype in families with the Li-Fraumeni syndrome. Oncogene 1998;17(9):1061–8.

14. Sidransky D, Tokino T, Helzlsouer K, et al. Inherited p53 gene mutations in breast cancer. Cancer Res 1992;52(10):2984–6.

15. Li FP, Fraumeni JF Jr. Soft-tissue sarcomas, breast cancer, and other neoplasms. A familial syndrome? Ann Intern Med 1969;71(4):747–52.

16. Li FP, Fraumeni JF Jr, Mulvihill JJ, et al. A cancer family syndrome in twenty-four kindreds. Cancer Res 1988;48(18):5358–62.

17. Masciari S, Dillon DA, Rath M, et al. Breast cancer phenotype in women with TP53 germline mutations: a Li-Fraumeni syndrome consortium effort. Breast Cancer Res Treat 2012;133(3):1125–30.

18. Shen WH, Balajee AS, Wang J, et al. Essential role for nuclear PTEN in maintaining chromosomal integrity. Cell 2007;128(1):157–70.

19. Hobert JA, Eng C. PTEN hamartoma tumor syndrome: an overview. Genet Med 2009;11(10):687–94.

20. Tan MH, Mester JL, Ngeow J, et al. Lifetime cancer risks in individuals with germline PTEN mutations. Clin Cancer Res 2012;18(2):400–7.

21. Pilarski R. Cowden syndrome: a critical review of the clinical literature. J Genet Couns 2009;18(1): 13–27.

22. Schrager CA, Schneider D, Gruener AC, et al. Similarities of cutaneous and breast pathology in Cowden's Syndrome. Exp Dermatol 1998;7(6):380–90.

23. Schrager CA, Schneider D, Gruener AC, et al. Clinical and pathological features of breast disease in Cowden's syndrome: an underrecognized syndrome with an increased risk of breast cancer. Hum Pathol 1998;29(1):47–53.

24. Starink TM, van der Veen JP, Arwert F, et al. The Cowden syndrome: a clinical and genetic study in 21 patients. Clin Genet 1986;29(3):222–33.

25. Kaurah P, MacMillan A, Boyd N, et al. Founder and recurrent CDH1 mutations in families with hereditary diffuse gastric cancer. JAMA 2007;297(21):2360–72.

26. Schrader KA, Masciari S, Boyd N, et al. Germline mutations in CDH1 are infrequent in women with early-onset or familial lobular breast cancers. J Med Genet 2011;48(1):64–8.

27. Hearle N, Schumacher V, Menko FH, et al. Frequency and spectrum of cancers in the Peutz-Jeghers syndrome. Clin Cancer Res 2006;12(10):3209–15.

28. Antoniou AC, Casadei S, Heikkinen T, et al. Breast-cancer risk in families with mutations in PALB2. N Engl J Med 2014;371(6):497–506.

29. Heyne HO, Karjalainen J, Karczewski KJ, et al. Mono- and biallelic variant effects on disease at biobank scale. Nature 2023;613(7944):519–25.

30. Shimelis H, LaDuca H, Hu C, et al. Triple-Negative Breast Cancer Risk Genes Identified by Multigene Hereditary Cancer Panel Testing. J Natl Cancer Inst 2018;110(8):855–62.

31. Yadav S, Boddicker NJ, Na J, et al. Contralateral Breast Cancer Risk Among Carriers of Germline Pathogenic Variants in ATM, BRCA1, BRCA2, CHEK2, and PALB2. J Clin Oncol 2023;41(9):1703–13.

32. Filippini SE, Vega A. Breast cancer genes: beyond BRCA1 and BRCA2. Front Biosci (Landmark Ed) 2013;18(4):1358–72.

33. Apostolou P, Papasotiriou I. Current perspectives on CHEK2 mutations in breast cancer. Breast Cancer 2017;9:331–5.

34. Caswell-Jin JL, Gupta T, Hall E, et al. Racial/ethnic differences in multiple-gene sequencing results for hereditary cancer risk. Genet Med 2018;20(2): 234–9.

35. Weischer M, Bojesen SE, Ellervik C, et al. CHEK2*1100delC genotyping for clinical assessment of breast cancer risk: meta-analyses of 26,000 patient cases and 27,000 controls. J Clin Oncol 2008;26(4): 542–8.

36. Cybulski C, Wokołorczyk D, Jakubowska A, et al. Risk of breast cancer in women with a CHEK2 mutation with and without a family history of breast cancer. J Clin Oncol 2011;29(28):3747–52.

37. Nurmi A, Muranen TA, Pelttari LM, et al. Recurrent moderate-risk mutations in Finnish breast and ovarian cancer patients. Int J Cancer 2019;145(10):2692–700.

38. Stolarova L, Kleiblova P, Janatova M, et al. CHEK2 Germline Variants in Cancer Predisposition: Stalemate Rather than Checkmate. Cells 2020;9(12):2675.

39. van Os NJ, Roeleveld N, Weemaes CM, et al. Health risks for ataxia-telangiectasia mutated heterozygotes: a systematic review, meta-analysis and evidence-based guideline. Clin Genet 2016;90(2):105–17.

40. Hu C, Hart SN, Gnanaolivu R, et al. A Population-Based Study of Genes Previously Implicated in Breast Cancer. N Engl J Med 2021;384(5):440–51.

41. De Brakeleer S, De Grève J, Loris R, et al. Cancer predisposing missense and protein truncating BARD1 mutations in non-BRCA1 or BRCA2 breast cancer families. Hum Mutat 2010;31(3):E1175–85.

42. Alenezi WM, Fierheller CT, Recio N, et al. Literature Review of BARD1 as a Cancer Predisposing Gene with a Focus on Breast and Ovarian Cancers. Genes 2020;11(8):856.

43. Weber-Lassalle N, Borde J, Weber-Lassalle K, et al. Germline loss-of-function variants in the BARD1 gene are associated with early-onset familial breast cancer but not ovarian cancer. Breast Cancer Res 2019;21(1):55.

44. Yang X, Song H, Leslie G, et al. Ovarian and Breast Cancer Risks Associated with Pathogenic Variants in RAD51C and RAD51D. J Natl Cancer Inst 2020; 112(12):1242–50.

45. Fanale D, Incorvaia L, Filorizzo C, et al. Detection of Germline Mutations in a Cohort of 139 Patients with

Bilateral Breast Cancer by Multi-Gene Panel Testing: Impact of Pathogenic Variants in Other Genes beyond *BRCA1/2*. Cancers 2020;12(9):2415.

46. Evans DG, Howard E, Giblin C, et al. Birth incidence and prevalence of tumor-prone syndromes: estimates from a UK family genetic register service. Am J Med Genet 2010;152A(2):327–32.

47. Landry JP, Schertz KL, Chiang YJ, et al. Comparison of Cancer Prevalence in Patients With Neurofibromatosis Type 1 at an Academic Cancer Center vs in the General Population From 1985 to 2020. JAMA Netw Open 2021;4(3):e210945.

48. Yap YS, Munusamy P, Lim C, et al. Breast cancer in women with neurofibromatosis type 1 (NF1): a comprehensive case series with molecular insights into its aggressive phenotype. Breast Cancer Res Treat 2018;171(3):719–35.

49. Suarez-Kelly LP, Yu L, Kline D, et al. Increased breast cancer risk in women with neurofibromatosis type 1: a meta-analysis and systematic review of the literature. Hered Cancer Clin Pract 2019;17:12.

50. Seminog OO, Goldacre MJ. Age-specific risk of breast cancer in women with neurofibromatosis type 1. Br J Cancer 2015;112(9):1546–8.

51. Sardanelli F, Podo F, Santoro F, et al. Multicenter surveillance of women at high genetic breast cancer risk using mammography, ultrasonography, and contrast-enhanced magnetic resonance imaging (the high breast cancer risk italian 1 study): final results. Invest Radiol 2011;46(2):94–105.

52. Lord SJ, Lei W, Craft P, et al. A systematic review of the effectiveness of magnetic resonance imaging (MRI) as an addition to mammography and ultrasound in screening young women at high risk of breast cancer. Eur J Cancer 2007;43(13):1905–17.

53. Komenaka IK, Ditkoff BA, Joseph KA, et al. The development of interval breast malignancies in patients with BRCA mutations. Cancer 2004;100(10):2079–83.

54. Vasen HF, Tesfay E, Boonstra H, et al. Early detection of breast and ovarian cancer in families with BRCA mutations. Eur J Cancer 2005;41(4):549–54.

55. Brekelmans CT, Seynaeve C, Bartels CC, et al. Effectiveness of breast cancer surveillance in BRCA1/2 gene mutation carriers and women with high familial risk. J Clin Oncol 2001;19(4):924–30.

56. Bahl M, Gaffney S, McCarthy AM, et al. Breast Cancer Characteristics Associated with 2D Digital Mammography versus Digital Breast Tomosynthesis for Screening-detected and Interval Cancers. Radiology 2018;287(1):49–57.

57. Hovda T, Holen ÅS, Lång K, et al. Interval and Consecutive Round Breast Cancer after Digital Breast Tomosynthesis and Synthetic 2D Mammography versus Standard 2D Digital Mammography in BreastScreen Norway. Radiology 2020;294(2):256–64.

58. Pattacini P, Nitrosi A, Giorgi Rossi P, et al. A Randomized Trial Comparing Breast Cancer Incidence and Interval Cancers after Tomosynthesis Plus Mammography versus Mammography Alone. Radiology 2022;303(2):256–66.

59. Heywang-Köbrunner SH, Jänsch A, Hacker A, et al. Tomosynthesis with synthesised two-dimensional mammography yields higher cancer detection compared to digital mammography alone, also in dense breasts and in younger women: A systematic review and meta-analysis. Eur J Radiol 2022;152: 110324.

60. Johnson K, Zackrisson S, Rosso A, et al. Tumor Characteristics and Molecular Subtypes in Breast Cancer Screening with Digital Breast Tomosynthesis: The Malmö Breast Tomosynthesis Screening Trial. Radiology 2019;293(2):273–81.

61. Bahl M, Mercaldo S, McCarthy AM, et al. Imaging Surveillance of Breast Cancer Survivors with Digital Mammography versus Digital Breast Tomosynthesis. Radiology 2021;298(2):308–16.

62. Sprague BL, Coley RY, Lowry KP, et al. Digital Breast Tomosynthesis versus Digital Mammography Screening Performance on Successive Screening Rounds from the Breast Cancer Surveillance Consortium. Radiology 2023;307(5):e223142.

63. Jansen-van der Weide MC, Greuter MJ, Jansen L, et al. Exposure to low-dose radiation and the risk of breast cancer among women with a familial or genetic predisposition: a meta-analysis. Eur Radiol 2010;20(11):2547–56.

64. Pijpe A, Andrieu N, Easton DF, et al. Exposure to diagnostic radiation and risk of breast cancer among carriers of BRCA1/2 mutations: retrospective cohort study (GENE-RAD-RISK). BMJ 2012;345: e5660.

65. Riedl CC, Luft N, Bernhart C, et al. Triple-modality screening trial for familial breast cancer underlines the importance of magnetic resonance imaging and questions the role of mammography and ultrasound regardless of patient mutation status, age, and breast density. J Clin Oncol 2015;33(10):1128–35.

66. Chiarelli AM, Blackmore KM, Muradali D, et al. Performance Measures of Magnetic Resonance Imaging Plus Mammography in the High Risk Ontario Breast Screening Program. J Natl Cancer Inst 2020;112(2):136–44.

67. Obdeijn IM, Mann RM, Loo CCE, et al. The supplemental value of mammographic screening over breast MRI alone in BRCA2 mutation carriers. Breast Cancer Res Treat 2020;181(3):581–8.

68. Monticciolo DL, Newell MS, Moy L, et al. Breast Cancer Screening for Women at Higher-Than-Average Risk: Updated Recommendations From the ACR [published online ahead of print, 2023 May 5]. J Am Coll Radiol 2023. https://doi.org/10.1016/j.jacr.2023.04.002. S1546-1440(23)00334-4.

69. Warner E, Messersmith H, Causer P, et al. Systematic review: using magnetic resonance imaging to

screen women at high risk for breast cancer. Ann Intern Med 2008;148(9):671–9.

70. Kriege M, Brekelmans CT, Peterse H, et al. Tumor characteristics and detection method in the MRISC screening program for the early detection of hereditary breast cancer. Breast Cancer Res Treat 2007; 102(3):357–63.

71. Saadatmand S, Geuzinge HA, Rutgers EJT, et al. MRI versus mammography for breast cancer screening in women with familial risk (FaMRIsc): a multicentre, randomised, controlled trial. Lancet Oncol 2019;20(8):1136–47.

72. Phi XA, Houssami N, Hooning MJ, et al. Accuracy of screening women at familial risk of breast cancer without a known gene mutation: Individual patient data meta-analysis. Eur J Cancer 2017;85:31–8.

73. Leach MO, Boggis CR, Dixon AK, et al. Screening with magnetic resonance imaging and mammography of a UK population at high familial risk of breast cancer: a prospective multicentre cohort study (MARIBS) [published correction appears in Lancet. 2005 May 28-Jun 3;365(9474):1848]. Lancet 2005;365(9473):1769–78.

74. Lo G, Scaranelo AM, Aboras H, et al. Evaluation of the Utility of Screening Mammography for High-Risk Women Undergoing Screening Breast MR Imaging. Radiology 2017;285(1):36–43.

75. Hoxhaj A, Drissen MMCM, Vos JR, et al. The yield and effectiveness of breast cancer surveillance in women with PTEN Hamartoma Tumor Syndrome. Cancer 2022;128(15):2883–91.

76. Lowry KP, Geuzinge HA, Stout NK, et al. Breast Cancer Screening Strategies for Women With ATM, CHEK2, and PALB2 Pathogenic Variants: A Comparative Modeling Analysis. JAMA Oncol 2022;8(4):587–96.

77. Heller SL, Moy L. MRI breast screening revisited. J Magn Reson Imaging 2019;49(5):1212–21.

78. Harvey SC, Di Carlo PA, Lee B, et al. An Abbreviated Protocol for High-Risk Screening Breast MRI Saves Time and Resources. J Am Coll Radiol 2016; 13(11S):R74–80.

79. Kuhl CK, Schrading S, Strobel K, et al. Abbreviated breast magnetic resonance imaging (MRI): first postcontrast subtracted images and maximum-intensity projection-a novel approach to breast cancer screening with MRI. J Clin Oncol 2014;32(22): 2304–10.

80. Naranjo ID, Sogani J, Saccarelli C, et al. MRI Screening of BRCA Mutation Carriers: Comparison of Standard Protocol and Abbreviated Protocols With and Without T2-Weighted Images. AJR Am J Roentgenol 2022;218(5):810–20.

81. Kwon MR, Choi JS, Won H, et al. Breast Cancer Screening with Abbreviated Breast MRI: 3-year Outcome Analysis. Radiology 2021;299(1):73–83.

82. Plaza MJ, Perea E, Sanchez-Gonzalez MA. Abbreviated Screening Breast MRI in Women at Higher-than-Average Risk for Breast Cancer with Prior Normal Full Protocol MRI. Journal of Breast Imaging 2020;2(4):343–51.

83. Sogani J, Mango VL, Keating D, et al. Contrast-enhanced mammography: past, present, and future. Clin Imaging 2021;69:269–79.

84. Sung JS, Lebron L, Keating D, et al. Performance of Dual-Energy Contrast-enhanced Digital Mammography for Screening Women at Increased Risk of Breast Cancer. Radiology 2019;293(1):81–8.

85. ClinicalTrials.gov. U.S. National Library of Medicine. Screening contrast-enhnaced mammography as an alternative to MRI (SCEMAM). Updated 17 Jan 2023. Available at: https://classic.clinicaltrials.gov/ct2/show/NCT04764292. Accessed 10 August 2023.

86. van Zelst JCM, Mus RDM, Woldringh G, et al. Surveillance of Women with the BRCA1 or BRCA2 Mutation by Using Biannual Automated Breast US, MR Imaging, and Mammography. Radiology 2017; 285(2):376–88.

Practice Advances

Contrast-enhanced Mammography versus MR Imaging of the Breast

Ritse M. Mann, MD, PhD[a,b,*], Valentina Longo, MD[c]

KEYWORDS

- Contrast-enhanced mammography • Breast MR imaging • BI-RADS lexicon

KEY POINTS

- Contrast-enhanced imaging improves diagnostic accuracy over conventional imaging techniques.
- Dynamic contrast-enhanced breast MR imaging is the most sensitive imaging modality currently available.
- Contrast-enhanced mammography has in general a slightly inferior performance but is in many situations a viable alternative for breast MR imaging.

INTRODUCTION

Breast cancer is the most frequently diagnosed cancer in women, with approximately 1 in 3 malignancies being of breast origin, representing the leading cause of cancer death among women worldwide.[1]

Mammography is the standard of care in the detection of breast cancer in screening programs and in symptomatic women. It is moderately effective in diagnosing breast cancer at an early stage and yields an associated breast cancer-specific mortality reduction of 16% to 35%, based on randomized trials.[2–5]

Nevertheless, many breast cancers are not diagnosed in a timely fashion on mammography. Moreover, mammography is also associated with a relatively high percentage of false positives.[6] Especially in women with extremely dense breast, the reduced contrast between tumors and surrounding tissue leads to masking of breast cancer and underdiagnosis of relevant cancers (ie, cancers that will do more harm when detected late). The program sensitivity of mammographic screening in women with very dense breasts declines from 86% to 62% to 68%.[7–9]

Therefore, over the years, efforts have focused on the development of alternative techniques for breast evaluation that may be able to overcome the limitations of standard mammography. Supplemental ultrasound (US) is widely regarded as the first potential technique to improve the screening yield. However, its added value is limited, and it has a high rate of false-positive findings, long examination times, and consequently high actual costs.

Contrast-enhanced techniques provide functional information on tumor vascularity and leakiness of the vessels that strongly boost the cancer detection rate in screening and also improve staging of breast cancer. Several functional techniques are currently available, including breast MR imaging and contrast-enhanced mammography (CEM) that will be discussed in this article, but this also includes for example, breast-specific gamma imaging. While the physiologic principles of tumor detection in contrast-enhanced methods are similar, they each have advantages and disadvantages.

[a] Department of Imaging, Radboud University Medical Center, Nijmegen, the Netherlands; [b] Department of Radiology, the Netherlands Cancer Institute, Amsterdam, the Netherlands; [c] Department of Bioimaging, Radiation Oncology and Hematology, UOC of Radiodiagnostica Presidio Columbus, Fondazione Policlinico Universitario A. Gemelli IRCSS, Largo A. Gemelli 8, Rome 00168, Italy
* Corresponding author. Department of Imaging, Radboud University Medical Center, 776, P.O. Box 9101, 6500HB Nijmegen, the Netherlands
E-mail address: ritse.mann@radboudumc.nl

Radiol Clin N Am 62 (2024) 643–659
https://doi.org/10.1016/j.rcl.2024.02.003
0033-8389/24/

Dynamic contrast-enhanced breast MR imaging is the standard contrast-enhanced imaging technique for breast evaluation and has been available since 1984. It requires a state-of-the-art MR imaging scanner, a dedicated breast coil, and the use of a gadolinium-based intravenously administered contrast agent.

CEM was introduced in 2011 and has only recently gained popularity as a diagnostic tool for breast imaging to improve the detection and characterization of breast lesions. Like breast MR imaging, it relies on the administration of an intravenous contrast agent in the examination, albeit the used contrast agent is iodine-based.

BREAST MR IMAGING: IMAGING PROTOCOL AND ACQUISITION

The crucial parts of breast MR imaging are the precontrast and early postcontrast T1-weighted acquisitions. These document the morphology of the breast and the presence of enhancing structures within the breast parenchyma. Prerequisites of these scans are a spatial resolution of below $1 \times 1 \times 2.5$ mm and some form of fat-suppression either during the administration or in the postprocessing phase by subtraction of precontrast and postcontrast series. It should be noted that virtually all modern scanners can easily produce T1-weighted images at a (near) isotropic resolution below 1 mm in any plane, and this is therefore recommended.

The contrast administered is a gadolinium chelate at a dose of 0.1 mmol/kg, usually through an intravenous-cannula placed in the cubital vein. Different from CEM, contrast administration in breast MR imaging is performed during the study, as it is not possible to create images that are unaffected by the contrast medium when this has been provided, and contrast administration should thus be performed with a power injector.

Peak enhancement of potentially malignant lesions within the breast usually occurs within 90 to 120 seconds, and therefore the early postcontrast acquisition should be obtained around that timepoint.

In postprocessing, the generation of subtraction images is highly recommended to discern real enhancement from structures that have a high T1 signal already before contrast administration. In addition, the generation of a maximum intensity projection (MIP) from the subtractions is deemed of importance, as this provides an overview of all enhancing structures in the breasts and axillae on a single image, thus preventing overlook errors and speeding up interpretation. The major strength of breast MR imaging is that it is a fully

three-dimensional (3D) imaging technique that can cover all parts of the breast (including the axillary tail and the medial aspects of the breasts that are difficult to image with mammographic techniques), and even in case of a nonsuspicious MIP image, evaluation of the (subtracted) slices may be of value to ascertain that, for example, motion artifacts did not obscure lesions in the MIP. The very basic protocol described above requires no more than 3 minutes of magnet time and is often referred to as abbreviated breast MR imaging. It can be supplemented with additional sequences that may improve predominantly specificity. In between the precontrast and postcontrast scan, so-called ultrafast acquisitions may be acquired.[10] These are highly undersampled T1-weighted images with a temporal resolution that is preferentially below 5 seconds. With modern image reconstruction algorithms, even these images can meet the spatial demands described earlier. Due to the leaky vasculature in malignant lesions, these tend to enhance earlier and faster than other structures and the breast parenchyma, which makes them standout as a lightbulb in an otherwise quiescent breast early during the contrast inflow phase. This also helps in discerning background parenchymal enhancement (BPE; see later discussion) from lesions. Since ultrafast images are obtained between the precontrast and postcontrast acquisition, they can be obtained without lengthening of the scan protocol. Use of such an approach is therefore possible even in screening.

Other additions to the MR imaging protocol include delayed phase T1-weighted images, where contrast behavior over time is evaluated after peak enhancement. Imaging may be done up to 7 minutes after contrast administration (usually consisting of several timepoint acquisitions). Lesions with leaky vessels will in this period show "wash-out," that is, the amount of contrast in the lesion declines after peak enhancement, which is consequently a sign of malignancy. In general, this information is similar to what can be obtained with ultrafast acquisitions during inflow (fast and early enhancing lesions also tend to show eventual wash-out), and the delayed phase is somewhat hampered by increasing the BPE over time in the normal breast parenchyma, which might obscure findings. Nonetheless, the delayed phase is crucial in women treated with neoadjuvant systemic treatment, as this may also affect the vessels and reduce permeability, thus leading to nonenhancement of residual lesions in the early postcontrast phase.

Further additions to the MR imaging protocol consist of T2 and diffusion-weighted imaging

(DWI) or diffusion-weighted sequences. Like delayed phase imaging, these lengthen the MR imaging protocol, and their use should consequently be balanced against the potential added value. In general, in problem-solving, cancer staging, and therapy evaluation, their use is recommended. T2-weighted acquisitions should preferably be obtained at the same spatial resolution as T1-weighted images to optimize cross correlation. They are generally used to assess the signal intensity in breast lesions (most breast cancers are relatively dark on T2, whereas myxoid fibroadenomas are typically homogeneously bright), as well as the presence of edema within the breast (either perifocal or diffuse). DWI should be obtained using b0 and b800 acquisitions and include generation of an ADC map. Spatial resolution in DWI is still limited but should not be over $2 \times 2 \times 4$ mm. Visual inspection of the b800 images may reveal potential lesions with diffusion restriction in the breast; however, the apparent diffucion coefficient (ADC) value should always be measured. Typical ADC values for malignant lesions are below 1.2×10^{-3} mm²/s, whereas typical ADC values for benign lesions exceed 1.5×10^{-3} mm²/s.[11] However, as always, imaging features should be interpreted in conjunction with each other and use of strict cutoffs is not recommended. In the presence of breast implants, silicone sequences may be used to evaluate implant integrity. A full breast MR imaging protocol including all sequences described above can be obtained in approximately 15 to 20 minutes of scanner time.

CONTRAST-ENHANCED MAMMOGRAPHY: IMAGING PROTOCOL AND ACQUISITION

CEM is a method that combines the morphologic information of digital mammography (DM) and functional information thanks to the use of iodinated contrast medium injected intravenously, which allows the evaluation of tumor neoangiogenesis similarly to what occurs in breast MR imaging.[4–6] The necessary equipment for CEM is a mammography machine, which is augmented by a specific filter for acquiring the high-energy image. The acquired images are then postprocessed for diagnostic purposes. As of now, there is no consensus within the scientific community regarding clear-cut optimal parameters for CEM, including contrast medium concentration, dose, flow rate, and the interval between contrast medium administration and image acquisition. However, despite this lack of consensus, generally accepted guidelines are available, and in clinical practice, reference is largely made to the publication by Dromain and colleagues in 2009.[12–16]

Before beginning the examination, patients undergo screening for any history of allergic-like and physiologic reactions to iodinated contrast, following the guidelines established by the American College of Radiology.[17] During the CEM procedure, the patient is positioned similarly as for a standard mammogram, with the breast compressed in various projections such as craniocaudal (CC), lateral, and medio-lateral-oblique. The resolution is the same as in a standard mammogram and therefore in the range of 80 μm in plane. CEM is, however, a two-dimensional (2D) technique, so the through plane resolution is similar to the breast thickness. Targeted compressions and enlargements may also be performed if necessary. The presence of breast implants does not restrict the feasibility of performing CEM, although it might lead to some distortion and artifacts. The procedure can be effectively conducted using the classic Eklund projections, which are routinely utilized for imaging breasts with implants.[18] Nevertheless, it is crucial to acknowledge that CEM has not been extensively studied in patients with implants. Despite being feasible in patients with implants, CEM is not considered a reliable method for assessing the integrity of silicone implants.

The iodinated contrast medium can be administered manually, but it is preferably done using an automatic injection pump, which ensures a controlled and consistent rate of injection of 3 mL/s, followed by a bolus of physiologic saline solution to help flush the contrast agent through the bloodstream. The total time available to obtain images before contrast washes out is between 7 and 10 minutes, so ideally the entire CEM should performed within that time frame.[19]

The acquisition of the images typically starts about 2 to 2.5 minutes after contrast administration to allow the contrast to circulate and reach the breast adequately. During the CEM procedure, the patient is positioned similarly to during a standard mammography examination. In a bilateral study, typically, the same view is alternated between the breasts (ie, mediolateral oblique [MLO] left, MLO right, CC left, and CC right) to ensure that at least 1 view of each breast is acquired while the contrast is at its maximum. Similar to breast MR imaging, the accumulation of contrast in the healthy breast tissue increases over time and hence later obtained images will have higher level of BPE than early obtained images. In cases where specific attention is needed for 1 breast, such as a newly diagnosed breast cancer, both views of that particular breast can be obtained first (ie, MLO left, CC left, MLO right, and CC right) to minimize BPE.

If needed, additional projections, such as magnifications or targeted compressions, can be performed in the remaining minutes after acquiring the standard projections to obtain more detailed information about specific areas of concern. The total acquisition time for a CEM examination is approximately 8 to 15 minutes, including the time required for the injection of the contrast medium. This duration is similar to that of a standard 4-view screen mammogram, although the total room time may be slightly longer due to the additional preparation time needed for the contrast medium injection. Overall, it is slightly shorter than a full breast MR imaging and lengthier than an abbreviated breast MR imaging protocol.

Following the intravenous administration of the iodinated contrast medium, the system automatically acquires 2 consecutive images for each mammographic projection: one at low energy (26–33 kVp) and one at high energy (44–50 kVp), which is higher than the iodine k edge. The filter used to acquire the high-energy image is usually made out of titanium or copper. The acquisition time for each projection may vary depending on the breast thickness and the specific mammography machine used, ranging from 2 to 20 seconds.[20]

The high-energy image alone cannot be used for diagnostic purposes, but it is processed by dedicated software along with the low-energy (LE) image to create a "recombined" (RC) image. This RC image highlights areas with contrast enhancement and is similar to the MIPs generated from MR imaging scans, effectively minimizing overlapping breast tissue. For each mammographic projection, the diagnostic images obtained from CEM also include a "low-energy" image, which can be compared with standard mammography.[21,22]

It should be noted that also x-ray-based contrast-enhanced breast imaging can be performed in pseudo- or full 3D. Preliminary studies explored the value of contrast-enhanced digital breast tomosynthesis (CE-DBT) and contrast-enhanced dedicated breast CT (CE-BCT). Due to the increasing number of projections for these techniques, the radiation doses are somewhat higher than for CEM.

Digital breast tomosynthesis generates sequential tomographic images, reconstructing a 3D representation of the breast from a limited number of projections taken at different angles. This approach aims to enhance lesion visibility by minimizing the superimposition of overlying breast tissue inherent in 2D mammographic images. Whether that is also advantageous for contrast-enhanced imaging remains to be seen as the depth resolution is not very good, and hence, the likelihood of improving the visibility of enhancing structures on the high-energy images may be limited. However, initial results are promising. CE-DBT can potentially also provide a dose reduction when both DBT and CEM are planned to be acquired (as all images can be generated from the same acquisition). CE-DBT's integration of 3D contrast enhancement and anatomic information may also facilitate improved biopsy guidance.

Different from CE-DBT, CE-BCT performs acquisition of the breast by obtaining data from all sides, thus showing a detailed location of eventual contrast enhancement in true 3D fashion.[23–25] Images resemble those of breast MR imaging while achieving a much higher spatial resolution, which is particularly good for margin assessment in mass lesions. Like in CEM, the lower contrast signal appears to reduce the visibility of nonmass lesions, and while this may improve specificity, it may also slightly reduce sensitivity. Both CE-DBT and CE-BCT do not overcome the field of view limitations of mammography, which means that posterior lesions and lesions in the axillary tail may not be visualized. However, both methods appear to strongly outperform conventional noncontrast-enhanced imaging techniques and are reported to be on par with CEM and breast MR imaging. It is consequently expected that these techniques will also gain a place in breast imaging, potentially replacing CEM eventually with 3D techniques. Nonetheless, these techniques have thus far not been sufficiently tested to be recommended in everyday practice. Therefore, the remainder of this article will focus on CEM and breast MR imaging.

IMAGE INTERPRETATION AND BI-RADS LEXICON

Interpretation and reporting of both MR imaging and CEM should be performed using the Breast Imaging - Reporting and Data System (BI-RADS) lexicon. For MR imaging, this has been available since 2003, with only minor changes over time. Predominantly, it focuses on the morphologic description of enhancing lesions within the breast (the functional aspect is covered by the fact that these lesions are enhancing), discerning between mass and nonmass lesions. Masses are further characterized by shape, margin, and internal enhancement pattern, whereas nonmass enhancement is characterized by distribution and pattern. BI-RADS acknowledges the value of many of the other sequences described above and provides also descriptors for curve assessment and T2-weighted imaging, but these are not mandatory. It should also be noted that there are many other descriptors for MR imaging that are of value to discern between benign and malignant abnormalities. Some of these are used for the so-called Kaiser score, a standardized interpretation algorithm that enables even novice readers to classify lesions at expert level.[26] Hallmarks of the Kaiser score are the presence of a "root" sign, which is an anatomic spiculation, the curve type, and the presence of edema within the breast.

In 2022, the American College of Radiology (ACR) introduced the BI-RADS lexicon (**Table 1**) specific to CEM. This publication aimed to standardize imaging reporting for CEM findings, providing a dedicated set of descriptors for interpreting each finding in both LE and RC images.[27] A significant finding on a CEM examination might be visible on the LE images only, the RC images only, or on both. Therefore, it is essential to include separate descriptions of the LE and RC images, as well as an overall description, to comprehensively report and interpret the findings. Furthermore, it is of utmost importance to clearly state in the report whether a finding is seen solely on the LE images, solely on the RC images, or if it appears on both image sets. In cases where there are distinct findings on both the LE and RC images, these separate findings should also be explicitly mentioned in the report. This detailed approach enhances the clarity and accuracy of the diagnostic report, facilitating effective communication between health care providers and ensuring appropriate patient management. The lexicon employed to report findings observed on the LE and RC images of CEM examinations is adapted from descriptors commonly used in conventional mammography and breast MR imaging.

Finding on Low-energy Images

In CEM, the LE provides the essential morphologic information about the breast tissue and any potential abnormalities, similar to what is observed in the standard digital mammogram. Consequently, reporting for this portion of the CEM examination should be conducted no differently than reporting for a standard mammogram.

Enhancement on Recombined Images

The postprocessed combination of LE and high-energy images should be referred to as the RC images. Before the 2022 ACR document, radiologists used to interpret CEM findings in the RC images using the MR imaging lexicon.[28,29]

However, the CEM lexicon incorporates fewer descriptors than the MR imaging lexicon, mainly due to the 2D nature of CEM. The new BI-RADS lexicon specifically designed for CEM provides precise descriptors tailored to this imaging

modality, ensuring accurate and consistent interpretation and reporting of CEM results.

The descriptors provided by the 2013 edition of the MR imaging lexicon for breast imaging include "focus," which refers to a small dot of enhancement that does not represent a space-occupying lesion; "mass," which describes a space-occupying lesion with recognizable margins and shape; and "nonmass enhancement," which denotes an area of enhancement that does not meet the criteria for a mass.[30,31] The distinction between focus and mass may evolve in future development of the MR imaging lexicon to reflect superior image resolution on modern scanners.

The new BI-RADS lexicon specifically designed for CEM also includes "mass" (a 3D space-occupying lesion with a convex-outward contour) and "nonmass enhancement" (similar to MR imaging, an area of enhancement that does not meet the criteria for a mass). The term "Focus," used in the MR imaging lexicon to describe dots of enhancement that are too small to further characterize in terms of margins or kinetics, is not part of the mammography lexicon and will not be retained in the new version of the MR imaging lexicon. Therefore, the term "mass" should be used, regardless of size, to describe these findings. Small areas of enhancement will be referred to as small masses, in analogy to what is seen on standard mammography or be regarded as part of the BPE. The fact that CEM does not allow kinetic assessment may make this differentiation somewhat more difficult than in MR imaging.

The 2022 BI-RADS CEM lexicon introduces an additional category called "enhancing asymmetries" (Eas; **Fig. 1**). These are findings visible on only one view in the RC images, specifically on either CC or MLO views.[27] The inclusion of "Eas" as a descriptor in the BI-RADS lexicon for CEM provides a specific term for identifying and characterizing subtle areas of enhancement that may be significant despite not presenting as a typical mass or nonmass enhancement.

The document introduces another significant concept, lesion conspicuity (**Fig. 2**) in CEM, which pertains to the degree of enhancement relative to the BPE. This assessment is described using subjective qualitative descriptors, including "low," "moderate," or "high." When the enhancement is similar to or slightly greater than BPE, it is categorized as "low." If the enhancement is much greater than BPE, it is labeled as "high," and if it falls in between "low" and "high," it is termed "moderate." It is important to note that, as of now, there are no available data to establish a correlation between lesion conspicuity and the likelihood of malignancy in CEM. However, terms for conspicuity have been

Table 1
CEM Lexicon (2022 ACR BI-RADSATLAS—Contrast-enhanced mammography—CEM)

Breast Tissue	Terms
A. Breast composition	a. Almost entirely fatty b. Scattered areas of fibroglandular density c. Heterogeneously dense d. Extremely dense
B. BPE	Level • Minimal • Mild • Moderate • Marked Symmetry • Symmetric • Asymmetric

RC Images Only

Findings	Terms
A. Mass enhancement	• Shape a. Oval b. Round c. Irregular • Margins a. Circumscribed b. Noncircumscribed • Irregular • Spiculated • Internal enhancement characteristics a. Homogeneous b. Heterogeneous c. Rim enhancement
B. Nonmass enhancement	• Distribution a. Focal b. Linear c. Segmental d. Regional e. Multiple regions f. Diffuse • Internal pattern a. Homogeneous b. Heterogeneous c. Clumped
C. Enhancing asymmetry	• Internal pattern a. Homogeneous b. Heterogeneous
D. Lesion conspicuity	a. Low b. Moderate c. High

Low-energy Findings with Associated Enhancement on RC Images

Finding	Terms
A. Morphology	Refer to mammography BI-RADS lexicon

(continued on next page)

Table 1
(continued)

Low-energy Findings with Associated Enhancement on RC Images

Finding	Terms
B. Internal enhancement pattern	a. Homogeneous b. Heterogeneous c. Rim enhancement
C. Extend of enhancement	a. Partial enhancement of ML b. Complete enhancement of ML c. Enhancement extends beyond ML d. No enhancement of the ML but enhancement in the adjacent tissue
D. Lesion conspicuity	a. Low b. Moderate c. High

Associated Features
Nipple retraction
Nipple invasion
Skin retraction
Skin thickening
Skin invasion
Axillary adenopathy

LE Imaged Only
Terms → Refer to mammography BI-RADS lexicon

incorporated into the lexicon to facilitate future research in this area.

BACKGROUND PARENCHYMAL ENHANCEMENT AND MENSTRUAL CYCLE

Understanding BPE on both CEM and MR imaging is crucial for successful interpretation. BPE is defined as the normal enhancement of glandular elements of the breast.

The current descriptors of BPE in CEM are adapted from the MR imaging BI-RADS lexicon, which includes the categories minimal, mild, moderate, and marked (**Fig. 3**). Notably, a study with over 200 patients has shown significant interreader agreement in characterizing background enhancement in both CEM and MR imaging, demonstrating consistency across the modalities.[32]

The available literature indicates that the majority of women who undergo CEM exhibit minimal or mild BPE.[32,33] However, in cases where BPE appears to be moderate or marked, there is a possibility that enhancing lesions may be missed. Due to the impossibility of optimal timing of imaging

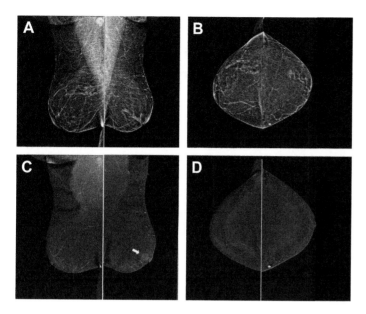

Fig. 1. Enhancing asymmetry. Contrast-enhanced DM was performed in a woman recalled for an asymmetry on the baseline screening mammogram (not shown) for further evaluation. In the early RC images (C, D), there is an enhancing asymmetry, only visible in MLO (arrow), in the retroareolar parenchyma of the left breast with moderate conspicuity. The enhancing asymmetry did not correspond to a clear finding in the LE images (A, B). The patient underwent US, which excluded the presence of suspicious findings.

in CEM, the ability to minimize BPE in the setting of CEM is more limited than with MR imaging.

Differentiating BPE from artifacts seen on RC images can also present challenges. One common artifact known as the "rim artifact," (see **Fig. 3B**) "breast-within-a-breast," or "halo artifact," is the result of scattered radiation during image acquisition. This artifact creates an apparent enhancing halo just beneath the skin surface, often observed in the upper breast, and may obscure small lesions.

In MR imaging reports, it is important to specify the composition of the breast and the amount of BPE.[34]

Higher fractions of both factors have been associated with an increased likelihood of malignancy being present.[35,36] However, the relationship between the amount of fibroglandular tissue, the extent of BPE, and the risk of developing breast cancer in future remains incompletely understood. Additionally, a higher fraction of BPE is linked to an increased risk of false-positive findings on DCE-MR imaging.[37] It was shown that the use of high-spatial, high-temporal acquisitions during the wash-in phase of contrast administration improves the cancer detection rate in breast MR imaging, once again showing that dynamic imaging during the inflow of contrast may improve both sensitivity and specificity of breast MR imaging.

Ongoing studies are investigating whether BPE is related to false-negative CEM examinations (cancer not identified on CEM) and false-positive CEM examinations. In cases where there is moderate or marked BPE, there is a possibility that enhancing lesions might be missed.[16,38] Until more data are available, it is important to keep in mind that CEM is a planar imaging technique, which means that small benign or malignant abnormalities may blend with BPE, especially when BPE is moderate or marked. As a result, any enhancement that stands out above the BPE on CEM should not be disregarded (**Fig. 4**). To maximize the detection of abnormal enhancement in the presence of increased BPE, the RC image can be viewed as an MIP. Special attention should be given to areas of asymmetric enhancement between the 2 breasts, focusing on regions separate from the BPE. Correlation with the LE images is critical to determine if there is an associated morphologic abnormality. If none is evident, additional evaluation with targeted US and possibly MR imaging may be recommended.

Currently, there are limited data supporting the timing of CEM during a specific phase of the menstrual cycle. In contrast, for MR imaging, the recommendation has been to schedule the examination during week 2 of the menstrual cycle.

However, several studies have indicated that the outcomes of MR imaging may not be significantly influenced by the stage of the menstrual cycle, and the use of dynamic evaluation during inflow further reduces this importance. This could also hold true for CEM, albeit dynamic imaging is lacking.[39,40] Available data do not suggest any significant influence of the menstrual cycle stage on the outcomes of CEM. Nevertheless, the degree of BPE observed in CEM seems to be less affected by the timing during the menstrual cycle, than in dynamic contrast-enhanced MR (DCE-MR) imaging.[16,41]

In summary, current data do not strongly support any specific timing of CEM during the

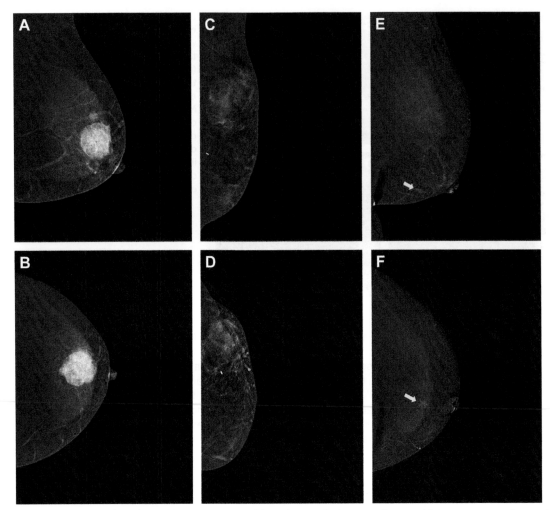

Fig. 2. Lesion conspicuity in CEM. (*A, B.* MLO/CC view) *High conspicuity.* Round mass with homogeneous internal enhancement pattern in the left breast. A small satellite is observed in the MLO view. (*C, D.* MLO/CC view) *Moderate conspicuity.* Regional area of nonmass enhancement with heterogeneous internal enhancement pattern in the left breast. (*E, F.* MLO/CC view) *Low conspicuity.* A 7 mm circumscribed oval mass demonstrating mild homogeneous enhancement (*arrows*) and corresponding to biopsy proven fibroepithelial lesion compatible with fibroadenoma.

menstrual cycle, and timing in breast MR imaging is also not critical. Nonetheless, BPE may significantly reduce sensitivity and specificity in both modalities. In MR imaging, this can be partly overcome by rapid dynamic imaging, and in CEM, lesion conspicuity scores may potentially help to optimize sensitivity.

CLINICAL APPLICATIONS: COMPARISON OF VALUE OF CONTRAST-ENHANCED MAMMOGRAPHY AND BREAST MR IMAGING FOR DIAGNOSTIC WORKUP

Functional contrast-enhanced imaging is valuable in various applications, including preoperative assessment in newly diagnosed breast cancer, monitoring response to neoadjuvant chemotherapy, problem-solving in suspicious findings, and screening for intermediate and high-risk individuals. CEM is mainly suggested as an alternative to MR imaging when MR imaging is not feasible for a patient. When choosing between CEM and MR imaging, consider that MR imaging has higher sensitivity for detecting breast cancer but may have lower or comparable specificity compared to CEM. MR imaging excels at visualizing areas not well seen on mammography, such as far posterior locations or the axilla. However, MR imaging is more expensive and not always covered by insurance. Screening with MR imaging is especially

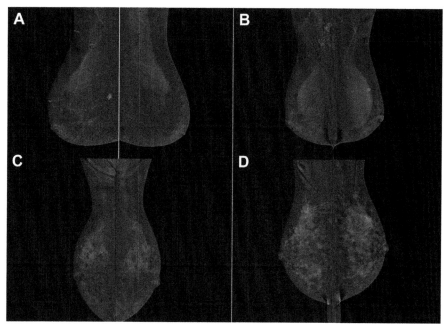

Fig. 3. Different degrees of BPE of the breast on CEM (RC images, MLO views). (*A*) CEM images show minimal BPE. There is a small area of mass enhancement in the right breast. (*B*) CEM images show mild BPE. Small area of mass enhancement in the left breast with metallic clip. A halo artifact is observed in both right and left images. (*C*) CEM images show moderate BPE. (*D*) CEM images show marked BPE.

recommended for very high-risk patients, such as BRCA mutation carriers, as they begin screening at a young age and may be more susceptible to the negative effects of ionizing radiation. It is important to note that CEM is currently not Food and Drug Administration-approved for screening, hence its use in this context is considered off-label. Facilities using CEM for screening should have strict screening criteria and conduct thorough result audits.[27]

Preoperative Staging

CEM has emerged as a valuable tool in preoperative staging for breast cancer and is a recognized alternative method to MR imaging for staging in

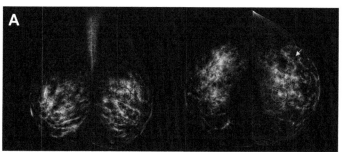

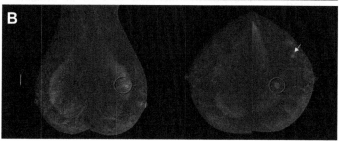

Fig. 4. Contrast-enhanced DM performed as staging for B5 microcalcification located supra-areolar in the left breast, subjected to stereotactic biopsy ductal carcinoma in situ (DCIS). In a context of high BPE, residual microcalcifications and an area of nonmass enhancement with adjacent magnetic clip are visible at the site of the previous biopsy (red circle) (*A,B*). Also, in the early RC image, there is an enhancing asymmetry in the outer quadrant of the left breast with high conspicuity, only visible in CC (*arrow*) associated to microcalcifications with linear distribution visible in the LE CC image (*B*). The patient underwent a second stereotactic biopsy of the microcalcifications in the upper outer quadrant, which confirmed a second location of DCIS.

European guidelines.[42] CEM has shown high precision in measuring the index malignancy, with a minimal difference in diameter (ranging from 0.03 mm to 5 mm) compared to the measurement taken from the surgical specimen.[19,21,43] This indicates that CEM provides reliable and close estimates of the actual tumor size, aiding in preoperative planning and treatment decisions. CEM has also proven to be effective in identifying multifocality and multicentricity of lesions. It is comparable to MR imaging in tumor size measurements but is somewhat less sensitive in showing nonmass enhancement, thereby offering slightly superior specificity, resulting in fewer false-positive findings during preoperative staging, but poorer documentation of more diffuse tumor extension (eg, extensive intraductal components).[44–46]

One of the primary limitations of CEM when compared to MR imaging is its inability to adequately study the axillary regions. This limitation arises from the field of view in CEM, which is superimposable on the mammographic image and does not provide the comprehensive 3D imaging necessary to completely assess the axilla. As a consequence, MR imaging remains superior in its sensitivity for evaluating both the chest wall and axilla. Also, the most medial part of the breast, the prepectoral zone, and the nipple areolar complex are areas prone to overlooking breast cancers on CEM. Overall, the 3D capabilities of MR imaging allow for a more detailed and comprehensive examination of the tumor extent and the relation to surrounding structures, providing valuable information about potential tumor spread and lymph node involvement.[47] This may be particularly important when oncoplastic breast surgery is attempted.

The combination of CEM and US of the axilla may overcome some of the shortcoming of CEM alone in the axillary tail, particularly when assessing the lymph node status for which US is the gold standard. This approach allows for a comprehensive assessment of the breast and axillary regions in a single session, streamlining the diagnostic process for patients.

In patients with implants, breast MR imaging should be considered as it can assess implant integrity in parallel and it suffers less from image distortion. Patients with allergies to iodinated contrast agents or renal insufficiency are also better suited for breast MR imaging. Invasive lobular carcinomas may be challenging to assess with full-field DM due to weak enhancement on CEM.[48] Breast MR imaging provides more accurate diameter measurements for this particular tumor type. Since evidence for invasive lobular cancer size measurements in CEM is limited, breast MR imaging may be the safer option.

Problem-solving

Problem-solving with CEM is valuable in cases of discrepancies between mammographic imaging and clinical or US findings. Problem-solving is, however, a nondescript term that is used for a variety of clinical settings including potential mammographic findings without a clear US correlate, clinical findings without an imaging correlate, or findings by any means that cannot readily be biopsied. Sometimes problem-solving is also used to further assess lesions after inconclusive biopsy results. The use of CEM for problem-solving was one of the earliest applications, driven by the small but realistic probability of cancer in discordant cases and the imminent need for a diagnostic answer. It is of particular value if it can be offered straight away, preventing uncertainty and anxiety in patients.

CEM for problem-solving may be used in clinical practice in select cases, often suggested for recalls due to suspicious findings on screening mammography that cannot easily be clarified with diagnostic mammogram and US examination. It should not be used for all screening recalls as many can be solved by targeted US alone.

Studies have shown that CEM offers a sensitivity ranging from 93% to 100% and a specificity ranging from 63% to 88% in the context of problem-solving. Compared to standard mammography, CEM demonstrates an increase of 5% to 46% in sensitivity and 3% to 15% in specificity, highlighting its potential to enhance diagnostic accuracy in problem-solving scenarios.[44,47,49]

Using CEM as the initial method of investigation in the detection of palpable masses significantly improves sensitivity and specificity compared to using DM alone. Specifically, the sensitivity of CEM was found to be 95%, a considerable increase compared to the sensitivity of 84% for DM alone. Similarly, the specificity of CEM was 81%, significantly higher than the specificity of 63% for DM alone.[50] However, this does not account for the routine use of US in this setting, which already overcomes the limited sensitivity of conventional mammography and may yield a definitive (benign) diagnosis in many patients. Therefore, the standard of care in evaluating palpable masses remains mammography and US as the initial examinations, with CEM as a possible adjunct examination if findings of mammogram and US are uncertain. When CEM is considered as a potential replacement for mammography in the analysis of palpable masses, it may be more practical to first perform US and choose between regular mammography and CEM based upon US findings.

Previous studies showed that breast MR imaging may also be of value in problem-solving, virtually ruling out malignancy in noncalcified nonenhancing masses and improving assessment of calcified lesions. Moreover, MR imaging is of exceptional value in the detection of carcinomas of unknown primary with a potential origin in the breast.

Three meta-analyses have directly compared the diagnostic accuracy of CEM to that of breast MR imaging.[51] Findings of Pötsch and colleagues' study suggest that CE-MR imaging may be more reliable compared to CEM in detecting breast cancer and ruling out malignancy, especially in cases where there is a higher likelihood of the disease.[52]

Likewise, a systematic review and meta-analysis conducted by the group of Maastricht University in 2023 that focused specifically on women with suspicious breast lesions identified through prior imaging or physical examination, revealed that both CEM and breast MR imaging had high sensitivity and moderate specificity. However, breast MR imaging exhibited higher overall diagnostic performance based on pooled estimates of the diagnostic odds ratio.[53]

Nevertheless, the observed differences in diagnostic performance are small, and practical considerations may prevail over minor differences in diagnostic accuracy. Further research and evidence are needed to establish the strengths and limitations of each imaging modality, especially in specific patient populations and clinical scenarios.

Neoadjuvant Chemotherapy Response

After neoadjuvant chemotherapy, the evaluation of treatment response and residual disease is crucial in guiding surgical management for patients with breast cancer. The current standard practice includes clinical examination and multiple imaging modalities, with MR imaging being the most accurate method. MR imaging plays a vital role in patient selection for neoadjuvant chemotherapy[34,54] and helps modify therapeutic strategies. It is the preferred imaging modality for assessing residual tumor size to determine eligibility for breast-conserving surgery and predicting pathologic complete response (pCR).

Various MR imaging parameters, including changes in tumor size, volume, and enhancement kinetics, are investigated to assess chemotherapy response. Researchers are also exploring functional methods like diverse DWI approaches and molecular imaging techniques to further understand and predict treatment response.

In recent years, with the emergence of targeted therapies, the rates of pCR have significantly increased, particularly for HER2-positive and triple-negative breast cancers.[55] This has sparked interest in exploring the feasibility of omitting surgery in patients achieving pCR based on imaging findings. MR imaging has demonstrated high sensitivity (83%–92%) in accurately identifying residual cancer and intermediate specificity (47%–63%) in accurately identifying pCR, which is also highly dependent on the molecular subtype of the treated cancer.[56,57]

Visual assessment of the absence of enhancement in the tumor bed is a commonly used imaging criterion for pCR. As CEM performs similarly to MR imaging in evaluating disease extent, there is growing interest in investigating its potential in evaluating treatment response. Overall, while there are still relatively few studies evaluating CEM's diagnostic performance in identifying residual disease after NAC, the results are encouraging and consistent.

CEM may be an especially useful tool in locations where MR imaging is not readily available.

The meta-analysis conducted by Cozzi and colleagues in 2022 showed promising results for CEM in identifying residual disease at the end of NAC. The study reported a sensitivity of 80.7% and specificity of 94% for CEM.[58]

When compared to MR imaging, which is currently considered the standard method for assessing NAC response,[57,59] CEM showed a comparable if not better sensitivity and specificity to MR imaging.

Iotti and colleagues found that CEM demonstrated a better prediction of pCR compared to MR imaging.[60]

Patel and colleagues reported comparable positive predictive values (PPVs) and sensitivity for CEM and MR imaging in detecting residual disease.[61]

Despite few available studies currently evaluating CEM's ability to identify residual disease after neoadjuvant chemotherapy, they show consistent and encouraging results. While CEM offers valuable insights, it cannot replace MR imaging due to the wealth of additional information MR imaging provides, including DWI and kinetic changes. Instead, CEM should be considered as an alternative when MR imaging is unavailable or contraindicated. It is important to emphasize that, based on current data, MRI's specificity is insufficient to entirely rule out residual disease postneoadjuvant treatment, and a similar scenario likely applies to CEM.

HIGH-RISK AND INTERMEDIATE-RISK SCREENING

Breast cancer lifetime risk is assessed by using one of multiple models that include factors like the presence of pathogenic hereditary gene mutations, family history, prior breast cancer, exposure to estrogens, high breast density, and high-risk conditions such as atypia or lobular carcinoma in situ. Breast density is an additional independent risk factor for breast cancer that simultaneously diminishes the sensitivity of mammography.[62] Particularly for women at intermediate and high risk (>15% lifetime risk), the analysis of neoangiogenesis, as is done with breast MR imaging, has led to a significant improvement of the quality of breast cancer screening.

Since the release of the American cancer society guidelines in 2007, annual breast MR imaging with or without supplemental mammography has become the advocated surveillance approach for these women. Breast MR imaging also demonstrates exceptional sensitivity in identifying concealed cancers, regardless of breast density, and the gain of MR imaging screening is greatest in dense breasts.[34]

Recently, the use of contrast-enhanced breast MR imaging for women with dense breasts even in the absence of other risk factors has been strongly advocated. Two pivotal trials played a significant role in shaping this approach: the DENSE trial and the EA1411 ECOG-ACRIN study. The DENSE trial, a multicenter randomized trial conducted in the Netherlands, encompassed women with extremely dense breast tissue.[63–65] Furthermore, the EA1411 ECOG-ACRIN study, which was an international effort mainly conducted in the United States, was carried out across 48 sites spanning academic, community hospital, and private practice settings. These trials show that breast MR imaging outperforms mammography and digital breast tomosynthesis, respectively, in women with dense breasts.[66] Further analysis of outcomes is demonstrating the potential to substantially reduce breast cancer mortality while providing a cost-effective intervention.

Many organizations place great importance on educating women about their breast density and promoting the sharing of density information during mammography screenings. The European Society of Breast Imaging (EUSOBI) also suggests informing women about the implications of individual breast density and endorsing supplemental screening for those with extremely dense breasts. In line with this, and following the trial outcomes, EUSOBI currently recommends incorporating screening breast MR imaging every 2 to 4 years for women aged 50 to 70 years with extremely dense breasts either as a supplemental or standalone screening test. The ACR and the Brazilian society of breast radiology have made similar recommendations that women with dense breasts who desire supplemental screening should have breast MR imaging. Given the diversity of individual preferences, the principle of shared decision-making is pivotal in the realm of screening. Women should be adequately informed about the advantages and disadvantages of both mammography and MR imaging-based screening, empowering them to make well-informed choices. This principle gains special significance in areas where national health care programs lack the provision of MR imaging screening. However, the financial implications and limited accessibility of MR imaging scanners present challenges for widespread adoption. To address this, abbreviated MR imaging protocols with shorter scan times could contribute to improved availability and cost-effectiveness, thus expanding the reach of effective breast cancer screening strategies.

Amid the challenge of accommodating a large number of patients for MR imaging, CEM emerges as a potential alternative that can be used to overcome the limited accessibility of MR imaging. Early findings in the use of CEM for screening are promising, though they are still in the initial phases of investigation.[67–69] Recent studies indicate that contrast-enhanced spectral mammography surpasses the combination of mammography and US in terms of cancer detection. For women with intermediate breast cancer risk and dense breasts, an additional cancer detection rate of 13.1 per 1000 screens over conventional mammography was reported.[14,70–72] Similarly, in a study of 904 patients, contrast-enhanced spectral mammography detected 6 additional cancers compared to LE images, resulting in a supplemental detection rate of 6.6 per 1000.[73] Likewise, CEM was shown to strongly improve the detection of recurrent cancers in women with a personal history of breast cancer, with a PPV of almost 50%. Of note, postoperative changes may sometimes lead to nonvisualization of the original tumor bed on mammographic imaging, in which case MR imaging provides a better evaluation option.

When compared to standard mammography, CEM showcased improved sensitivity (90.5% vs 52.4%) but also reduced specificity (76.1% vs 90.5%). Like with MR imaging, the incorporation of US to CEM did not lead to a substantial improvement in diagnostic performance; instead, it seemed to potentially elevate unnecessary biopsy rates.[67] The intensity of lesion enhancement is notably diminished on CEM compared to MR imaging. Whether this reduces the sensitivity compared to MR imaging is yet unknown.[68] The lower enhancement of benign lesions may potentially lead to a slightly higher PPV and a lower false-positive rate for CEM. Unfortunately, an accurate comparison of the performance of MR imaging and CEM has thus far not been performed, which makes it difficult to directly compare the techniques.

For screening, the use of CEM may potentially lead to substantial cost savings. However, economic analysis is quite variable. It was estimated that if CEM were employed for high-risk supplemental screening instead of MR imaging, the estimated annual cost savings could be as high as US$1.1 billion for US health care,[69] whereas another economic evaluation found that the use of abbreviated MR imaging had the lowest incremental cost-effectiveness ratio.[74]

It is worth noting that compared to MR imaging, CEM does introduce an increased radiation dose, which could be a limitation for high-risk patients with an elevated lifetime risk. This is particularly important in young high-risk patients due to the heightened radiosensitivity of this population and the associated potential for radiation-induced tumors.[73,75–77]

In summary, both MR imaging and CEM present valuable options for breast cancer screening. Considering the large numbers of women that would benefit from contrast-enhanced screening tools, in practice likely both techniques are necessary to meet the needs of all eligible women. While MR imaging, especially when using abbreviated protocols, exhibits high efficiency, CEM offers a potentially more accessible alternative, particularly for women with low BPE (eg, postsurgery, after 60 years of age). There is ongoing research to advance breast cancer screening techniques. As interest in risk assessment and personalized screening grows, a significant development is the ongoing randomized clinical trial in the United Kingdom, which involves enrolling 13,200 women with elevated risk due to mammary glandular density. In this trial, CEM is integrated into the screening protocol as an adjunct to mammography and is being compared with the addition of US or MR imaging. This trial, known as breast screening - risk adaptive imaging for density (BRAID), reflects the commitment to refining breast cancer screening through tailored approaches.[78]

Another pivotal trial is the ongoing Contrast-Enhanced Mammography Imaging Screening Trial (CMIST). This trial aims to compare the effectiveness of CEM with 3D mammography for women with dense breasts. The results of CMIST, anticipated in 2025, hold the promise of enhanced cancer detection and a reduction in false-positive results, thus contributing to improved breast cancer screening outcomes.[79]

FURTHER CONSIDERATIONS: AVAILABILITY, COST, CONTRAST, RADIATION EXPOSURE, COMPRESSION, CLAUSTROPHOBIA, AND NOISE

While the current availability of MR imaging scanners is much higher than that of CEM, accessibility to breast MR imaging is limited due to competition for neuro, cardiac, and musculoskeletal applications. Although for none of these applications, evidence of benefit in terms of improved clinical outcome and even mortality reduction is as strong as for breast imaging, this necessitates a need to advocate for scanner time. In larger breast imaging centers placing a dedicated breast MR imaging scanner may be of value due to increasing demand. CEM only applies to breast imaging and, therefore, the only competition is the performance of a normal mammogram or DBT examination. Modern mammography machines can be equipped with a CEM license at relatively low cost, thus reducing the start-up costs. However, it should be noted that older machines need to be fully replaced. For the latter, CEM has the advantage that the same footprint can be used, although it is advantageous to slightly enlarge examination rooms to accommodate the placement of a contrast pump. Costs are extremely variable across the world, and are therefore difficult to compare, but are in general somewhat higher for MR imaging than for CEM due to these factors and the lower costs for iodine-compared to gadolinium-based contrast agents. Still, in high throughput facilities, actual costs are mainly dominated by personnel requirements, which are similar for both modalities.

Iodine-based contrast agents are associated with a roughly 7 times higher risk of allergic reactions than gadolinium-based agents, but serious reactions are rare with both types of agents. Concerns surrounding prolonged gadolinium deposition associated with MR imaging have surfaced in recent years.[80] However, in screening of healthy women this does not appear to be of concern as no effects were noted at all in women who underwent multiple breast MR imaging screening rounds.[81]

MR imaging does not use x-rays, so patients are not exposed to the harmful effects of ionizing radiation. CEM is an x-ray-based method and, consequently, depends on ionizing radiation. The dual-energy method used in CEM involves a double exposure for each single projection, which even results in increased radiation dose compared to standard mammography. Specifically, the high-energy exposure in CEM leads to an additional radiation dose compared to DM, while the LE exposure dose is comparable to that of DM. The overall radiation dose increase with CEM typically ranges from 20% to 80%, depending on factors such as the type of equipment, system settings, and breast thickness.[20,82,83] Despite this increase in radiation dose, studies have shown that the values remain below the safety thresholds set by European guidelines for screening mammography[42] and the guidelines of the Mammography Quality Standards Act.[84] While the increased radiation dose might be a concern in standard diagnostic settings and, particularly, screening scenarios, it becomes less relevant when using CEM for preoperative staging in women diagnosed with breast cancer.[85] CEM also relies on standard breast compression during acquisition, which is the factor least well tolerated by women undergoing mammography. In MR imaging, breast compression is not necessary and, therefore, does not disincentivize screening participation. However, prone positioning in MR imaging is not feasible for all women. In addition, due to the design of common breast coils, the weight on the sternum is substantial, and this can be uncomfortable in longer examinations. MR imaging scanners are also noisy, and this in combination with the tube like configuration can provoke anxiety, especially in women with claustrophobia. As such it is important to weigh benefits and disadvantages of both techniques on an individual basis, allowing women the opportunity for informed decision-making.

SUMMARY

In summary, any form of contrast-enhanced imaging currently outperforms any noncontrast enhanced alternative. Breast MR imaging is the current gold standard. However, the performance of CEM is only slightly inferior and this consequently provides a viable alternative in many settings. For screening, data on CEM is still limited and performance is consequently uncertain, however it certainly outperforms conventional mammography. Reporting is analogous in both modalities, using a similar lexicon to describe similar features, albeit for CEM the lexicon is adjusted to the 2D nature and taking into account corresponding features on the LE images (that resemble a standard mammography examination). Factors to take into account when choosing between modalities include the likelihood of strong BPE (that can be better managed with MR imaging, the importance of radiation (particularly relevant in young women), the availability of the equipment, and women's preferences (due to claustrophobia, compression, noise, and so forth).

CLINICS CARE POINTS

- CEM is useful as an alternative to breast MR imaging in many clinical scenarios including problem-solving, breast cancer staging, and neoadjuvant chemotherapy monitoring.
- The dynamic nature of breast MR imaging makes interpretation of imaging easier in cases with strong BPE.
- Due to the increasing indications for contrast-enhanced screening and surveillance, both breast MR imaging and CEM are likely required to meet the demands. CEM may be particularly useful in postoperative follow-up as BPE in the affected breast is minimized by previous radiotherapy.
- When choosing an imaging modality, it is important to take women's preferences into account.

REFERENCES

1. Siegel R, Miller K, Fuchs H, et al. Cancer Statistics, 2021. CA. Cancer J. Clin. 2021;71:7–33.
2. Humphrey L, Helfand M, Chan B, et al. Breast cancer screening: a summary of the evidence for the U.S. Preventive Services Task Force. Ann Intern Med 2002;137:347–360».
3. Marmot M, Altman D, Cameron D, et al. The benefits and harms of breast cancer screening: an independent review. Lancet 2012;380(9855):1778–1786».
4. Lauby-Secretan B, Scoccianti C, Loomis D, et al. Breast cancer screening–viewpoint of the IARC Working Group. N Engl J Med 2015;372(24):2353–2358».
5. Paci E, Broeders M, Hofvind S, et al. European breast Cancer service screening outcomes: a first balance sheet of the benefits and harms. Cancer Epidemiol Biomark Prev 2014;23(7):1159–1163».
6. E. Pisano, C. Gatsonis, E. Hendrick et al., Digital Mammographic Imaging Screening Trial (DMIST) Investigators Group, Diagnostic performance of digital vers».
7. Wanders J, Holland K, Veldhuis W, et al. Volumetric breast density affects performance of digital screening mammography. Breast Cancer Res Treat 2017;162(1):95–103».
8. Kolb T, Lichy J, Newhouse J. Comparison of the performance of screening mammography, physical examination, and breast US and evaluation of factors that influence them: an analysis of 27,825 patient evaluations. Radiology 2002;225:165–175».
9. Emaus M, Bakker M, Peeters P, et al. MR Imaging as an additional screening modality for the detection of

breast cancer in women aged 50-75 years with extremely dense breasts: the DENSE trial study design. Radiology 2015;0:141827».

10. M. Tsarouchi, A. Hoxhaj e R. Mann, New Approaches and Recommendations for Risk-Adapted Breast Cancer Screening.».

11. Baltzer P, Mann R, Iima M, et al. EUSOBI international Breast Diffusion-Weighted Imaging working group. Diffusion-weighted imaging of the breast-a consensus and mission statement from the EUSOBI International Breast Diffusion-Weighted Imaging working group. Eur Radiol 2020;30(3):1436».

12. Dromain C, Balleyguier C, Adler G, et al. Contrast-enhanced digital mammography. Eur J Radiol 2009;69:34–42.

13. Lobbes M, Smidt M, Houwers J, et al. Contrast enhanced mammography: techniques, current results, and potential indications. Clin Radiol 2013; 68(9):935–44.

14. Dromain C, Thibault F, Diekmann F, et al. Dual-energy contrastenhanced digital mammography: initial clinical results of a multireader, multicase study. Breast Cancer Res 2012;14(3):R94.

15. Patel B, Lobbes M, Lewin J. Contrast enhanced spectral mammography: a review. Semin Ultrasound CT MR 2018;39(1):70–9.

16. Perry H, Phillips J, Dialani V, et al. Contrast-enhanced mammography: a systematic guide to interpretation and reporting. AJR Am J Roentgenol 2019;212(1):222–31.

17. ACR Committee on drugs and contrast Media. ACR Manual on Contrast Media. ACR Man Contrast Media – Version 9, 2013 105:128».

18. Carnahan M, Pockaj B, Pizzitola V, et al. Contrast-Enhanced Mammography for Newly Diagnosed Breast Cancer in Women With Breast Augmentation: Preliminary Findings. AJR Am J Roentgenol 2021; 217(4):855–6.

19. Jochelson M, Dershaw D, Sung J, et al. Bilateral contrast enhanced dual-energy digital mammography: feasibility and comparison with conventional digital mammography and MR imaging in women with known breast carcinoma. Radiology 2013;266:743–51.

20. Jochelson M, Lobbes M. Contrast-enhanced Mammography: State of the Art. Radiology 2021; 299:36–48.

21. Lobbes M, Lalji U, Nelemans P, et al. The quality of tumor size assessment by contrast-enhanced spectral mammography and the benefit of additional breast MRI. J Cancer 2015;6(2):144–50.

22. Francescone M, Jochelson M, Dershaw D, et al. Low energy mammogram obtained in contrast-enhanced digital mammography (CEDM) is comparable to routine full-field digital mammography (FFDM). Eur J Radiol 2014;83(8):1350–5.

23. Zhu Y, O'Connell A, Ma Y, et al. Dedicated breast CT: state of the art-Part II. Clinical application and future outlook. Eur Radiol 2022 Apr;32(4):2286–300 [Erratum in: Eur Radiol. 2022 Feb 14].

24. Berger N, Marcon M, Wieler J, et al. Contrast Media-Enhanced Breast Computed Tomography With a Photon-Counting Detector: Initial Experiences on In Vivo Image Quality and Correlation to Histology. Invest Radiol 2022;57(10):704–9.

25. Wienbeck S, Lotz J, Fischer U. Review of clinical studies and first clinical experiences with a commercially available cone-beam breast CT in Europe. Clin Imaging 2017;42:50–9.

26. Dietzel B. How to use the kaiser score as a clinical decision rule for diagnosis in multiparametric breast MRI: a pictorial essay. Insights Imaging 2018;9(3): 325–35.

27. Lee C, Phillips J, Sung J, et al. ACR BI-RADS® ATLAS-MAMMOGRAPHY CONTRAST ENHANCED MAMMOGRAPHY (CEM); A supplement to ACR BI-RADS®Mammography 2013. Reston (VA): American College of Radiology; 2022.

28. Knogler T, Homolka P, Hoernig M, et al. Application of BI-RADS Descriptors in Contrast-Enhanced Dual-Energy Mammography: Comparison with MRI. Breast Care 2017;12:212–216».

29. Kamal R, Helal M, Mansour S, et al. Can we apply the MRI BI-RADS lexicon morphology descriptors on contrast-enhanced spectral mammography? Br J Radiol 2016;89:20160157».

30. Morris E, Comstock C, Lee C, et al. ACR BI-RADS® Magnetic Resonance Imaging. In: Morris E, Comstock C, Lee C, editors. *ACR BI-RADS® Atlas, breast imaging reporting and data system*. Reston, VA: American College of Radiology; 2013.

31. Spak D, Plaxco J, Santiago L, et al. BI-RADS® fifth edition: A summary of changes. Diagn. Interv. Imaging 2017;98:179–90.

32. Sogani J, Morris E, Kaplan J, et al. Comparison of background parenchymal enhancement at contrast-enhanced spectral mammography and breast MR imaging. Radiology 2017;282:63–73.

33. Sorin V, Yagil Y, Shalmon A, et al. Background Parenchymal Enhancement at Contrast-Enhanced Spectral Mammography (CESM) as a Breast Cancer Risk Factor. Acad Radiol 2019;27(9):1234–40.

34. Mann RM, Cho N, Moy L. Breast MRI: State of the Art. Radiology 2019;292:520–36.

35. King V, Brooks J, Bernstein J, et al. Background parenchymal enhancement at breast MR imaging and breast cancer risk. Radiology 2011;260(1):50–60.

36. Dontchos B, Rahbar H, Partridge S, et al. Are qualitative assessments of background parenchymal enhancement, amount of fibroglandular tissue on MR images, and mammographic density associated with breast cancer risk? Radiology 2015;276(2): 371–380».

37. Ray K, Kerlikowske K, Lobach I, et al. Effect of background parenchymal enhancement on breast MR

imaging interpretive performance in community-based practices. Radiology 2018;286(3):822–829».

38. Nori J, Kaur KKA, Meenal D, et al. Atlas of contrast-enhanced mammography. 1st edition. Springer; 2021.

39. DeMartini WLF, Peacock S, Eby P, et al. Background Parenchymal Enhancement on Breast MRI: Impact on Diagnostic Performance. AJR 2012;198:W373–W380».

40. Lee C, Bryce Y, Zheng JSJ, et al. Outcome of screening MRI in premenopausal women as a function of the week of the menstrual cycle. AJR 2020; 214:1175–1181».

41. Bhimani C, Matta D, Roth RG, et al. Contrast-enhanced spectral mammography: technique, indications, and clinical applications. Acad Radiol 2017;24(1):84–8.

42. Perry N, Broeders M, de Wolf C, et al. European guidelines for quality assurance in breast cancer screening and diagnosis. Fourth edition–summary document. Ann. Oncol. Off. J. Eur. Soc. Med. Oncol. 2008;19:614–622».

43. M. Travieso-Aja, P. Naranjo-Santana, C. Fernández-Ruiz et al., Factors affecting the precision of lesion sizing with contrast-enhanced spectral mammography, Clin».

44. Åhsberg K, Gardfjell A, Nimeus E, et al. Added value of contrast-enhanced mammography (CEM) in staging of malignant breast lesions-a feasibility study. World J Surg Oncol 2020;18:100.

45. E. Kim, I. Youn, K. Lee, J.-S. Yun et al., Diagnostic Value of Contrast-Enhanced Digital Mammography versus Contrast-Enhanced Magnetic Resonance Imaging for the Preoperative Evaluatio».

46. Amato F, Bicchierai G, Cirone D, et al. Preoperative loco-regional staging of invasive lobular carcinoma with contrast-enhanced digital mammography (CEDM). Radiol Med 2019;124(12):1229–37.

47. Lalji U, Houben I, Prevos e R, et al. Contrast-enhanced spectral mammography in recalls from the Dutch breast cancer screening program: validation of results in a large multireader, multicase study. Eur Radiol 2016;26:4371–9.

48. van Nijnatten T, Jochelson M, Pinker K. Differences in degree of lesion enhancement on CEM between ILC and IDC. BJR Open 2019;5:20180046.

49. Tardivel A-M, Balleyguier C, Dunant A, et al. Added Value of Contrast-Enhanced Spectral Mammography in Postscreening Assessment. Breast J 2016;22:520–8.

50. Tennant S, James J, Cornford E, et al. Contrast-enhanced spectral mammography improves diagnostic accuracy in the symptomatic setting. Clin Radiol 2016;71:1148–55.

51. Xiang W, Rao H, Zhou L. A meta-analysis of contrast-enhanced spectral mammography versus MRI in the diagnosis of breast cancer. Thorac Cancer 2020;11:1423–1432».

52. Pötsch N, Vatteroni G, Clauser P, et al. Contrast-enhanced mammography versus contrast-enhanced breast MRI : a systematic review and meta-analysis. Radiology 2022;305:94–103».

53. Neeter L, Robbe Q, van Nijnatten T, et al. Comparing the Diagnostic Performance of Contrast- Enhanced Mammography and Breast MRI: a Systematic Review and Meta-Analysis. J Cancer 2023;14(1): 174–82.

54. Le-Petross H, Lim B. Role of MR imaging in neoadjuvant therapy monitoring. Magn Reson Imaging Clin N Am 2018;26(2):207–220».

55. von Minckwitz G, Untch M, JU B, et al. Definition and impact of pathologic complete response on prognosis after neoadjuvant chemotherapy in various intrinsic breast cancer subtypes. J Clin Oncol 2012;30(15):1796–1804».

56. Marinovich M, Houssami N, Macaskill P, et al. Meta-analysis of magnetic resonance imaging in detecting residual breast cancer after neoadjuvant therapy. J Natl Cancer Inst 2013;105(5):321–33, 132.

57. Scheel J, Kim E, Partridge S, et al. MRI, clinical examination, and mammography for preoperative assessment of residual disease and pathologic complete response after neoadjuvant chemotherapy for breast cancer: ACRIN 6657 trial. AJR Am J Roentgenol 2018;210(6):1376–85.

58. Cozzi A, Magni V, Zanardo M, et al. Contrast-enhanced Mammography: A Systematic Review and Meta-Analysis of Diagnostic Performance. Radiology 2022;302:568–81.

59. Marinovich M, Macaskill P, Irwig L, et al. Agreement between MRI and pathologic breast tumor size after neoadjuvant chemotherapy, and comparison with alternative tests: individual patient data meta-analysis. BMC Cancer 2015;15(1):662.

60. Iotti V, Ravaioli S, Vacondio R, et al. Contrast-enhanced spectral mammography in neoadjuvant chemotherapy monitoring: a comparison with breast magnetic resonance imaging. Breast Cancer Res 2017;19(1):106».

61. Patel B, Hilal T, Covington M, et al. Contrast-enhanced spectral mammography is comparable to MRI in the assessment of residual breast cancer following neoadjuvant systemic therapy. Ann Surg Oncol 2018;25(5):1350–1356».

62. Breast cancer screening in women with extremely dense breasts recommendations of the European Society of Breast Imaging (EUSOBI)».

63. Bakker M, de Lange S, Pijnappel R, et al. Supplemental MRI screening for women with extremely dense breast tissue. N Engl J Med 2019;381(22): 2091–2102».

64. Veenhuizen S, de Lange S, Bakker M, et al. Supplemental breast MRI for women with extremely dense breasts: results of the second screening round of the DENSE trial. Radiology 2021;299(2):278–286».

65. Geuzinge H, Bakker M, Heijnsdijk E, et al. Costeffectiveness of MRI screening for women with extremely dense breast tissue. J Natl Cancer Inst 2021; 113(11):1476–1483».

66. Comstock C, Gatsonis C, Newstead G. Comparison of abbreviated breast MRI vs digital breast tomosynthesis for breast cancer detection among women with dense breasts undergoing screening. JAMA 2020;323(8):746–56.

67. Covington M. Contrast-Enhanced Mammography Implementation, Performance, and Use for Supplemental Breast Cancer Screening. Radiol. Clin. North Am. 2021;59:113–28.

68. Li L, Roth R, Germaine P, et al. Contrast-enhanced spectral mammography (CESM) versus breast magnetic resonance imaging (MRI): a retrospective comparison in 66 breast lesions. Diagn Interv Imaging 2017;98:113–23.

69. Patel B, Gray R, Pockaj B. Potential cost savings of contrastenhanced digital mammography. Am J Roentgenol 2017;208:W231–7.

70. Cheung Y, Lin Y, Wan Y, et al. Diagnostic performance of dual-energy contrast-enhanced subtracted mammography in dense breasts compared to mammography alone: interobserver blind-reading analysis. Eur Radiol 2014;24(10):2394–403.

71. Tagliafico A, Bignotti B, Rossi F, et al. Diagnostic performance of contrastenhanced spectral mammography: Systematic review and meta-analysis. Breast 2016;28:13–19».

72. B. Patel, S. Garza, S. Eversman, Y. Lopez-Alvarez et al., Assessing tumor extent on contrast-enhanced spectral mammography versus full-field.».

73. Sung J, Lebron LKD, et al. Performance of Dual-Energy Contrastenhanced Digital Mammography for Screening Women at Increased Risk of Breast Cancer. Radiology 2019;293(1):81–8.

74. Blankenburg M, Sánchez-Collado I, Soyemi BO, et al. Economic evaluation of supplemental breast cancer screening modalities to mammography or digital breast tomosynthesis in women with heterogeneously and extremely dense breasts and average or intermediate breast cancer risk in US healthcare. J Med Econ 2021;26(1):850–61.

75. Hogan M, Amir T, Sevilimedu V, et al. Contrast-Enhanced Digital Mammography Screening for Intermediate-Risk Women With a History of Lobular Neoplasia. AJR Am J Roentgenol 2021;216: 1486–91.

76. Phi X-A, Saadatmand S, De Bock G, et al. Contribution of mammography to MRI screening in BRCA mutation carriers by BRCA status and age : Individual patient data meta-analysis. Br J Cancer 2016; 114(6):631–7.

77. F. Sardanelli, F. Podo e F. Santoro, Multicenter surveillance of women at high genetic breast cancer risk using mammography, ultrasonography, and contrast-enhanced magnetic resonance imaging (the high breast cancer risk italian 1 study): final results».

78. S. Vinnicombe, Harvey, H. et al., Introduction of an abbreviated breast MRI service in the UK as part of the BRAID trial: practicalities, challenges, and future directions».

79. Available at: www.acr.org. Accessed March 1, 2024.

80. Gulani V, Calamante F, Shellock F, et al. Gadolinium deposition in the brain: summary of evidence and recommendations. Lancet Neurol 2017;16:564–70.

81. Bennani-Baiti B, Krug B, Giese D, et al. Evaluation of 3.0-T MRI Brain Signal after Exposure to Gadoterate Meglumine in Women with High Breast Cancer Risk and Screening Breast MRI. Radiology 2019;293(3): 523–30.

82. Zanardo M, Cozzi A, Trimboli R, et al. Technique, protocols and adverse reactions for contrast-enhanced spectral mammography (CESM): a systematic review. Insights Imaging 2019;10:76.

83. Sensakovic W, Carnahan M, Czaplicki C. Contrast-enhanced Mammography: How Does It Work? Radiogr. Rev. Publ. Radiol. Soc. N. Am. Inc. 2021;41: 829–39.

84. James J, Pavlicek W, Hanson J, et al. Breast Radiation Dose With CESM Compared With 2D FFDM and 3D Tomosynthesis Mammography. AJR Am J Roentgenol 2017;208:362–72.

85. L. M.B. et al., Contrast enhanced mammography (CEM) versus magnetic resonance imaging (MRI) for staging of breast cancer: The pro CEM perspective.».

Non-contrast Breast MR Imaging

Jin You Kim, MD, PhD[a], Savannah C. Partridge, PhD[b,c],*

KEYWORDS

- Diffusion-weighted magnetic resonance imaging • Breast cancer • Diagnosis • Biomarkers
- Supplemental screening

KEY POINTS

- Diffusion-weighted MR imaging (DWI) is a fast, unenhanced technique that can demonstrate breast malignancy based on reduced water diffusivity in tumors compared to normal fibroglandular tissue.
- DWI has wide clinical applications in breast cancer detection, characterization, prognosis, and predicting treatment response as both an adjunct and alternative modality to dynamic contrast-enhanced MR imaging.
- DWI has shown the potential to serve as a stand-alone unenhanced MR imaging screening method.
- Standardization of DWI protocols and interpretation strategies is essential to optimize image quality and reliability and further enhance the clinical role of DWI for breast imaging.

INTRODUCTION

Dynamic contrast-enhanced (DCE) MR imaging of the breast is a well-established MR imaging technique with high sensitivity for the detection and characterization of breast cancer.[1] DCE MR imaging is recommended by the American Cancer Society as an adjunct to screening mammography in women with a lifetime breast cancer risk ≥ 20% based on family history or genetic mutation.[2] However, the use of DCE MR imaging is limited by the need for administration of contrast agents, its long scan time, and its high cost. Variable risks of gadolinium-based contrast agents have been reported and there have been growing concerns about the deposition of gadolinium in bone, skin, and solid organs as well as central nervous system tissue.[3–5] Furthermore, a high-risk screening population might be at higher risk of gadolinium retention due to repeated annual DCE MR imaging screening starting at a relatively young age. Therefore, there is increasing interest in identifying a non-contrast (ie, unenhanced) MR imaging approach that might be potentially safer, more rapid, and less expensive than DCE MR imaging for clinical use.

DIFFUSION-WEIGHTED IMAGING

The most promising non-contrast MR imaging technique to date for breast cancer detection and characterization is diffusion-weighted imaging (DWI). DWI is a fast, non-contrast MR imaging technique that is widely available on MR imaging systems and commonly used in clinical practice. DWI was first applied for breast imaging by Englander and colleagues in 1997,[6] and there have been numerous studies exploring the clinical utility of DWI as a supplement to conventional DCE MR imaging or as a stand-alone modality. In this article, the authors review the basic principles of DWI, technical considerations including b-value selection, and focus on the various applications of DWI in the clinical setting. They also briefly review a variety of other non-contrast MR imaging techniques that are currently under investigation.

Funding: This work was supported in-part by NIH grants R01CA207290.
[a] Department of Radiology and Medical Research Institute, Pusan National University Hospital, Pusan National University School of Medicine, Busan, Republic of Korea; [b] Department of Radiology, University of Washington, Seattle, WA, USA; [c] Fred Hutchinson Cancer Center, Seattle, WA, USA
* Corresponding author. Department of Radiology, University of Washington, 1144 Eastlake Avenue East, Seattle, WA 98109.
E-mail address: scp3@uw.edu

Basics of Diffusion-Weighted Imaging

DWI measures the degree of water movement within tissues. Motion-sensitizing gradients are applied during DWI image acquisition, and the reduction in the signal intensity of DWI is proportional to the water mobility, as described by the monoexponential equation;

$$S_D = S_0\, e^{-b*ADC}$$

where S_D is the signal intensity, S_0 is the signal intensity without diffusion weighting, b is the diffusion sensitization factor, which is defined by the strength and timing of the applied diffusion gradients (s/mm^2), and the apparent diffusion coefficient (ADC) is the rate of diffusion, which is defined as the average area occupied by a water molecule per unit time (mm^2/s).

ADC can be calculated using the image acquisitions at 2 or more different b-values and quantitatively reflects underlying tissue microenvironment including cellularity and cell membrane integrity. In general, malignant breast lesions demonstrate reduced diffusivity with respect to normal fibroglandular tissue and benign breast lesions due to high cellularity, which causes them to appear bright on the diffusion-weighted images and dark on the gray-scale ADC map (**Figs. 1** and **2**). Regarding normal breast tissue, there is a wide range of reported ADC values from 1.51×10^{-3} mm^2/s to 2.09×10^{-3} mm^2/s (with maximum b-values ranging from 600 to 1000 s/mm^2).[7] Although the breast is a hormonally responsive organ, normal fluctuation of breast ADC during a menstrual cycle is relatively small.[8–10] A recent study reported that ADC values in not only normal breast tissue but also breast cancer were not affected significantly by menstrual cycle.[10]

B-value Selection

In terms of technical considerations, one of the most critical factors affecting DWI performance is the level of diffusion sensitization, described by the "b-value." B-value selection affects the ADC value, signal-to-noise ratio (SNR), and the lesion contrast-to-noise ratio.[11–13] Differences in signal decay rates between tumor and normal breast tissue result in greater relative signal difference and lesion contrast-to-noise ratio as the b-value increases, which could improve cancer visibility and specificity for cancer detection. However, SNR decreases as the b-value increases, and imaging acquisition at a higher b-value leads to increased distortions due to susceptibility effects and eddy currents and lengthens the scan time.[14] Furthermore, it is well-recognized that in vivo ADC values are directly influenced by the maximum b-value used for measurement. Increased non-Gaussian diffusion behavior (ie, kurtosis effect) evident at higher b-values (>1000 s/mm^2) reflecting tissue microstructural complexity, along with reduced perfusion influence at higher b-values,

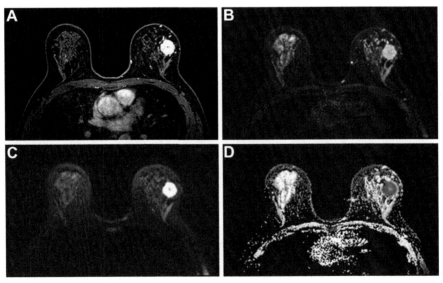

Fig. 1. Example breast diffusion-weighted MR imaging (DWI) obtained in a 49-year-old woman with grade III triple negative invasive ductal carcinoma in the left breast. Shown are corresponding axial images from (A) postcontrast T1-weighted DCE image as reference, (B) DWI with b = 0 s/mm^2, (C) DWI with b = 800 s/mm^2, and (D) apparent diffusion coefficient (ADC) map. The invasive breast cancer exhibits reduced diffusivity on DWI, appearing hyperintense on the b = 800 s/mm^2 and hypointense on the ADC map (mean ADC = 0.78×10^{-3} mm^2/s) compared to normal breast tissue (mean ADC = 1.88×10^{-3} mm^2/s).

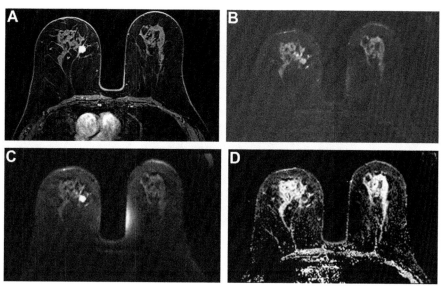

Fig. 2. Example breast DWI obtained in an 82-year-old woman with grade II triple negative invasive ductal carcinoma in the right breast. Shown are corresponding axial images from (*A*) postcontrast T1-weighted DCE image as reference, (*B*) DWI with $b = 0$ s/mm^2, (*C*) DWI with $b = 800$ s/mm^2, and (*D*) ADC map. The invasive breast cancer exhibits reduced diffusivity on DWI, appearing hyperintense on the $b = 800$ s/mm^2 and hypointense on the ADC map (mean ADC = 0.82×10^{-3} mm^2/s) compared to normal breast tissue (mean ADC = 1.96×10^{-3} mm^2/s).

causes ADC to be lower with higher maximum b-values.[15] Therefore, optimal b-value selection for breast DWI is essential for improving cancer detection as well as standardization and interpretation of the ADC (**Table 1**). Previous studies evaluating the optimal b-value selection have shown variable results.[11–13,16] A maximum b-value of 800 s/mm^2 is recommended as a good compromise for standardization of breast ADC measurements according to the European Society of Breast Imaging (EUSOBI)International Breast DWI working group.[17] However, in a screening setting, a very high b-value of 1200 to 1500 s/mm^2 may be optimal to maximize lesion contrast and visibility,[18–20] despite the lower SNR and longer scan time. Hence, adding another high b-value and thus DWI acquisitions with 3 different b-values (ie, 0–50 sec/mm^2, 800 sec/mm^2, and 1200–1500 sec/mm^2) may be ideal for breast cancer screening purposes. In theory, b-value selection is independent of field strength, although lower overall SNR at

lower field strength (eg, 1.5 T vs 3T) may necessitate more signal averages at higher b-values for acceptable quality, adding to scan time.

CLINICAL APPLICATION OF DIFFUSION-WEIGHTED IMAGING
Diffusion-Weighted Imaging in Combination with Standard MR Imaging

Diagnosis of suspicious breast lesions
The most widely used clinical application of DWI for breast imaging is as a supplemental diagnostic tool to DCE MR imaging to improve differential diagnosis (malignant from benign breast lesions). Numerous studies have shown that ADC values in malignant breast lesions are commonly lower than those in benign breast lesions (**Fig. 3**),[21–23] although a specific ADC cut-off value has not been established (false-negative DWI findings will be discussed later in this review). Meta-analysis pooling data across studies demonstrated that the diagnostic specificity

Table 1
DWI tissue microenvironmental sensitivity by b-value

B-values (s/mm^2)	Predominant Tissue Microenvironment Factor	Breast Imaging Application
0–200	Vascularity	Perfusion, microcirculation assessment
400–1000	Cellularity	Lesion characterization; standardized ADC measurement
> 1200	Tissue microstructure	Cancer detection (vs. normal, benign tissues)

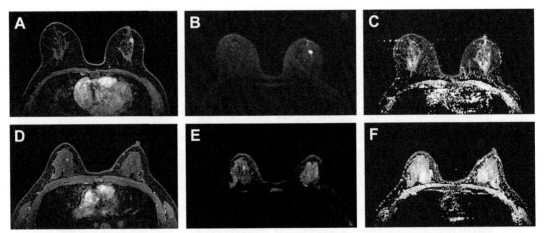

Fig. 3. DWI for characterization of suspicious (Breast Imaging Reporting and Data System [BI-RADS]) lesions detected on DCE-MR imaging. Each enhanced on postcontrast T1-weighted Dynamic contrast-enhanced(DCE) MR imaging (*A, D*). (*A–C*) Invasive ductal carcinoma detected in the left breast in a 64-year-old woman. The lesion exhibits high signal intensity on (*B*) DWI (*b* = 800 s/mm^2) with low ADC of 0.82 × 10^{-3} mm^2/s on (*C*) the corresponding ADC map. (*D–F*) Fibroadenoma detected in the right breast in a 42-year-old woman. The lesion exhibits high signal intensity on (*E*) DWI (*b* = 800 s/mm^2) and a relatively high ADC of 1.84 × 10^{-3} mm^2/s on (*F*) the corresponding ADC map.

of DWI ranges between 76% and 82%, which is superior compared to 71% for DCE-MR imaging.[24,25] The improved specificity can result in the reduction of the number of unnecessary biopsies. A prospective multicenter trial reported that using an ADC cutoff of 1.53 × 10^{-3} mm^2/s could prevent 35.9% of false-positive MR imaging findings and reduce the number of biopsies by 20.9% without affecting the sensitivity.[26]

There is a wide range of reported cut-off values of ADC (from 0.66 × 10^{-3} mm^2/s to 1.50 × 10^{-3} mm^2/s) to discriminate between benign and malignant breast lesions.[24] Non-standardized, variable acquisition parameters of DWI used in the prior studies require caution in interpreting the results and applying the ADC threshold in clinical practice. Recently, the need for standardization and quality controls in breast DWI has been emphasized and consensus recommendations for DWI acquisition and ADC measurement of breast lesions were published by an international working group.[17] Research on the reproducibility of quantitative ADC measurements of breast tumors is ongoing.[27,28] Furthermore, development of a breast ADC categorization system for the assessment, documentation, and reporting of ADC has been proposed to complement Breast Imaging Reporting and Data System (BI-RADS) criteria.[29] These efforts are expected to contribute to the implementation of breast DWI in clinical routine.

Characterization of breast cancer
Preoperative characterization of breast cancer based on established prognostic factors or molecular subtypes is essential for individualized

treatment strategies. Research has increasingly addressed the association between tumor ADC values and biomarkers of breast cancer and suggested the potential of ADC as a non-invasive imaging biomarker. Overall, an inverse correlation has generally been shown between ADC values and tumor aggressivity, with the mean ADC of invasive disease being lower than that of in situ disease.[30,31] It is suggested that ADC assessment can help prediction of pathologic upstaging, from high-risk to malignant lesions or in situ to invasive disease (**Fig. 4**).[32–35] In a recent study, maximum ADC less than 1.19 × 10^{-3} mm^2/s was reported to be an independent predictor of upstaging in women with biopsy-proven ductal carcinoma in situ (DCIS) and a predictive model based on the DWI feature and clinicopathologic factors showed good performance for prediction of upstaging.[32]

Within invasive carcinoma, ADC values have shown to negatively correlate with tumor grade.[36–39] Increased cellularity of higher grade tumors may result in more restricted diffusion, leading to low signal intensity on the ADC map. Similar correlations have been shown with proliferation marker Ki-67,[31,38,40,41] with high Ki-67 lesions exhibiting lower ADC than low Ki-67 lesions. Although a large meta-analysis reported that ADC could not predict tumor grade and Ki-67 status, there were limitations to the meta-analysis because it was conducted from the data collected from variable prior studies using different MR imaging equipment and protocols.[42] In addition, tumor cellularity may decrease due to central necrosis in a highly proliferative tumor, and the decreased cellularity would be a potential confounder for the high Ki-67 lesions. An inverse

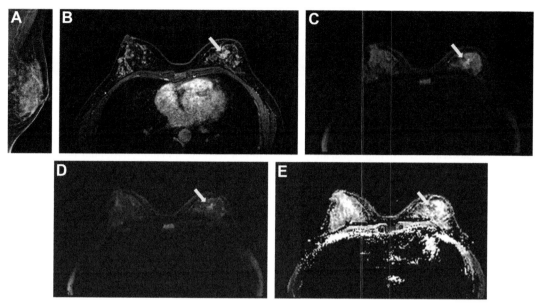

Fig. 4. Example breast DWI obtained in a 44-year-old asymptomatic woman who was diagnosed with low-grade ductal carcinoma in situ by 14-gauge needle biopsy. (*A*) Left mediolateral oblique view of the screening mammogram shows negative findings in the background of the extremely heterogeneously dense breast. (*B*) Postcontrast T1-weighted DCE image shows an irregular enhancing mass in the left breast (*arrow*). (*C*) DWI with $b = 800$ s/mm^2 and (*D*) computed DWI with $b = 1500$ s/mm^2 show high signal intensity (*arrow*) in the area corresponding to the enhanced lesion. (*E*) The lesion exhibits low ADC value of 0.92×10^{-3} mm^2/s (*arrow*); ADC map was calculated using b values 0, 800 s/mm^2. Breast-conserving surgery was performed and the pathologic findings showed 1.0 cm invasive ductal carcinoma with histologic grade 3.

correlation was also shown between tumor ADC values and the presence of lymphovascular invasion, another marker of cancer aggressiveness.[43–45] Regarding tumor size, larger tumors have been shown to have lower ADC values in several studies,[38,39,46] but other studies did not find any correlations.[44,47–49] Larger tumors tend to be more heterogeneous due to necrosis or hemorrhage and more frequently present as nonmass enhancement. These characteristics cause variability in ADC measurement and may explain the reason for the weak correlation of tumor size with ADC values. In regard to receptor status and tumor subtypes, estrogen receptor (ER) and/or progesterone receptor-positive tumors tended to have lower ADC values than those that are negative, and human epidermal growth factor receptor 2 (HER2)-positive and triple-negative tumors exhibited the higher ADC values.[49–51] However, in a meta-analysis involving 2990 breast tumors from 28 studies, the ADC values in different breast cancer subtypes overlapped significantly.[52] Recently, radiomic features on DWI and heterogeneity on the ADC map, both reflecting microstructural heterogeneity, have been proposed to discriminate the triple-negative subtype from other subtypes[53,54] based on higher level of intratumoral ADC heterogeneity (**Fig. 5**).[54] Further validation studies are needed.

Within in situ carcinoma, research into the value of ADC for DCIS grading has been inconclusive. Several studies suggested that ADC values could help identify low-grade DCIS lesions.[55,56] Iima and colleagues reported that the specificity and positive predictive value were 100% with a threshold of minimum ADC value of 1.30×10^{-3} mm^2/s in the diagnosis of low-grade DCIS (median size of region of interest (ROI) = 63.5 mm^2, range: 24.5–272.0 mm^2).[55] However, in the studies by Rahbar and colleagues, ADC value did not show differences between high-grade and non-high-grade DCIS.[57,58]

Monitoring of treatment response

Neoadjuvant chemotherapy is increasingly being used to downstage primary breast cancers and axilla, which may potentially permit breast-conserving surgery or obviate the need for axillary dissection. DWI has been widely explored to predict tumor response and evaluate the efficacy of neoadjuvant chemotherapy. The supporting rationale is that chemotherapy-induced cytotoxic effects cause disruption of cell membrane and decrease cellularity of the tumor, resulting in less diffusion restriction and higher ADC values. Studies in women undergoing neoadjuvant treatment for breast cancer have shown that tumor ADC values usually increase in response to treatment and post-treatment ADC

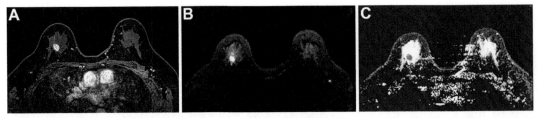

Fig. 5. Preoperative breast MR imaging in a 54-year-old woman with invasive ductal carcinoma. (*A*) Postcontrast T1-weighted DCE MR imaging shows an irregular heterogeneously enhancing mass in the right breast. (*B*) DWI with $b = 800$ s/mm^2 shows a mass with high signal intensity. (*C*) On ADC map, the minimum, maximum, and mean ADC values were 0.57×10^{-3} mm^2/s, 1.32×10^{-3} mm^2/s, and 0.81×10^{-3} mm^2/s, respectively. The ADC heterogeneity* value was 0.93. Breast-conserving surgery was performed and the pathologic findings showed 1.6 cm invasive ductal carcinoma with a histologic grade of 3 that was ER-negative, PR-negative, and HER2-negative (triple negative breast cancer). *ADC heterogeneity was calculated using the following formula: (ADC$_{max}$ − ADC $_{min}$)/ADC $_{mean}$.

measurement could be used to evaluate residual disease.[59] Predicting a pathologic complete response (pCR) is essential for tailoring therapies because patients achieving a pCR (defined as no residual invasive cancer in the breast and/or axillary lymph nodes) experience improved overall and disease-free survival outcomes, making pCR a useful short-term surrogate for therapeutic efficacy.[60] The change in ADC value after treatment has been reported to be greater in patients with pCR versus non-pCR outcomes.[61–63] Multiple meta-analyses have reported the sensitivity and specificity of DWI in predicting therapeutic response (pCR or near-pCR) as 88%–93% (95% CI, 0.53–0.99) and 72%–85% (95% CI, 0.68–0.94), respectively.[59,64,65] Change in tumor ADC value may predict pCR early in the course of treatment, offering opportunity to adjust preoperative treatment strategies (**Fig. 6**). Notably, the American College of Radiology Imaging Network 6698, the first, large-scale, multicenter trial of breast DWI for monitoring therapy demonstrated that an increase in breast tumor ADC on DWI performed at mid-treatment (12 weeks) of chemotherapy could predict a pCR to neoadjuvant chemotherapy,[61] with predictive value varying by tumor subtype. Data from another large multicenter study showed early change in tumor ADC, even after the first cycle (3 weeks) of treatment, is predictive of pathologic response both for standard chemotherapy regimens and newer immunotherapy-based regimens.[66] Some studies have also suggested that pretreatment ADC values may help to identify tumors more likely to respond to treatment,[62,67,68] but mixed results have been reported regarding the value of pretreatment ADC in predicting pCR.[61,69–71]

Before translating the study results into real practice for guiding treatment, there are some issues that need to be considered. Considerable variabilities in DWI acquisition techniques, timing of follow-up examinations, ADC measurement

methods, treatment regimens, definition of pCR, as well as biological heterogeneity due to various tumor subtypes across the studies may cause variability in performance of DWI for predicting pCR and hamper successful clinical implementation of DWI.[72] Further multicenter clinical trials are warranted to validate ADC as a biomarker for monitoring of treatment response.

Axillary lymph node metastasis

Axillary lymph node metastasis is one of the most powerful prognostic factors in patients with breast cancer and prediction of axillary nodal status before surgery could help in the choice of therapeutic strategies. Many studies have investigated the associations between nodal status of breast cancer and ADC values of primary tumor and axillary lymph node. Based on direct lymph node ADC measurement, a meta-analysis reported pooled sensitivity and specificity of DWI in differentiating between metastatic and nonmetastatic axillary lymph node of 83% (95% CI, 80%–86%) and 82% (95% CI, 79%–85%).[73] These values are comparable to the reported sensitivity of 74% (95% CI, 70%–78%) and 88% (95% CI, 84%–91%), but lower than the specificity of 82% and 100% of ultrasound-guided fine-needle aspiration and core-needle biopsy, respectively.[74] However, negative results were also reported; among morphologically suspicious axillary lymph nodes identified on breast MR imaging, ADC measurement showed little value in discriminating between malignant and benign outcomes or improving accuracy over conventional morphologic assessment.[75]

Studies regarding the associations of primary tumor ADC with axillary nodal status produced mixed outcomes, with generally lower ADC values in breast cancer with positive lymph node status than with negative lymph node status (**Fig. 7**).[39,46,47,76] A recent meta-analysis of 23 different studies including

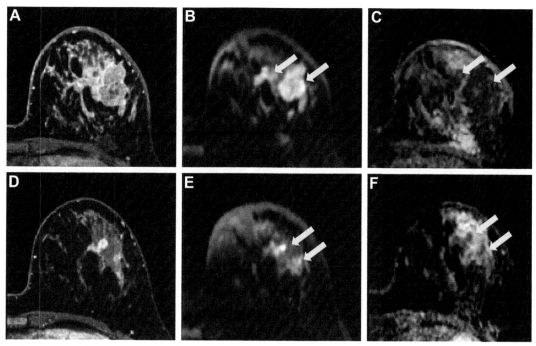

Fig. 6. Example of response to neoadjuvant chemotherapy treatment observed on DWI. MR images in a 31-year-old woman with grade 3, triple negative (estrogen receptor [ER]-/progesterone receptor[PR]-/human epidermal growth factor receptor 2 [HER2]-) invasive ductal carcinoma. (*A–C*) Prior to treatment, postcontrast T1-weighted DCE image (*A*) shows multiple similar appearing adjacent irregular masses spanning 72 mm in the left breast corresponding to the biopsy-proven cancer. (*B*) On DWI (*b* = 800 s/mm^2), the tumor region is hyperintense to adjacent breast tissue (*arrows*). (*C*) ADC map shows low diffusivity in the tumor (ADC = 1.16×10^{-3} mm^2/s) (*arrows*). (*D–F*) Mid-treatment (8 weeks, after 4 dose-dense cycles of doxorubicin-cyclophosphamide (AC) chemotherapy), postcontrast T1-weighted DCE image (*D*) shows reduction in primary tumor size to 54 mm total extent. (*B*) On DWI (*b* = 800 s/mm^2), areas of the tumor region remain hyperintense to adjacent breast tissue (*arrows*). (*C*) ADC map indicates increased lesion diffusivity in the remaining tumor (ADC = 1.63×10^{-3} mm^2/s) (*arrows*) versus pre-treatment values. At the end of neoadjuvant treatment, the patient underwent mastectomy and pathologic assessment revealed no residual invasive disease indicating a pathologic complete response.

1669 breast cancers and 1423 axillary lymph nodes (876 benign and 547 malignant) demonstrated the mean ADC values of metastatic axillary lymph nodes to be lower than benign nodes (0.90×10^{-3} mm^2/s and 1.17×10^{-3} mm^2/s, respectively), and the mean ADC of primary tumors was lower for those with positive versus negative nodal status (0.89×10^{-3} mm^2/s and 0.96×10^{-3} mm^2/s, respectively). The authors suggest ADC values of both axillary lymph node and primary tumor may help predict axillary nodal status of breast cancer.[52]

Overall, more studies are still needed to determine the role and optimal interpretation strategy of DWI in axillary lymph node staging in breast cancer.

Potential surrogate marker for recurrence

The Oncotype DX genomic assay provides prognostic information for 10-year risk of distant recurrence in women with ER-positive, lymph node–negative breast cancer treated with tamoxifen.[77] Quantitative ADC values have been proposed as potential markers for recurrence risk stratified using Oncotype DX recurrence score, and several studies have reported ADC values in lesions at high risk for recurrence to be lower than those at low and intermediate risk.[78–80] Furthermore, intratumor microstructural heterogeneity reflected on DWI may be a hallmark of more aggressive disease at increased risk for recurrence. One study by Kim and colleagues analyzed tumor ADC parameters using whole-lesion histogram analysis, and the results showed that lower ADC difference value (a measure of intratumor heterogeneity, calculated as difference between the 5th and 95th percentiles of ADCs) was associated with a low risk of recurrence of breast cancer in women with ER-positive, HER2-negative, node-negative breast cancer who underwent the Oncotype DX assay.[80] Similarly, another retrospective study involving 258 patients with

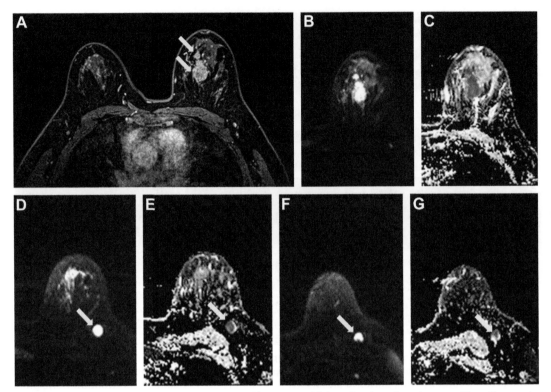

Fig. 7. Example breast DWI obtained in a 42-year-old woman with invasive ductal carcinoma with axillary metastasis. (*A*) Postcontrast T1-weighted DCE MR imaging shows 2 irregular enhancing masses in the left breast (*arrows*). (*B, C*) The breast lesions exhibit restricted diffusion on DWI ($b = 800$ s/mm^2; *B*) with low ADC (*C*). (*D–G*) Multiple abnormal level 1 axillary lymph nodes exhibit reduced diffusivity on DWI, appearing hyperintense on the $b = 800$ s/mm^2 images (*arrows, D, F*) and hypointense on the corresponding ADC maps (*arrows, E, G*).

invasive breast cancers found the ADC difference value (calculated as the difference between minimum and maximum ADCs) was higher in women with distant metastasis than in those without distant metastasis and a higher ADC difference value ($>0.698 \times 10^{-3}$ mm^2/s) was associated with poorer distant-metastasis-free survival at multivariate analysis (adjusted HR, 4.5; $P < .001$).[81]

Although the results aforementioned have been obtained from a single-center and/or small-sized cohorts with retrospective study design, the potential role of DWI as a prognostic biomarker for breast cancer is promising and remains an active area of research.

Diffusion-Weighted MR Imaging as a Stand-Alone Unenhanced Approach

Unenhanced MR imaging for breast cancer screening

Considering the inherent limitations of DCE MR imaging (gadolinium-related safety concerns, long scan time, high cost), DWI presents a compelling alternative tool for supplemental screening in women with elevated breast cancer risk. Preliminary studies suggest unenhanced MR imaging with DWI holds promise in detecting and discriminating MR imaging-detected mammographically occult breast cancer. In a study of 118 mammographically and clinically occult breast lesions (sizes ranging from 0.4 – 5.5 cm, median, 1.1 cm), 89% of the DCE MR imaging-detected mammographically occult breast cancers could be detected on DWI.[82] Also, benign and malignant lesions could be discriminated by ADC measures and the diagnostic performances of DWI were 96% sensitivity, 55% specificity, 39% positive predictive value, and 98% negative predictive value for an ADC threshold of 1.60×10^{-3} mm^2/s. Another study investigated the relative visibility of mammographically occult breast cancer on DWI compared to ultrasound and the results showed that more cancers were visible on DWI than targeted ultrasound (78% vs 63%; $P = .049$).[83] However, in these aforementioned studies, the readers were not blinded to DCE MR imaging images for DWI or ultrasound interpretations but guided by the lesion location on DCE MR imaging, which limits ability to adequately assess the relative performance of DWI for supplemental screening.

Diffusion-weighted imaging performance in breast cancer detection

Many blinded DWI reader studies have been conducted to evaluate the performance of DWI for non-contrast cancer detection in clinical setting. Readers assessed DWI with or without T1-or T2-weighted images in these studies, which demonstrated that the sensitivity of DWI ranges between 45% and 94%, and specificity between 79% and 95%.[84–88] When the performance of DWI for stand-alone breast cancer detection was compared with other imaging modalities, the sensitivity and/or accuracy of DWI was reported to be higher than that of mammography[88,89] and combined mammography and ultrasound,[90] lower than that of DCE MR imaging,[87,88,91,92] and comparable to abbreviated MR imaging.[84] Notably, a wide range of reported performance of DWI among the prior studies may be due to the differences in study population as well as acquisition protocols. The lowest sensitivity of 45% was reported by McDonald et al., likely due to the focus on only mammographically and clinically occult cancers, and also that DWI was obtained using a relatively low b-value (600 s/mm^2) limiting lesion contrast-to-noise.[85] In a reader study of 343 asymptomatic patients with personal history of breast cancer, fused DWI using T1-weighted imaging with DWI maximum-intensity projection (obtained at b-value of 1000 s/mm^2) showed sensitivities of 89%–100% and specificities of 93%–95% across readers.[84] Although promising results have been obtained in the blinded reader studies, evidence from large prospective multicenter studies using standardized DWI protocols is needed to facilitate the clinical use of DWI for breast cancer screening. Currently, prospective clinical trials are ongoing to investigate the role of DWI in screening high-risk women (NCT03835897) or women with dense breasts (NCT03607552), using standardized and optimized DW MR imaging protocols.

False-negative findings on diffusion-weighted imaging

Examples of frequently missed or misinterpreted lesions on DWI include DCIS, small breast cancers (<10–12 mm), nonmass enhancement lesions, and tumors with high water content (ie, mucinous carcinomas, triple-negative breast cancer with significant necrosis), as shown in **Figs. 8** and **9**.

DCIS, which commonly presents as nonmass enhancement on MR imaging, constitutes 18% to 25% of the total number of newly diagnosed breast cancers,[93] and screening-detected breast cancers are more often tumors of smaller size.[94] To improve the diagnostic performance of noncontrast MR imaging screening for breast cancer, these particular false-negatives should be addressed. Fortunately, there are a number of technologic advancements that may overcome current image quality shortcomings of DWI and improve sensitivity. It is reported that emerging DWI techniques such as multishot echo-planar imaging acquisitions, reduced field-of-view echo-planar imaging, and simultaneous multislice imaging could help to detect smaller features by both improving the image quality and spatial resolution.[95]

Image Analysis of Diffusion-Weighted Imaging

Quantitative apparent diffusion coefficient analysis

DWI assessment includes both qualitative interpretation of DWI for lesion detection and quantitative measurement of ADC for lesion characterization. Areas of restricted diffusion demonstrate higher signal intensity on high b-value DWI that is distinct from background signal, and lower signal intensity on ADC map. After visual inspection of high b-value DWI and ADC map, an ADC value of the suspicious breast lesion should be measured. In general, tumor ADC values are measured by manually placing a ROI on the ADC map. When placing a ROI, care should be taken to avoid surrounding normal breast tissues or fat, hemorrhagic or necrotic parts of the lesion, and artifacts. As the methodology for ADC measurement in breast lesions has not been standardized and established, different ROI placement methods have been used for quantitative ADC analysis. Hence, the cut-off values of ADC to discriminate malignant from benign breast lesion may differ based on the measurement methods, which should be recognized when comparing the results from the literature. The most common methods of ROI placement are whole lesion ROI and focused ROI placement. Whole lesion ROI is drawn as large as possible to encompass the entire cross section of the lesion, while focused ROI (or 'hot-spot') is applied to the most restricting portion of the lesion, identified as the darkest tumor region on the ADC map. It has been shown that ROI size and positioning could significantly affect ADC values and reproducibility.[28,96,97] Bickel and colleagues reported that a small ROI method (ie, focused ROI) in a single-slice had better diagnostic performance than a large ROI in a single-slice or 3-dimensional ROI in multiple slices.[96] However, in other studies, the focused ROI method to sample the lowest ADC did not show higher performance in differentiating between benign and malignant breast lesions.[98,99] In the ACRIN 6698 multicenter trial, whole tumor ADC method was used for the ADC quantification[61] and its excellent reproducibility

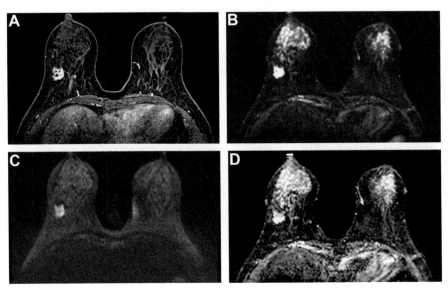

Fig. 8. Example of common false-negative finding on DWI. MR images in a 63-year-old woman with mucinous carcinoma. (*A*) Postcontrast T1-weighted DCE MR imaging shows an irregular heterogeneously mass in the right breast. (*B, C*) On DWI with $b = 0$ s/mm^2 and $b = 1000$ s/mm^2, the mass is hyperintense (*D*) but also exhibits very high ADC (ADC $= 2.01 \times 10^{-3}$ mm^2/s); ADC map was calculated using b values 0, 1000 s/mm^2.

was reported in a study by Newitt and colleagues[27] In clinical practice, the multisection whole tumor ROI method is less feasible as it is time-consuming and needs a dedicated software tool, although new tools to automate the measure would make this a more viable approach. Recently, the EUSOBI DWI working group suggests the use of focused ROI as the preferred method for ADC measurement because it may reduce inter-reader and intra-reader variability.[17] A better understanding of the potential effects from quantification methods on ADC measures would facilitate clinical interpretation of breast DWI.

Background diffusion signal

The signal intensity of normal breast parenchymal tissues on high b-value DWI, termed "background diffusion signal," may vary individually in terms of degree and distribution. It can be visually assessed according to the 4-point scale of minimum, mild, moderate, and marked (**Fig. 10**),[100] similar to background parenchymal enhancement on DCE MR imaging. The associations between background diffusion signals and breast cancer detection have been reported.[101,102] In a recent blind-reader study involving 316 breast cancer patients, the degree of background diffusion signal was scored as follows: minimal in 114 patients (36.1%), mild in 115 (36.4%), moderate in 52 (16.5%), and marked in 35 (11.1%). The results showed that a higher (moderate/marked) degree of background diffusion signal was associated with increased false-negative results in the diagnosis of invasive breast cancer using fused high b-value DWI and unenhanced T1-weighted imaging,[101] which supports previous results showing that high background parenchymal

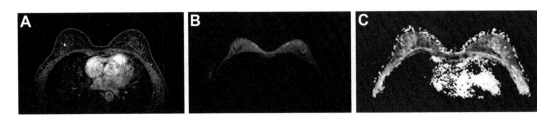

Fig. 9. Example of common false-negative finding on DWI. MR images in a 60-year-old woman with small invasive breast cancer. (*A*) Postcontrast T1-weighted DCE image shows a 5 mm lobulated enhancing mass in the right breast. (*B*) On DWI ($b = 1000$ s/mm^2), the lesion is isointense to adjacent breast tissue and exhibits low signal contrast. (*C*) ADC map shows no abnormal signal intensity in the corresponding lesion; ADC map was calculated using b values 0, 1000 s/mm^2.

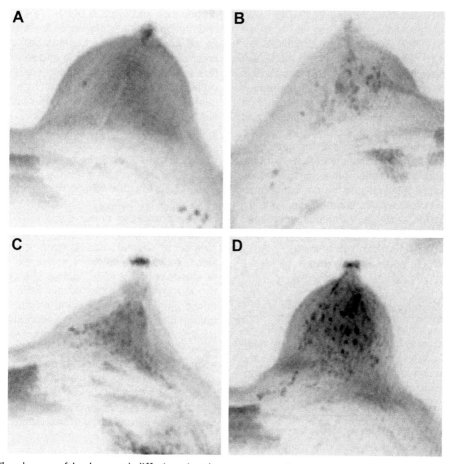

Fig. 10. The degree of background diffusion signals on DWI. Maximum intensity projection (MIP) diffusion-weighted images in 4 different women show varying degrees of background diffusion signal: (*A*) minimal, (*B*) mild, (*C*) moderate, and (*D*) marked. Note: MIPs are displayed using inverted grayscale technique where highest signal is black and lowest signal is white, which is sometimes preferred for clarity.

enhancement was a factor in false-negative MR imaging interpretation.[103]

EMERGING ALTERNATIVE NON-CONTRAST MR IMAGING TECHNIQUES
Simulated Contrast-Enhanced MRI

Recent studies have investigated artificial intelligence (AI) applications to reduce the amount of contrast media needed for breast DCE MR imaging.[104,105] With use of deep learning, simulated contrast-enhanced T1-weighted MR imaging scans were generated from precontrast MR imaging sequences in patients with breast cancer and simulated MR imaging scans were quantitatively similar to real contrast-enhanced MR imaging scans, with a high mean structural similarity index (0.88 ± 0.05).[105] Additional studies are warranted to investigate the potential role of simulated contrast-enhanced MR imaging in breast cancer screening.

Magnetic Resonance Spectroscopy

A variety of other commercially available non-contrast MR imaging techniques have been explored for breast imaging, but remain further away from clinical integration. Perhaps the most well-studied is proton magnetic resonance (MR) spectroscopy (^{1}H-MRS), a noninvasive technique for investigation of tissue metabolism. Rather than images, MRS techniques produce spatially localized signal spectra, with spectral peaks representing the structure and concentration of different chemical compounds in that region. Proton MRS studies have shown that breast cancers typically exhibit elevated levels of the metabolite choline, which is thought to be a marker of cell proliferation. MRS holds potential primarily as an adjunct tool to conventional breast MR imaging, where choline measures have shown value as a marker of malignancy and for evaluating response to therapy.[106] For evaluating suspicious breast lesions, MRS sensitivity ranges 71%–74% with specificity of 78%–88%, comparing well to those reported for DWI (84%–91% and 75%–84%, respectively.)[107] Both single voxel and multivoxel (ie, MR Spectroscopic Imaging [MRSI]) techniques are possible (**Fig. 11**)[108]; MRSI offers advantages of higher spatial resolution and wider breast coverage, but is more technically challenging and less widely used. Despite promising diagnostic performance, there are several obstacles to routine clinical use of MRS of the breast, including (i) relatively long acquisition times, (ii) low sensitivity for choline detection and frequent data quality issues, (iii) challenging standardization, and (iv) requirement for accurate voxel placement and high-quality shimming during acquisition, necessitating additional technologist training.[109] As a result, MRS currently remains more or less a research tool.

Magnetic Resonance Elastography

Magnetic resonance elastography (MRE) is another emerging non-contrast MR imaging technique that is widely used for liver assessment and has also shown promise for breast cancer diagnosis and characterization. MRE quantitatively interrogates the mechanical properties of tissue, which can provide important insights into tissue disease status, as changes in the composition and cytoarchitecture of tissue often accompany disease progression. In MRE, a mechanical driver is used on the surface of the patient's body to generate tissue penetrating shear waves while an MR imaging acquisition sequence measures the propagation and velocity of the waves. From this information, tissue stiffness and elasticity maps (ie, elastograms) can be quantitatively derived. In preliminary studies, MRE has shown promise for use in multiparametric imaging assessment of breast disease generally based on higher stiffness (perhaps reflecting collagen deposition) associated with malignancy (**Fig. 12**).[110] However, some subtypes of malignancies, including those with more aggressive features, have been shown to exhibit more "liquid-like behavior" and so stiffness alone may not be a reliable characteristic of malignancy. In a study of suspicious breast lesions in 43 patients, Balleyguier and colleagues found MRE viscosity and phase angle were increased in malignant lesions and that phase angle, a combination of several viscoelastic properties of lesions, could more reliably improve the specificity of standard breast MR imaging.[111] More work is needed to determine the value of MRE as a prognostic biomarker in malignant lesions, for monitoring therapy, and for non-contrast cancer detection. There is also interest to assess the relationship between breast density and MRE-based stiffness as a possible novel indicator of breast cancer risk. Developing technical advancements for MRE acquisition to improve spatial resolution and decrease scan time will facilitate further exploration of the clinical utility of this technique.[110]

Other Non-contrast MR Techniques

There are a variety of other functional MR imaging approaches at earlier stages of development that have shown promise for advancing breast cancer

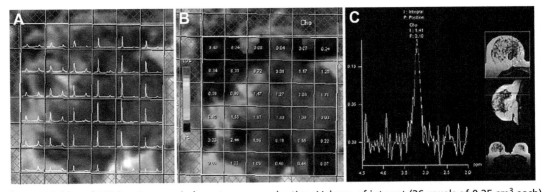

Fig. 11. Multivoxel MR Spectroscopy in breast cancer evaluation. Volume of interest (36 voxels of 0.25 cm³ each) centered on an invasive lobular carcinoma in the right breast of a 67-year-old patient and spectral map showing intense water and minor fat peaks in the lesion (*A*). This array of unsuppressed spectra is shown for the chemical shift range of 0 to 6 ppm. After application of water and fat suppression intense, Cho signals are detected in the whole lesion as shown in green on the metabolic map (*B*). The highest detected Cho level (the red voxel on the metabolic map) is used for quantification. The sum of all tumor MR spectra together is shown in (*C*) where the fit for Cho is shown in red (range 2–4.5 ppm). (Figure reprinted from Dorrius MD, Pijnappel RM, van der Weide Jansen MC, et al. The added value of quantitative multi-voxel MR spectroscopy in breast magnetic resonance imaging. Eur Radiol. 2012;22:915-22.)

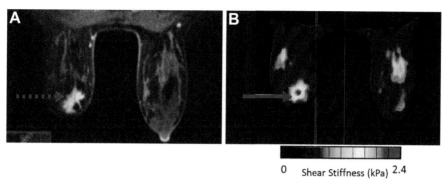

0   Shear Stiffness (kPa) 2.4

Fig. 12. MR elastography (MRE) of the breast. A 41-year-old female with biopsy-proven invasive ductal carcinoma. (A) Post-contrast axial image demonstrates an irregular enhancing mass (*dashed arrow*) in the right retro-areolar region, compatible with biopsy-proven malignancy. (B) MREstiffness values were calculated within the mass, in the surrounding fibroglandular tissue, as well as the adipose tissue. Color maps demonstrate stiffness in various parts of the breast bilaterally. Stiffness in adipose tissue was measured as 0.41 ± 0.10 kPa, stiffness in glandular tissue was measured as 0.90 ± 0.18 kPa, and stiffness in the invasive ductal carcinoma (*solid arrow*) was measured as 1.42 ± 0.17 kPa. (Figure reprinted from Patel BK, Samreen N, Zhou Y, et al. MR Elastography of the Breast: Evolution of Technique, Case Examples, and Future Directions. *Clin Breast Cancer*. 2021;21:e102-e111, with permission from Elsevier.)

detection and characterization in preliminary investigations. These include ^{23}Na (sodium)-MR imaging reflecting altered cellular metabolism associated with disease initiation and progression,[112] chemical exchange saturation transfer , a molecular imaging technique enabling detection of biomolecules in vivo,[113] arterial spin labeling for non-contrast perfusion imaging,[114] and high spectral and spatial imaging for mapping variations in breast tissue composition based on features of water and fat resonance spectra,[115,116] which for now remain less widely available and beyond the scope of this review.

SUMMARY

DWI has wide clinical applications as a non-contrast tool for breast imaging. As a supplement to DCE MR imaging, DWI could help in diagnosis and characterization of breast cancer, prediction of treatment response, and evaluation of axillary nodal status. DWI could also serve as a potential prognostic biomarker for breast cancer. As a stand-alone unenhanced modality, DWI has shown promise in detecting and differentiating mammographically occult breast cancer. DWI could serve as an alternative supplemental breast cancer screening tool with sensitivity lower than that of DCE MR imaging but superior to that of mammography. However, DWI has not been yet incorporated into BI-RADS. Standardized and optimized DWI protocols and interpretation are essential to further enhance the clinical applications of DWI for breast imaging and more data are needed to support these efforts. A variety of other non-

contrast MR imaging techniques are under investigation, but these have not yet gained much traction in breast imaging primarily due to technical complexities and limited availability slowing progress for clinical evaluation. Beyond novel acquisitions, AI-enhanced post-processing techniques show compelling potential to dramatically advance the utility of low-dose and non-contrast MR imaging for cancer detection, warranting further study.

CLINICS CARE POINTS

- A DWI approach might be potentially safer, more rapid, and less expensive than DCE MR imaging for clinical use.

- As an adjunct modality, DWI provides complementary information to DCE MR imaging and ADC measures show clear value in diagnosis and treatment of breast cancer.

- DWI holds potential to serve as an alternative supplemental breast cancer screening tool with sensitivity lower than that of DCE MR imaging but superior to that of mammography.

- Breast DWI needs standardization to be generalized and to enable reliable use of ADC measures in routine clinical practice.

DISCLOSURE

This work was supported in-part by National Institutes of Health grant R01CA207290.

REFERENCES

1. Peters NH, Borel Rinkes IH, Zuithoff NPA, et al. Meta-analysis of MR imaging in the diagnosis of breast lesions. Radiology 2008;246:116–24.

2. Saslow D, Boetes C, Burke W, et al. American Cancer Society guidelines for breast screening with MRI as an adjunct to mammography. CA: a cancer journal for clinicians 2007;57:75–89.

3. Kanda T, Fukusato T, Matsuda M, et al. Gadolinium-based contrast agent accumulates in the brain even in subjects without severe renal dysfunction: evaluation of autopsy brain specimens with inductively coupled plasma mass spectroscopy. Radiology 2015;276:228–32.

4. McDonald RJ, McDonald JS, Kallmes DF, et al. Intracranial gadolinium deposition after contrast-enhanced MR imaging. Radiology 2015;275:772–82.

5. McDonald JS, McDonald RJ. MR Imaging Safety Considerations of Gadolinium-Based Contrast Agents: Gadolinium Retention and Nephrogenic Systemic Fibrosis. Magn Reson Imaging Clin N Am 2020;28:497–507.

6. Stejskal EO, Tanner JE. Spin diffusion measurements: spin echoes in the presence of a time-dependent field gradient. J Chem Phys 1965;42: 288–92.

7. Partridge SC, McDonald ES. Diffusion Weighted Magnetic Resonance Imaging of the Breast: protocol optimization, interpretation, and clinical applications Magn Reson Imaging Clin N Am 2013;21: 601–24.

8. O'Flynn EA, Morgan VA, Giles SL, et al. Diffusion weighted imaging of the normal breast: reproducibility of apparent diffusion coefficient measurements and variation with menstrual cycle and menopausal status. Eur Radiol 2012;22:1512–8.

9. Partridge SC, McKinnon GC, Henry RG, et al. Menstrual cycle variation of apparent diffusion coefficients measured in the normal breast using MRI. J Magn Reson Imaging 2001;14:433–8.

10. Kim JY, Suh HB, Kang HJ, et al. Apparent diffusion coefficient of breast cancer and normal fibroglandular tissue in diffusion-weighted imaging: the effects of menstrual cycle and menopausal status. Breast Cancer Res Treat 2016;157:31–40.

11. Han X, Li J, Wang X. Comparison and Optimization of 3.0 T Breast Images Quality of Diffusion-Weighted Imaging with Multiple B-Values. Acad Radiol 2017;24:418–25.

12. Peters NH, Vincken KL, van den Bosch MA, et al. Quantitative diffusion weighted imaging for differentiation of benign and malignant breast lesions: the influence of the choice of b-values. J Magn Reson Imaging 2010;31:1100–5.

13. Tamura T, Murakami S, Naito K, et al. Investigation of the optimal b-value to detect breast tumors with diffusion weighted imaging by 1.5-T MRI. Cancer Imag 2014;14:11.

14. Nilsson M, Szczepankiewicz F, Van Westen D, et al. Extrapolation-Based References Improve Motion and Eddy-Current Correction of High B-Value DWI Data: Application in Parkinson's Disease Dementia. PLoS One 2015;10(11):e0141825.

15. Tang L, Zhou XJ. Diffusion MRI of cancer: From low to high b-values. J Magn Reson Imaging 2019;49: 23–40.

16. Bogner W, Gruber S, Pinker K, et al. Diffusion-weighted MR for differentiation of breast lesions at 3.0 T: how does selection of diffusion protocols affect diagnosis? Radiology 2009;253:341–51.

17. Baltzer P, Mann RM, Iima M, et al. Diffusion-weighted imaging of the breast-a consensus and mission statement from the EUSOBI International Breast Diffusion-Weighted Imaging working group. Eur Radiol 2020;30:1436–50.

18. Amornsiripanitch N, Bickelhaupt S, Shin HJ, et al. Diffusion-weighted MRI for Unenhanced Breast Cancer Screening. Radiology 2019;293:504–20.

19. DelPriore MR, Biswas D, Hippe DS, et al. Breast cancer conspicuity on computed versus acquired high b-value diffusion-weighted MRI. Acad Radiol 2021;28:1108–17.

20. Choi BH, Baek HJ, Ha JY, et al. Feasibility study of synthetic diffusion-weighted MRI in patients with breast cancer in comparison with conventional diffusion-weighted MRI. Korean J Radiol 2020;21: 1036–44.

21. Park MJ, Cha ES, Kang BJ, et al. The role of diffusion-weighted imaging and the apparent diffusion coefficient (ADC) values for breast tumors. Korean J Radiol 2007;8:390–6.

22. Suo S, Cheng F, Cao M, et al. Multiparametric diffusion-weighted imaging in breast lesions: Association with pathologic diagnosis and prognostic factors. J Magn Reson Imaging 2017;46:740–50.

23. Maric J, Boban J, Ivkovic-Kapicl T, et al. Differentiation of breast lesions and distinguishing their histological subtypes using diffusion-weighted imaging and ADC values. Front Oncol 2020;10:332.

24. Zhang L, Tang M, Min Z, et al. Accuracy of combined dynamic contrast-enhanced magnetic resonance imaging and diffusion-weighted imaging for breast cancer detection: a meta-analysis. Acta Radiol 2016;57:651–60.

25. Baxter GC, Graves MJ, Gilbert FJ, et al. A Meta-analysis of the Diagnostic Performance of Diffusion MRI for Breast Lesion Characterization. Radiology 2019;291:632–41.

26. Rahbar H, Zhang Z, Chenevert TL, et al. Utility of Diffusion-weighted Imaging to Decrease Unnecessary Biopsies Prompted by Breast MRI: A Trial of the ECOG-ACRIN Cancer Research Group (A6702). Clin Cancer Res 2019;25:1756–65.

27. Newitt DC, Zhang Z, Gibbs JE, et al. Test-retest repeatability and reproducibility of ADC measures by breast DWI: Results from the ACRIN 6698 trial. J Magn Reson Imaging 2019;49:1617–28.

28. Le NN, Li W, Onishi N, et al. Effect of inter-reader variability on diffusion-weighted MRI apparent diffusion coefficient measurements and prediction of pathologic complete response for breast cancer. Tomography 2022;8:1208–20.

29. Bickel H, Clauser P, Pinker K, et al. Introduction of a breast apparent diffusion coefficient category system (ADC-B) derived from a large multicenter MRI database. Eur Radiol 2023;33:5400–10.

30. Bickel H, Pinker-Domenig K, Bogner W, et al. Quantitative apparent diffusion coefficient as a noninvasive imaging biomarker for the differentiation of invasive breast cancer and ductal carcinoma in situ. Invest Radiol 2015;50:95–100.

31. Choi SY, Chang YW, Park HJ, et al. Correlation of the apparent diffusion coefficiency values on diffusion-weighted imaging with prognostic factors for breast cancer. Br J Radiol 2012;85:e474–9.

32. Lee SA, Lee Y, Ryu HS, et al. Diffusion-weighted breast MRI in prediction of upstaging in women with biopsy-proven ductal carcinoma in situ. Radiology 2022;305:307–16.

33. Cheeney S, Rahbar H, Dontchos BN, et al. Apparent diffusion coefficient values may help predict which MRI-detected high-risk breast lesions will upgrade at surgical excision. J Magn Reson Imaging 2017;46:1028–36.

34. Mori N, Ota H, Mugikura S, et al. Detection of invasive components in cases of breast ductal carcinoma in situ on biopsy by using apparent diffusion coefficient MR parameters. Eur Radiol 2013;23:2705–12.

35. Hussein SA, EL-Dhurani S, Abdelnaby Y, et al. High-risk breast lesions: role of multi-parametric DCE-MRI in detection and histopathological upgrade prediction. Egyptian Journal of Radiology and Nuclear Medicine 2022;53:1–12.

36. Costantini M, Belli P, Rinaldi P, et al. Diffusion-weighted imaging in breast cancer: relationship between apparent diffusion coefficient and tumour aggressiveness. Clin Radiol 2010;65:1005–12.

37. Cipolla V, Santucci D, Guerrieri D, et al. Correlation between 3 T apparent diffusion coefficient values and grading of invasive breast carcinoma. Eur J Radiol 2014;83:2144–50.

38. Shin JK, Kim JY. Dynamic contrast-enhanced and diffusion-weighted MRI of estrogen receptor-positive invasive breast cancers: Associations between quantitative MR parameters and Ki-67 proliferation status. J Magn Reson Imaging 2017; 45:94–102.

39. Razek AA, Gaballa G, Denewer A, et al. Invasive ductal carcinoma: correlation of apparent diffusion coefficient value with pathological prognostic factors. NMR Biomed 2010;23:619–23.

40. Mori N, Ota H, Mugikura S, et al. Luminal-type breast cancer: correlation of apparent diffusion coefficients with the Ki-67 labeling index. Radiology 2015;274:66–73.

41. Shen L, Zhou G, Tong T, et al. ADC at 3.0 T as a noninvasive biomarker for preoperative prediction of Ki67 expression in invasive ductal carcinoma of breast. Clin Imaging 2018;52:16–22.

42. Surov A, Clauser P, Chang YW, et al. Can diffusion-weighted imaging predict tumor grade and expression of Ki-67 in breast cancer? A multicenter analysis. Breast Cancer Res 2018;20:58.

43. Mori N, Mugikura S, Takasawa C, et al. Peritumoral apparent diffusion coefficients for prediction of lymphovascular invasion in clinically node-negative invasive breast cancer. Eur Radiol 2016; 26:331–9.

44. Durando M, Gennaro L, Cho GY, et al. Quantitative apparent diffusion coefficient measurement obtained by 3.0 Tesla MRI as a potential noninvasive marker of tumor aggressiveness in breast cancer. Eur J Radiol 2016;85:1651–8.

45. Igarashi T, Furube H, Ashida H, et al. Breast MRI for prediction of lymphovascular invasion in breast cancer patients with clinically negative axillary lymph nodes. Eur J Radiol 2018;107:111–8.

46. Kitajima K, Yamano T, Fukushima K, et al. Correlation of the SUVmax of FDG-PET and ADC values of diffusion-weighted MR imaging with pathologic prognostic factors in breast carcinoma. Eur J Radiol 2016;85:943–9.

47. Kim JY, Seo HB, Park S, et al. Early-stage invasive ductal carcinoma: Association of tumor apparent diffusion coefficient values with axillary lymph node metastasis. Eur J Radiol 2015;84:2137–43.

48. Kim EJ, Kim SH, Park GE, et al. Histogram analysis of apparent diffusion coefficient at 3.0 t: correlation with prognostic factors and subtypes of invasive ductal carcinoma. J Magn Reson Imaging 2015; 42:1666–78.

49. Jeh SK, Kim SH, Kim HS, et al. Correlation of the apparent diffusion coefficient value and dynamic magnetic resonance imaging findings with prognostic factors in invasive ductal carcinoma. J Magn Reson Imaging 2011;33:102–9.

50. Horvat JV, Bernard-Davila B, Helbich TH, et al. Diffusion-weighted imaging (DWI) with apparent diffusion coefficient (ADC) mapping as a quantitative imaging biomarker for prediction of immuno-histochemical receptor status, proliferation rate, and molecular subtypes of breast cancer. J Magn Reson Imaging 2019;50:836–46.

51. Suo S, Zhang D, Cheng F, et al. Added value of mean and entropy of apparent diffusion coefficient values for evaluating histologic phenotypes of

invasive ductal breast cancer with MR imaging. Eur Radiol 2019;29:1425–34.

52. Meyer HJ, Wienke A, Surov A. Diffusion weighted imaging to predict nodal status in breast cancer: A systematic review and meta-analysis. Breast J 2021;27:495–8.

53. Wang Q, Mao N, Liu M, et al. Radiomic analysis on magnetic resonance diffusion weighted image in distinguishing triple-negative breast cancer from other subtypes: a feasibility study. Clin Imaging 2021;72:136–41.

54. Kim JJ, Kim JY, Suh HB, et al. Characterization of breast cancer subtypes based on quantitative assessment of intratumoral heterogeneity using dynamic contrast-enhanced and diffusion-weighted magnetic resonance imaging. Eur Radiol 2022; 32(2):822–33.

55. Iima M, Le Bihan D, Okumura R, et al. Apparent diffusion coefficient as an MR imaging biomarker of low-risk ductal carcinoma in situ: a pilot study. Radiology 2011;260:364–72.

56. Kim JY, Kim JJ, Lee JW, et al. Risk stratification of ductal carcinoma in situ using whole-lesion histogram analysis of the apparent diffusion coefficient. Eur Radiol 2019;29:485–93.

57. Rahbar H, Partridge SC, DeMartini WB, et al. In vivo assessment of ductal carcinoma in situ grade: a model incorporating dynamic contrast-enhanced and diffusion-weighted breast MR imaging parameters. Radiology 2012;263:374–82.

58. Rahbar H, Partridge SC, Eby PR, et al. Characterization of ductal carcinoma in situ on diffusion weighted breast MRI. Eur Radiol 2011;21:2011–9.

59. Gu YL, Pan SM, Ren J, et al. Role of Magnetic Resonance Imaging in Detection of Pathologic Complete Remission in Breast Cancer Patients Treated With Neoadjuvant Chemotherapy: A Meta-analysis. Clin Breast Cancer 2017;17:245–55.

60. Asselain B, Barlow W, Bartlett J, et al. Long-term outcomes for neoadjuvant versus adjuvant chemotherapy in early breast cancer: meta-analysis of individual patient data from ten randomised trials. Lancet Oncol 2018;19:27–39.

61. Partridge SC, Zhang Z, Newitt DC, et al. Diffusion-weighted MRI Findings Predict Pathologic Response in Neoadjuvant Treatment of Breast Cancer: The ACRIN 6698 Multicenter Trial. Radiology 2018;289:618–27.

62. Shin HJ, Baek HM, Ahn JH, et al. Prediction of pathologic response to neoadjuvant chemotherapy in patients with breast cancer using diffusion-weighted imaging and MRS. NMR Biomed 2012; 25:1349–59.

63. Sharma U, Danishad KKA, Seenu V, et al. Longitudinal study of the assessment by MRI and diffusion-weighted imaging of tumor response in patients with locally advanced breast cancer undergoing neoadjuvant chemotherapy. NMR Biomed 2009;22:104–13.

64. Gao W, Guo N, Dong T. Diffusion-weighted imaging in monitoring the pathological response to neoadjuvant chemotherapy in patients with breast cancer: a meta-analysis. World J Surg Oncol 2018; 16:145.

65. Chu W, Jin W, Liu D, et al. Diffusion-weighted imaging in identifying breast cancer pathological response to neoadjuvant chemotherapy: a meta-analysis. Oncotarget 2018;9:7088.

66. Li W, Le NN, Onishi N, et al. Diffusion-Weighted MRI for Predicting Pathologic Complete Response in Neoadjuvant Immunotherapy. Cancers 2022;14: 4436.

67. Park SH, Moon WK, Cho N, et al. Diffusion-weighted MR imaging: pretreatment prediction of response to neoadjuvant chemotherapy in patients with breast cancer. Radiology 2010;257:56–63.

68. Richard R, Thomassin I, Chapellier M, et al. Diffusion-weighted MRI in pretreatment prediction of response to neoadjuvant chemotherapy in patients with breast cancer. Eur Radiol 2013;23: 2420–31.

69. Woodhams R, Kakita S, Hata H, et al. Identification of residual breast carcinoma following neoadjuvant chemotherapy: diffusion-weighted imaging—comparison with contrast-enhanced MR imaging and pathologic findings. Radiology 2010;254:357–66.

70. Fangberget A, Nilsen L, Hole KH, et al. Neoadjuvant chemotherapy in breast cancer-response evaluation and prediction of response to treatment using dynamic contrast-enhanced and diffusion-weighted MR imaging. Eur Radiol 2011;21: 1188–99.

71. Li W, Newitt DC, Wilmes LJ, et al. Additive value of diffusion-weighted MRI in the I-SPY 2 TRIAL. J Magn Reson Imaging 2019;50:1742–53.

72. van der Hoogt KJ, Schipper RJ, Winter-Warnars GA, et al. Factors affecting the value of diffusion-weighted imaging for identifying breast cancer patients with pathological complete response on neoadjuvant systemic therapy: a systematic review. Insights Imaging 2021;12:187.

73. Xing H, Song C-I, Li W-j. Meta analysis of lymph node metastasis of breast cancer patients: clinical value of DWI and ADC value. Eur J Radiol 2016;85: 1132–7.

74. Balasubramanian I, Fleming C, Corrigan M, et al. Meta-analysis of the diagnostic accuracy of ultrasound-guided fine-needle aspiration and core needle biopsy in diagnosing axillary lymph node metastasis. Br J Surg 2018;105:1244–53.

75. Rahbar H, Conlin JL, Parsian S, et al. Suspicious Axillary Lymph Nodes Identified on Clinical Breast MRI in Patients Newly Diagnosed with Breast Cancer. Acad Radiol 2015;22:430–8.

76. Kato F, Kudo K, Yamashita H, et al. Predicting metastasis in clinically negative axillary lymph nodes with minimum apparent diffusion coefficient value in luminal A-like breast cancer. Breast cancer 2019;26:628–36.

77. Paik S, Shak S, Tang G, et al. A multigene assay to predict recurrence of tamoxifen-treated, node-negative breast cancer. N Engl J Med 2004;351:2817–26.

78. Amornsiripanitch N, Nguyen VT, Rahbar H, et al. Diffusion-weighted MRI characteristics associated with prognostic pathological factors and recurrence risk in invasive ER+/HER2- breast cancers. J Magn Reson Imaging 2018;48:226–36.

79. Thakur SB, Durando M, Milans S, et al. Apparent diffusion coefficient in estrogen receptor-positive and lymph node-negative invasive breast cancers at 3.0 T DW-MRI: A potential predictor for an oncotype Dx test recurrence score. J Magn Reson Imaging 2018;47:401–9.

80. Kim JY, Kim JJ, Hwangbo L, et al. Diffusion-weighted MRI of estrogen receptor-positive, HER2-negative, node-negative breast cancer: association between intratumoral heterogeneity and recurrence risk. Eur Radiol 2020;30:66–76.

81. Kim JY, Kim JJ, Hwangbo L, et al. Diffusion-weighted imaging of invasive breast cancer: relationship to distant metastasis–free survival. Radiology 2019;291:300–7.

82. Partridge SC, Demartini WB, Kurland BF, et al. Differential diagnosis of mammographically and clinically occult breast lesions on diffusion-weighted MRI. J Magn Reson Imaging 2010;31:562–70.

83. Amornsiripanitch N, Rahbar H, Kitsch AE, et al. Visibility of mammographically occult breast cancer on diffusion-weighted MRI versus ultrasound. Clin Imaging 2018;49:37–43.

84. Kang JW, Shin HJ, Shin KC, et al. Unenhanced magnetic resonance screening using fused diffusion-weighted imaging and maximum-intensity projection in patients with a personal history of breast cancer: role of fused DWI for postoperative screening. Breast Cancer Res Treat 2017;165:119–28.

85. McDonald ES, Hammersley JA, Chou SH, et al. Performance of DWI as a Rapid Unenhanced Technique for Detecting Mammographically Occult Breast Cancer in Elevated-Risk Women With Dense Breasts. AJR Am J Roentgenol 2016;207:205–16.

86. Trimboli RM, Verardi N, Cartia F, et al. Breast cancer detection using double reading of unenhanced MRI including T1-weighted, T2-weighted STIR, and diffusion-weighted imaging: a proof of concept study. AJR Am J Roentgenol 2014;203:674–81.

87. Telegrafo M, Rella L, Ianora AAS, et al. Unenhanced breast MRI (STIR, T2-weighted TSE, DWIBS): An accurate and alternative strategy for detecting and differentiating breast lesions. Magn Reson Imaging 2015;33:951–5.

88. Yabuuchi H, Matsuo Y, Sunami S, et al. Detection of non-palpable breast cancer in asymptomatic women by using unenhanced diffusion-weighted and T2-weighted MR imaging: comparison with mammography and dynamic contrast-enhanced MR imaging. Eur Radiol 2011;21:11–7.

89. Kazama T, Kuroki Y, Kikuchi M, et al. Diffusion-weighted MRI as an adjunct to mammography in women under 50 years of age: An initial study. J Magn Reson Imaging 2012;36:139–44.

90. Ha SM, Chang JM, Lee SH, et al. Detection of contra-lateral breast cancer using diffusion-weighted magnetic resonance imaging in women with newly diagnosed breast cancer: comparison with combined mammography and whole-breast ultrasound. Korean J Radiol 2021;22:867–79.

91. Pinker K, Moy L, Sutton EJ, et al. Diffusion-Weighted Imaging With Apparent Diffusion Coefficient Mapping for Breast Cancer Detection as a Stand-Alone Parameter. Inves Radiol 2018;53:587–95.

92. Bu Y, Xia J, Joseph B, et al. Non-contrast MRI for breast screening: preliminary study on detectability of benign and malignant lesions in women with dense breasts. Breast Cancer Res Treat 2019;177:629–39.

93. Ward EM, DeSantis CE, Lin CC, et al. Cancer statistics: breast cancer in situ. CA: a cancer journal for clinicians 2015;65:481–95.

94. Welch HG, Prorok PC, O'Malley AJ, et al. Breast-cancer tumor size, overdiagnosis, and mammography screening effectiveness. N Engl J Med 2016;375:1438–47.

95. Amornsiripanitch N, Partridge S. Noncontrast MRI. Advances in magnetic resonance Technology and applications, vol. 5. Elsevier; 2022. p. 383–410.

96. Bickel H, Pinker K, Polanec S, et al. Diffusion-weighted imaging of breast lesions: Region-of-interest placement and different ADC parameters influence apparent diffusion coefficient values. Eur Radiol 2017;27:1883–92.

97. Giannotti E, Waugh S, Priba L, et al. Assessment and quantification of sources of variability in breast apparent diffusion coefficient (ADC) measurements at diffusion weighted imaging. Eur J Radiol 2015;84:1729–36.

98. Wielema M, Dorrius MD, Pijnappel RM, et al. Diagnostic performance of breast tumor tissue selection in diffusion weighted imaging: A systematic review and meta-analysis. PLoS One 2020;15:e0232856.

99. McDonald ES, Romanoff J, Rahbar H, et al. Mean Apparent Diffusion Coefficient Is a Sufficient Conventional Diffusion-weighted MRI Metric to Improve Breast MRI Diagnostic Performance: Results from the ECOG-ACRIN Cancer Research Group A6702 Diffusion Imaging Trial. Radiology 2021;298:60–70.

100. Lee SH, Shin HJ, Moon WK. Diffusion-Weighted Magnetic Resonance Imaging of the Breast: Standardization of Image Acquisition and Interpretation. Korean J Radiol 2021;22:9–22.

101. Kim JJ, Kim JY. Fusion of high b-value diffusion-weighted and unenhanced T1-weighted images to diagnose invasive breast cancer: factors associated with false-negative results. Eur Radiol 2021; 31:4860–71.

102. Hahn SY, Ko ES, Han BK, et al. Analysis of factors influencing the degree of detectability on diffusion-weighted MRI and diffusion background signals in patients with invasive breast cancer. Medicine (Baltim) 2016;95:e4086.

103. Uematsu T, Kasami M, Watanabe J. Does the degree of background enhancement in breast MRI affect the detection and staging of breast cancer? Eur Radiol 2011;21:2261–7.

104. Müller-Franzes G, Huck L, Tayebi Arasteh S, et al. Using machine learning to reduce the need for contrast agents in breast MRI through synthetic images. Radiology 2023;307:e222211.

105. Chung M, Calabrese E, Mongan J, et al. Deep learning to simulate contrast-enhanced breast MRI of invasive breast cancer. Radiology 2023; 306:e213199.

106. Fardanesh R, Marino MA, Avendano D, et al. Proton MR spectroscopy in the breast: Technical innovations and clinical applications. J Magn Reson Imaging 2019;50:1033–46.

107. Sardanelli F, Carbonaro LA, Montemezzi S, et al. Clinical breast MR using MRS or DWI: who is the winner? Front Oncol 2016;6:217.

108. Dorrius MD, Pijnappel RM, van der Weide Jansen MC, et al. The added value of quantitative multi-voxel MR spectroscopy in breast magnetic resonance imaging. Eur Radiol 2012;22:915–22.

109. Kazerouni AS, Dula AN, Jarrett AM, et al. Emerging techniques in breast MRI. Advances in Magnetic Resonance Technology and Applications 2022;5: 503–31.

110. Patel BK, Samreen N, Zhou Y, et al. MR Elastography of the Breast: Evolution of Technique, Case Examples, and Future Directions. Clin Breast Cancer 2021;21:e102–11.

111. Balleyguier C, Lakhdar AB, Dunant A, et al. Value of whole breast magnetic resonance elastography added to MRI for lesion characterization. NMR Biomed 2018;31:e3795.

112. Poku LO, Phil M, Cheng Y, et al. ^{23}Na-MRI as a Noninvasive Biomarker for Cancer Diagnosis and Prognosis. J Magn Reson Imaging 2021;53:995–1014.

113. Zhang S, Seiler S, Wang X, et al. CEST-Dixon for human breast lesion characterization at 3 T: A preliminary study. Magn Reson Med 2018;80:895–903.

114. Franklin SL, Voormolen N, Bones IK, et al. Feasibility of Velocity-Selective Arterial Spin Labeling in Breast Cancer Patients for Noncontrast-Enhanced Perfusion Imaging. J Magn Reson Imaging 2021; 54:1282–91.

115. Medved M, Fan X, Abe H, et al. Non-contrast enhanced MRI for evaluation of breast lesions: comparison of non-contrast enhanced high spectral and spatial resolution (HiSS) images versus contrast enhanced fat-suppressed images. Acad Radiol 2011;18:1467–74.

116. Medved M, Li H, Abe H, et al. Fast bilateral breast coverage with high spectral and spatial resolution (HiSS) MRI at 3T. J Magn Reson Imaging 2017; 46:1341–8.

Nonsurgical Management of High-Risk Lesions

Mariana Afonso Matias, MD, PG Cert Med Leadership, PG Cert Med Education,
Nisha Sharma, MBChB, MRCP, FRCR, MSc*

KEYWORDS

- High-risk lesions • Vacuum-assisted biopsy • Vacuum-assisted excision • Overdiagnosis
- Overtreatment

KEY POINTS

- High-risk lesions of the breast warrant further sampling due to the potential of upgrade to malignancy at the time of diagnosis.
- Vacuum-assisted excision is recognized as an acceptable alternative to surgery for managing high-risk lesions as per the United Kingdom and European Society of Breast Cancer Specialists (EUSOMA) guidelines.
- High-risk lesions are benign lesions, and it is recognized that we should minimize overtreatment by avoiding unnecessary benign surgical operations.

INTRODUCTION

Breast lesions that are routinely biopsied are histologically classified as B1—normal, through to B5—malignant, as per the United Kingdom pathology B-classification.[1] Although, most of these lesions can be definitively classified as normal, benign, or malignant, there is a proportion of lesions that based on their histologic heterogeneity are reported as B3—borderline or high-risk lesions.

High-risk lesions are defined as lesions of uncertain malignant potential with different increased risk of associated malignancy. These lesions are histologically categorized as B3 lesions based on their heterogenous morphology and behavior, and correspond to 7.9% of all breast lesions diagnosed in the United Kingdom.[1] Higher B3 rates have been reported in screening populations because of the use of new imaging techniques and increased availability of wide-bore vacuum-assisted needle biopsy techniques.[2,3] They are often identified as areas of calcification or small masses on screening mammography and are mostly asymptomatic.

This heterogeneous group include atypical intraductal epithelial proliferation (AIDEP); atypical ductal hyperplasia (ADH); classic lobular neoplasia (LN); flat epithelial atypia; radial scar (RS), with or without atypia; papillary lesion (PL), with and without atypia; cellular fibroepithelial lesion; phyllodes tumors; mucocele-like lesion; and spindle cell lesion.[3]

Their unifying characteristic is their low but significant risk of upgrade to malignancy. A meta-analysis reviewing the surgical management of B3 lesions showed an upgrade rate of 17% at excision.[4] Bianchi and colleagues conducted a multicentric study, including one of the largest series of nonpalpable breast lesions assessed with vacuum-assisted biopsy (VAB) with a B3 outcome, considering the prevalence and positive predictive value (PPV) on the surgical excision.[5] Their results showed a PPV of 21.2%, just below the average value from several other published studies, with upgrade rates ranging from 9.9% to 35.1%.[6,7]

The upgrade to malignancy is related to the heterogeneity of the lesion and is increased in the presence of cytologic ± architectural atypia. Griffiths and colleagues reported that up to 35.7% of atypia initially identified on needle biopsy is latter upgraded to malignancy on surgical excision.[8]

Breast Unit, Leeds Teaching Hospital NHS Trust, Level 1 Chancellor Wing, St James Hospital, Beckett Street, Leeds LS9 7TF
* Corresponding author.
E-mail address: nisha.sharma2@nhs.net

Radiol Clin N Am 62 (2024) 679–686
https://doi.org/10.1016/j.rcl.2023.12.005

Based on the above, a B3 diagnosis warrants further sampling due to concerns regarding possible undersampling of the area of concern and the uncertainty of potential-associated malignancy.

Traditionally, these lesions have been further sampled and managed with surgical diagnostic excision, an invasive procedure performed under general anesthesia that may result in complications and/or poor cosmetic outcomes, and potentially adversely affect patient's satisfaction and quality of life. Therefore, minimally invasive nonsurgical techniques have been explored in order to reduce the morbidity and complications associated with the so far standard surgical treatment. These may also greatly benefit the health-care system, including cost savings associated with the avoidance of surgery.

Throughout this article, we will discuss the implications of overdiagnosis and overtreatment of B3 lesions, current recommendations regarding B3 lesions sampling techniques, nonsurgical management and surveillance, and the role of risk-reducing therapies.

OVERDIAGNOSIS/OVERTREATMENT

Worldwide, cancer screening programs remain controversial due to their potential to overdetect or overdiagnose indolent cancers that would otherwise not become clinically apparent and not cause any harm through a person's lifetime in the absence of screening.[9] It is noted that overdetected cancers are histologically proven cancers and therefore should not be confused with false-positive screening outcomes because of an equivocal screening test.

Screening-associated cancer overdiagnosis includes both (1) indolent nonprogressive cancers and (2) slowly progressive cancers that would have not been detected in unscreened individuals before they had passed away due to another cause. Overdiagnosis in this context is particularly relevant for older screened individuals in comparison to younger individuals due to associated comorbidities that represent potential competing causes of death.[9]

However, breast cancer screening programs have proven to reduce morbidity and mortality up to 20% due to breast cancer by allowing an early detection and treatment of smaller cancers with overall better prognosis.[10] In the United Kingdom, the breast cancer screening program invites women from ages 50 to 70 years for a screening mammogram every 3 years, and more than 1300 breast cancer deaths are assumed to be prevented because of women attending the screening program.

In 2013, the Marmot review was published based on an independent panel review of the evidence on benefits and harms of breast screening in the context of the UK breast-screening program. The review concluded that breast screening indeed saves lives but one of the potential harms is related to overdiagnosis. The panel estimated that for 10,000 UK women invited to screening from age 50 for 20 years, about 681 cancers will be found of which 129 will represent overdiagnosis and 43 deaths from breast cancer will be prevented.[10]

The main detriment associated with screening overdiagnosis of breast cancer is overtreatment. The Marmot review highlighted the need to minimize overtreatment in the context of slowly progressive cancers with good prognosis. Minimizing overtreatment is crucial because overtreatment leads to women unnecessarily becoming patients with cancer, requiring surgery and subsequent adjuvant treatments, which can adversely have a psychological impact on women and their families, as well as significant costs to the health-care system.[10]

Overtreatment of breast cancer has been particularly concerning in the context of in situ disease. The gold standard treatment of ductal carcinoma in situ (DCIS) remains breast-conserving surgery, often followed by adjuvant radiotherapy and sometimes endocrine therapy. Recent data have shown that in cases of DCIS with low risk of recurrence, radiotherapy can safely be omitted as part of the treatment.[11] As a result, several randomized controlled trials have been set up across the world to evaluate if active surveillance with annual mammography of low-to-intermediate grade DCIS is safe, including the LOw RISk DCIS (LORIS) trial in the United Kingdom. The LORIS study is a phase III, multicenter study including 49 sites and it was open to recruitment from July 2014 to March 2020, with a 2-year internal feasibility phase. Since then, the LOw Risk DCIS (LORD) study was initiated in Netherlands, the Comparison of Operative versus Monitoring and Endocrine Therapy Trial (COMET) in the United States and the low-risk DCIS with endocrine therapy alone-tamoxifen (LORETTA) study in Japan.

The results from these trials, yet to be published, have the potential to not only change our current clinical practice regarding DCIS surgical management but also the management of B3 lesions because these high-risk lesions when upgraded to malignancy are predominantly associated with low-grade cancers such as low-grade DCIS. Therefore, the traditional surgical management of these lesions can also be considered overtreatment.

The NHS Breast-screening program set up a working group to assess how the potential overtreatment of high-risk lesions diagnosed within the breast-screening program could be minimized. The working group recommended vacuum-assisted excision (VAE) for thorough sampling to support secondary assessment of most B3 lesions, whether they had been initially diagnosed on needle core biopsy (NCB) or primary diagnostic VAB. Studies have shown that VAE can be deployed with appropriate training to all screening centers,[12] and the technique is overall well accepted by patients—in a survey of 189 female patients, 90% preferred VAB to surgical biopsy, costing them less time and providing "better cosmetic results."[13]

Less frequently, B3 lesions are upgraded to low-grade invasive carcinomas, often estrogen receptor-positive, that harbor a good prognosis.[7,12] Considering their potential overtreatment, VAE has also currently been evaluated as a valid alternative to the traditional breast-conserving surgical excision of these small, low-grade screen-detected invasive breast cancers as part of the SMALL trial.[14] This is a UK-based, prospective, phase III, multicenter randomized study, designed to support the safe surgical deescalation in the context of adjuvant radiotherapy and endocrine therapy, provided VAE is noninferior to completely excise the cancer when compared with traditional surgery, and there is an acceptable local recurrence risk post-VAE with long-term follow-up.

NONSURGICAL MANAGEMENT: VACUUM-ASSISTED EXCISION

High-risk B3 lesions are conventionally diagnosed on NCB with or without vacuum assistance. VAB was developed in the late 1990s by Fred Burbank to overcome the undersampling issues with the traditional 14G NCB. By using vacuum assistance, this device allows for multiple tissue specimens to be obtained contiguously from the targeted lesion with a single needle insertion. The needle gauges vary from 14G to 7G. A conventional 14G core will retrieve about 15 mg of tissue per core and a 7G VAB sample will retrieve about 300 mg of tissue per sample.[15] In the United Kingdom, VAB has replaced the 14G NCB for stereotactic procedures in most breast-screening units.

VAB can be used for both diagnostic and excision purposes with the latter being called VAE. VAE procedure is often chosen when a larger volume of tissue is required to avoid or replace a surgical diagnostic biopsy. This is still a diagnostic procedure. By using this vacuum technology, adequate tissue sampling can now be safely performed without the potential complications associated with a more invasive surgical procedure. Small breast lesions (less than 15 mm) have the potential to be completely excised by VAE.[16]

A meta-analysis of 26 studies investigating the efficacy and safety of VAE in benign breast lesions found the complete resection rate following VAE of 93% (95% CI; $P < .001$) and recurrence rate of 39% (95% CI; $P<.001$).[17] Studies have shown that the complete excision rate and recurrence rates were similar for VAE versus surgical excision.[18–20] The use of VAE in the excision of benign breast lesions has been supported by the National Institute for Health and Care Excellence since 2006.[21]

In the United Kingdom, VAE has been shown to reduce the rate of benign surgical biopsies in breast screening resulting in a better preoperative diagnostic rate with no impact on the cancer detection rate.

The achievable benign surgical biopsy rate for women screened for the first time (prevalent round) should be less than 1.0 out of 1000 and for women who have been screened before (incident round) the rate should be less than 0.75 out of 1000. This rate is achieved by the breast-screening units in the United Kingdom.

Mammographic surveillance after VAE has also proven to be more reliable than surveillance post-surgical excision by overcoming the difficult interpretation of postsurgical changes that often mimic asymmetrical architectural distortions and result in unnecessary further needle interventions.[16]

The use of VAE was extrapolated to the management of B3 lesions identified on NCB or diagnostic stereotactic VAB. The radiological–pathologic discordances in the context of B3 lesions can often be answered by obtaining more extensive representative sampling to exclude coexisting invasive or noninvasive malignancy, which can be achieved with VAE in the majority of the cases.[12]

Strachan and colleagues, published data from a single center where VAE was being use for secondary sampling of B3 lesions diagnosed on NCB or primary diagnostic VAB instead of surgery from 2009 to 2013.[22] Their results showed that of the 321 women who had VAE, no further intervention was required in 245 cases. Seventy-six women did go onto have surgical excision but in 43 cases, this was a therapeutic operation to treat malignancy diagnosed at VAE. This article highlighted that VAE can safely replace surgery in a large proportion of women with B3 lesion and additionally improved the preoperative diagnosis of malignancy in this cohort.[22]

In 2021, Yaziji and colleagues conducted a cost analysis using an economic decision model comparing the cost impact of VAE with diagnostic surgical excision on the management of B3 lesions, from the health-care provider point of view.[23] This modeling study was conducted in a breast unit in United Kingdom and included 398 women that were diagnosed with B3 lesions on either NCB or VAB. These women were split into 2 pathways according to a decision tree: one pathway using VAE as part of the B3 lesions management and the other one using diagnostic surgical excision. Further patient care was based on the current national standards.

Overall, this analysis showed that VAE is a cost-effective alternative to surgical diagnostic excision of B3 lesions, with an average cost reduction of £1510.75 per patient.[23]

CURRENT GUIDELINES FOR MANAGING B3 LESIONS

Internationally, different expert groups have published their recommendations for the diagnosis and management of B3 lesions including the American Society of Breast Surgeons (ASBS) consensus guidelines,[24] the European guidelines developed jointly by EUSOMA, EUSOBI, European Society of Pathology (Breast working group) (ESP [BWG]), and European Society of Surgical Oncology (ESSO),[25] the Third International Consensus Conference guidelines[26] and the NHS breast-screening multidisciplinary working group guidelines.[3]

The ASBS group recommends surgical excision of all B3 lesions without radiological–pathological concordance and encourages MDT discussion of the remaining lesions considering the estimated risk of upgrade to malignancy and patient's individual risk factors.

The remaining guidelines are mostly in agreement, recommending excision of all B3 lesions and suggesting VAE as a valid alternative to surgical excision provided there is radiological–pathological concordance and the lesion has been completely removed.

The main difference lies in the management of ADH lesions. The UK guidelines use the term AIDEP for core biopsy and the term ADH is used only for surgical diagnostic biopsies. Their argument is based on limited volume of tissue sampled in a core biopsy being insufficient to warrant the diagnosis of ADH. The authors consider this group as having a moderately increased risk of upgrade to malignancy with a PPV of 21% from VAB. Their proposed management pathway for AIDEP includes VAE after initial diagnosis on NCB or VAB. If no further atypia is seen on the excised specimen or if further atypia is seen but there is radiological and pathologic concordance, annual mammographic surveillance is advised for 5 years, following MDT discussion.

The international consensus conference guidelines recommend surgical excision of ADH after NCB (76%) or VAB (58%). If the lesion has been totally excised on VAB, only 34% of the group recommended observation and mammographic surveillance with 8% of the group advising VAE.

It is noted that the international consensus conference guidelines consider that the upgrade rate should not exceed 5% for invasive cancer and 10% for DCIS and yet the upgrade rate for ADH varies from 10% to 30%.[6] The UK guidelines therefore do not agree with this metric but instead aim to improve the preoperative diagnosis of breast cancer and reduce the number of women going through unnecessary surgery. The EUSOMA guidelines also recognize VAE as an alternative to surgery to help minimize overtreatment (Fig. 1).[25]

Recently published data showed that the implementation of UK guidelines had little impact on numbers of invasive cancers detected. Second-line VAE did not result in more cancers missed than surgery at 1 year (1.08 [0.11–5.9] vs 1.12 [0.24–3.9] cancers per 1000 women respectively) or 3 years (9.23 [4.1–18.4] vs 18.5 [12.8–25.8] cancers per 1000 women, respectively). This applied to all atypia types and was independent of the site of cancer. Once again emphasizing that VAE is a safe alternative to surgery and maintains cancer detection rate.[27]

Overall, the current European and UK guidelines recognize that VAE, as a cost-effective nonsurgical method, can adequately provide a thorough sample to further evaluate most B3 lesions. It is recognized that PLs with atypia seen in the initial NCB or VAB specimen requires surgical excision rather than VAE. The authors consider the extent of atypia of these lesions needs to be assessed in continuity and, therefore a histologic evaluation of the whole specimen is required rather than piecemeal samples.

The aim of VAE is to sample enough tissue that is representative of the nature of high-risk lesion (equivalent to the volume of a diagnostic surgical excision) and, ideally to completely excise it (eg, if < 15 mm). If the lesion cannot be totally excised by VAE, at least 12x7G cores are recommended, which represent approximately 4 g, depending on the nature (fatty or fibroglandular) of the tissue sampled. If using a 9G needle, then this would require 33 core samples.[15]

RSs with and without atypia that are larger than 25 mm may require surgical diagnostic excision due to the larger size of the lesion, which means that sampling with VAE will be limited regarding assessing the margin of the lesion. This is important because in RSs associated with DCIS, the DCIS is normally at the periphery (Fig. 2).[3]

Surgical excision rather than VAE is recommended for spindle cell lesions and fibroepithelial lesions.[3,25,26]

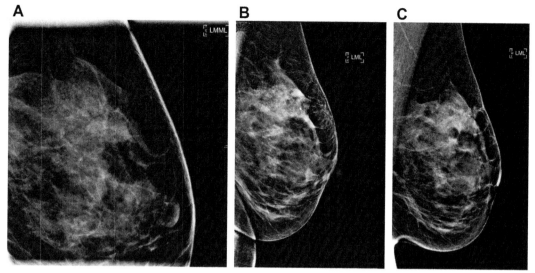

Fig. 1. A 55-year-old woman with a 25-mm focal cluster of calcifications UOQ left breast. Initial VAB 9G showed AIDEP, and she went onto have a VAE with 7Gx18 cores and diagnosed LGDCIS. Treated with left wide local excision. (*A*) Left lateral magnification view showing 25 mm focal cluster of calcifications left breast UOQ. (*B*) Post 9 G VAB with cores. Marker clip in a good position. (*C*) Post 7G VAE: 18x7G cores and diagnosed low-grade DCIS. LGDCIS, low grade ductal carcinoma insitu; UOQ, upper outer quadrant.

For extensive lesions, VAE from more than one area should be considered and guided by the mammographic features. The areas of greater radiological concern should be targeted on additional biopsies, ideally away from the site primarily sampled. Representative sampling should include at least one-third of an extensive area of concern.[28]

SURVEILLANCE

The risk of developing breast cancer after the diagnosis and treatment of a B3 lesion is extremely variably. Atypical epithelial lesions such as ADH, AIDEP, and classic LN confer a higher risk of breast cancer (up to 3–5 fold in the long term), high enough for surveillance to be consider as part of their management. Following clinical assessment women with a moderate risk of breast cancer will receive annual mammographic surveillance until 59 years of age.

Currently, for those women not eligible for moderate risk surveillance, there are no clear guidelines on surveillance, regarding the optimal frequency, duration, and methodology of surveillance that

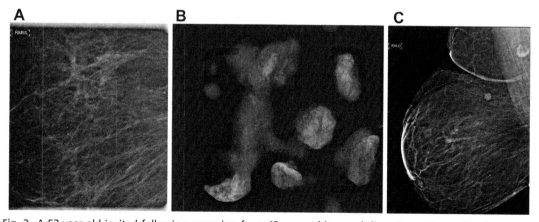

Fig. 2. A 52-year-old invited following screening for a 43-mm architectural distortion with calcifications upper half right breast. This was biopsied using a 10G VAB needle and 6 cores were taken. Pathology showed an RS with no atypia. Following MDT discussion, this was referred for a surgical excision due to the size. Surgery showed this to be an RS with no atypia. (*A*) Right lateral magnification view showing a 43-mm architectural distortion. (*B*) 10G VAB with 6 cores showing an RS, no atypia and postclip mammogram on the right MLO view. (*C*) Postclip mammogram on the right MLO view in good position. MLO, medio-lateral oblique view.

should be recommended. Annual surveillance is suggested to ensure that no breast cancers are missed at excision and allow for an early detection in this high-risk group although, this practice is not evidence based. In the United Kingdom, women diagnosed with epithelial atypia, similarly to women diagnosed with breast cancer, are offered 5-year annual mammographic surveillance. The ASBS guidelines recommend at least 2 years follow-up if a B3 lesion is not excised.

Recently, an expert group has made some recommendations based on the evidence from the English Slone atypia prospective project. The observational analysis of the Slone atypia cohort, that included more than 3000 women with screen detected atypia in the United Kingdom, showed that the number of invasive breast cancers diagnosed after atypia were low and similar in number to those in the general screening population, both ipsilateral and contralateral, regardless of the type of atypia, breast density or women's age.[27,29] Evidence suggests that some atypias may represent risk factors instead of signifying invasive breast cancer precursors. Based on this data, the group of experts does not support increased short-term mammographic surveillance and recommends that women diagnosed with atypia as part of the screening program should continue with their routine 3-yearly screening mammograms following VAE or surgical excision of the atypical lesions until the age of 70 years.[30]

RISK REDUCING THERAPY

Thomas reviewed the most recently published randomized trials considering the use of antiestrogen therapy in high-risk women including those with ADH and LN, as a preventative measure of both invasive breast cancer and DCIS.[6] These trials assessed the value of ER blockers (the National Surgical Adjuvant Project for Breast and Bowel Cancers [NSABP-1], International Breast Cancer Intervention Study [IBIS-I]) and, aramotase inhibitors (IBIS-II, Mammary Prevention 3 [MAP 3]) versus placebo in reducing the incidence of breast cancer among high-risk group of women, when taken daily for 5 years.

The NSABP-1 trial recruited more than 13,000 women, 6576 were randomized in the tamoxifen arm, and found that tamoxifen reduces the incidence of invasive and noninvasive breast cancer by 49% ($P < .0001$) and 50% ($P<.002$), respectively.[31] Within the subgroup of patients with high-risk lesions such as ADH and LN, which corresponded to 15% of the whole cohort, the risk reduction was as high as 86% (RR 0.14, 95% CI 0.03–0.47) and 56% (RR 0.44, 95% CI 0.16–1.06), respectively.

The IBIS-I trial equally showed a risk reduction in breast cancer in high-risk women taking tamoxifen for 5 years, including the small subgroup of women with atypia or LN.[32]

In 2019, DeCensi and colleagues, conducted a small randomized controlled trial assessing the value of a low-dose tamoxifen (5 mg instead of the standard 20 mg) taken for 3 years versus placebo in risk reducing ipsilateral and contralateral breast cancer in women with either DCIS, LN, or ADH. Their results showed similar efficacy to a full-dose with an overall reduced risk of invasive breast cancer (RR 0.48, 95% CI 0.26–0.92) and lower toxicity rates. They also reported reduced risk of contralateral breast cancer (RR 0.25, 95% CI 0.07–0.88).[33]

Considering tamoxifen's main side effects are increased risk of thromboembolic events and endometrial cancer, alternatives such as raloxifene, which does not carry these side effects, have also been tested during the Study of Tamoxifen and Raloxifene (STAR) trial.[34] Raloxifene was shown to be a valid alternative to tamoxifen at preventing both invasive disease and DCIS, particularly within the group of women with ADH and LN.

Similar results have been published regarding the use of anastrazole and exemestane as risk reducing therapy of both invasive cancers and DCIS, in postmenopausal high-risk women including women with ADH and LCIS. The IBIS II trial[32] showed a risk reduction of breast cancer of 0.31 (95% CI, 0.12%–0.84%) when patients took anastrozole for 5 years versus 0.61 (95% CI, 0.20–1.82) for exemestane as published by the MAP 3 trial.[35]

Overall, the drugs used in these trials are only effective in preventing ER-positive breast cancers, and they have no apparent benefit in terms of survival considering the long-term follow-up of some of these studies.

Litzenburger and colleagues have published data on the use of preventative drugs such as metformin, retinoids, and nonsteroidal anti-inflammatory drugs against nonestrogen-sensitive breast cancers although these are currently not in use and the study has not included patients with B3 lesions.[36]

Despite the undeniable benefits of these risk reduction therapies, the uptake of these drugs is generally very low (less than 4%).[25] Dedicated clinics focused on patient education and decision aid might help in future overcome this limitation.

Along with these therapies, lifestyle interventions, such as smoking cessation, increasing physical activity, reducing alcohol intake and weight loss, should also be encouraged because these can positively impact not only patient's physical and mental health but also breast cancer incidence and management outcomes.[25]

SUMMARY

Breast lesions that fall into the B3 category are the subject of a great deal of interest, partly because of their uncertain malignant potential but also due to the lack of clear guidance regarding their assessment and management.

During the last decade, several studies have been conducted covering this heterogeneous group that resulted in many guidelines being published across the world proposing different management strategies based on the current evidence.

Traditionally, a surgical diagnostic biopsy was required to obtain a representative sample and ensure there was no coexistent malignancy followed by an open surgical excision. However, new evidence has led to VAE being accepted as a valid, more conservative, and cost-effective alternative to the traditional surgical excision with good patient acceptance. VAE has proven to safely address the overtreatment issue associated with these high-risk lesions and simultaneously reduce the morbidity for patients without detriment to oncological outcomes.

Overall, these lesions associated with long-term moderate-to-high risk of development of malignancy should be managed and followed up as per updated national guidance, with VAE becoming a standard practice across most breast units in the United Kingdom and Europe.

CLINICS CARE POINTS

- VAE is different to VAB and care should be taken to manage the patient accordingly
- Multidisciplinary approach to managing the high-risk lesions is important to ensure safe deliverance of good quality of care
- Good communication with the patient is important for them to understand the immediate and long-term risks in terms of developing breast cancer

DISCLOSURE

Dr N. Sharma—speaker fees from BD and Hologic.

REFERENCES

1. Public Health England. UK National Health Service Breast Screening Programme Pathology Audit. Updated September, 2021. Accessed November 11, 2023.

2. Catanzariti F, Avendano D, Cicero G, et al. High-risk lesions of the breast: concurrent diagnostic tools and management recommendations. Insights Imaging 2021;12:63.

3. Pinder SE, Shaaban A, Deb R, et al. NHS Breast Screening multidisciplinary working group guidelines for the diagnosis and management of breast lesions of uncertain malignant potential on core biopsy (B3 lesions). Clin Radiol 2018;73:682–92.

4. Forester ND, Lowes S, Mitchell E, et al. High risk (B3) breast lesions: what is the incidence of malignancy for individual lesion subtypes? A systematic review and meta-analysis. Eur J Surg Oncol 2019; 45(4):519–27.

5. Bianchi S, Caini S, Renne G, et al. Positive predictive value for malignancy on surgical excision of breast lesions of uncertain malignant potential (B3) diagnosed by stereotactic vacuum-assisted needle core biopsy (VANCB): a large multi-institutional study in Italy. Breast 2011;20(3):264–70.

6. Thomas PS. Diagnosis and Management of High-Risk Breast Lesions. J Natl Compr Canc Netw 2018;16(11):1391–6.

7. Rageth CJ, O'Flynn EAM, Pinker K, et al. Second International Consensus Conference on lesions of uncertain malignant potential in the breast (B3 lesions). Breast Cancer Res Treat 2019;174(2):2 79–96.

8. Griffiths R, Kaur C, Alarcon L, et al. Three-year Trends in Diagnosis of B3 Breast Lesions and Their Upgrade Rates to Malignancy Lesions. Clin Breast Cancer 2020;20(3):e353–7.

9. Yaffe MJ, Mainprize JG. Overdetection of Breast Cancer. Curr Oncol 2022;29:3894–910.

10. Marmot MG, Altman DG, Cameron DA, et al. – The Independent UK Panel on Breast Cancer Screening. The benefits and harms of breast cancer screening: an independent review. Br J Cancer 2013;108:2205–40.

11. Collins LC, Laronga C, Wong JS. Ductal Carcinoma In Situ: Treatment and Prognosis. UpToDate. Wolters Kluwer; 2023. Updated July 31, 2023. Available at: https://www.uptodate.com/contents/ductal-carcinoma-in-situ-treatment-and-prognosis. Accessed November 11, 2023.

12. Sharma N, Wilkinson LS, Pinder SE. The B3 conundrum – the radiologist' perspective. Br J Radiol 2017;90(1071):20160595.

13. Eller A, Janka R, Lux M, et al. Stereotactic vacuum-assisted breast biopsy (VABB)—a patients' survey. Anticancer Res 2014;34:3831–7.

14. Morgan J, Potter S, Sharma N, et al. The SMALL Trial: A Big Change for Small Breast Cancers. Clin Oncol 2019;31:659–63.

15. Preibsch H, Baur A, Wietek BM, et al. Vacuum assisted breast biopsy with 7-gauge, 8-gauge, 9-gauge, 10-gauge, and 11-gauge needles: how many specimens are necessary? Acta Radiol 2015;56: 1078–84.

16. Shaaban AM, Sharma N. Management of B3 Lesions – Practical Issues. Current Breast Cancer Reports 2019;11(2):83–8.

17. Yoo HS, Kang W, Pyo J, et al. Efficacy and Safety of Vacuum-Assisted Excision for Benign Breast Mass Lesion: A Meta-Analysis. Medicina (Kaunas) 2021; 57(11):1260.

18. Wang WJ, Wang Q, Cai QP, et al. Ultrasonographically guided vacuum-assisted excision for multiple breast masses: Non-randomized comparison with conventional open excision. J Surg Oncol 2009; 100:675–80.

19. Ouyang Q, Li S, Tan C, et al. Benign Phyllodes Tumor of the Breast Diagnosed After Ultrasound-Guided Vacuum-Assisted Biopsy: Surgical Excision or Wait-and-Watch? Ann Surg Oncol 2016;23:1129–34.

20. Kim GR, Kim EK, Yoon JH, et al. Recurrence Rates of Benign Phyllodes Tumors After Surgical Excision and Ultrasonography-Guided Vacuum-Assisted Excision. Ultrasound Q 2016;32:151–6.

21. National Institute for Health and Care Excellence (NICE). Image-guided vacuum-assisted excision biopsy of benign lesions. Published February, 2006. Available at: https://www.nice.org.uk/guidance/ipg156/chapter/1-guidance. Accessed November 11, 2023.

22. Strachan C, Horgan K, Millican-Slater RA, et al. Outcome of a new patient pathway for managing B3 breast lesions by vacuum-assisted biopsy: time to change current UK practice? J Clin Pathol 2016; 69(3):248–54.

23. Yaziji N, Sharma N, Selfridge J, et al. Cost analysis of managing B3 breast lesions by vacuum excision at Leeds Breast Unit using a decision model. BMJ Open 2021;11(12):e054525.

24. The American Society of Breast Surgeons. Consensus Guideline on Concordance Assessment of Image-Guided Breast Biopsies and Management of Borderline or High-Risk Lesions. Published November, 2016. Available at: https://www.breastsurgeons.org/docs/statements/Consensus-Guideline-on-Concordance-Assessment-of-Image-Guided-Breast-Biopsies.pdf?v2. Accessed November 11, 2023.

25. Rubio IT, Wyld L, Marotti L, et al. European guidelines for the diagnosis, treatment and follow-up of breast lesions with uncertain malignant potential (B3 lesions) developed jointly by EUSOMA, EUSOBI, ESP (BWG) and ESSO. Eur J Surg Oncol 2023;50(1):107292.

26. Elfgen C, Leo C, Kubik-Huch RA, et al. Third International Consensus Conference on lesions of uncertain malignant potential in the breast (B3 lesions). Virchows Arch 2023;483:5–20.

27. Freeman K, Jenkinson D, Clements K, et al. Breast screening atypia and subsequent development of cancer: an observational analysis of the Slone atypia prospective cohort in England. BMJ 2023. https://doi.org/10.1136/bmj-2023-077039.

28. Public Health England. Breast Screening: clinical guidelines for screening assessment. Updated November 15, 2016. Accessed November 11, 2023.

29. Jenkinson D, Freeman K, Clements K, et al. Breast screening atypia and subsequent development of cancer: protocol for an observational analysis of the Sloane database in England (Sloane atypia cohort study). BMJ Open 2022;12(1):e058050.

30. Freeman K., Mansbridge A., Stobart H., et al., Evidence-informed recommendations on managing breast screening atypia: perspectives from an expert panel consensus meeting reviewing results from the Slone atypia project, BJR, 2023, https://doi.org/10.1093/bjr/tqad053.

31. Fisher B, Costantino JP, Wickerham DL, et al. Tamoxifen for prevention of breast cancer: report of the National Surgical Adjuvant Breast and Bowel Project P-1 Study. J Natl Cancer Inst 1998;90(18):1371–88.

32. Cuzick J, Forbes J, Sestak L, et al. Long-term results of tamoxifen prophylaxis for breast cancer – 96 month follow-up of the randomized IBIS-I trial. J Natl cancer Inst 2007;99(4):272–82.

33. DeCensi A, Puntoni M, Guerrieri-Gonzaga A, et al. Randomized Placebo Controlled Trial of Low-Dose Tamoxifen to prevent Local and Contralateral Recurrence in Breast Intraepithelial Neoplasia. J Clin Oncol 2019;37(19):1629–37.

34. Vogel VG, Costantino JP, Wickerham DL, et al. Effects of tamoxifen vs raloxifen on the risk of developing invasive breast cancer and other disease outcomes: the NSABP Study of Tamoxifen and Raloxifene (STAR) P-2 Trial. JAMA 2006;295(23):2727–41.

35. Goss PE, Ingle JN, Ales-Martinez JE, et al. Exemestane for breast-cancer prevention in postmenopausal women. N Engl J Med 2011;364(25):2381–91.

36. Litzenburger BC, Brown PH. Advances in Preventive Therapy for Estrogen-Receptor-Negative Breast Cancer. Curr Breast Cancer Rep 2014;6:96–109.

Practice Challenges

Auditing Abbreviated Breast MR Imaging
Clinical Considerations and Implications

Jean M. Seely, MD, FRCPC*, Victoria Domonkos, MD,
Raman Verma, MD, FRCPC

KEYWORDS

- Breast imaging • Breast MR imaging • Audit • Abbreviated MR imaging • Breast cancer
- Breast screening • Benchmarks

KEY POINTS

- Abbreviated breast MR (AB-MR) imaging is a relatively new breast imaging tool primarily used for women at elevated risk for breast cancer, which maintains diagnostic accuracy while reducing costs and image acquisition and interpretation times compared with full-protocol breast MR (FP-MR) imaging.
- Unlike FP-MR imaging, there are no established benchmarks for AB-MR imaging but studies demonstrate comparable performance for cancer detection rate, positive predictive value 3, sensitivity, and specificity if T2 imaging is added.
- Benchmarks for breast MR imaging provide a standard against which performance can be measured to identify strengths and areas for improvement.

INTRODUCTION

Breast cancer is the recognized leading cause of cancer deaths among women worldwide.[1] Many advancements have been made in the treatment of breast cancer but early detection remains the primary strategy to improve the prognosis of women with the disease.

Breast MR imaging is the most sensitive modality for the detection of breast cancer.[2] It can detect very small malignancies, which helps to establish an early-stage diagnosis that is linked to increased metastasis-free survival.[3] As a result, breast MR imaging has become the standard of care for screening women with a high lifetime risk of breast cancer[2] and women with dense breasts who have above-average risk.[4] There are, however, multiple drawbacks associated with full-protocol breast MR (FP-MR) imaging, including high monetary costs and long image acquisition and interpretation times compared with other screening modalities such as mammography.

Abbreviated breast MR (AB-MR) imaging is a relatively new tool increasingly used for screening and diagnostic purposes. Its shortened protocol substantially reduces image acquisition and interpretation times while maintaining diagnostic performance compared with FP-MR imaging.[5] AB-MR imaging is helping to increase access to MR imaging screening because the increased throughput from the shortened imaging time allows more women to be imaged. Shortened imaging times also improve patient comfort, thereby increasing patient acceptance of the test.

Performance benchmarks serve as a reference standard for high-quality diagnostic and screening programs. Audits are an essential tool to evaluate program and individual-level performance measures, which can then be compared with established benchmarks to determine if standards are

Department of Radiology, The Ottawa Hospital, General Campus, 501 Smyth Road, Ottawa, Ontario K1H 8L6, Canada
* Corresponding author.
E-mail address: jeseely@toh.ca
Twitter: @JeanSeely (J.M.S.); @RamanVermaMD (R.V.)

Radiol Clin N Am 62 (2024) 687–701
https://doi.org/10.1016/j.rcl.2023.12.010
0033-8389/24/© 2023 Elsevier Inc. All rights reserved.

being met. Although performance benchmarks for screening MR imaging have been established, benchmarks for AB-MR imaging have yet to be set. In this article, we will provide an overview of AB-MR imaging and the benefits and barriers to its implementation, including cost, time to acquisition, and interpretation. We will discuss the technical specifics of AB-MR imaging, including the protocol options, along with technical considerations for clinical implementation. This will be followed by a discussion of benchmarks for breast MR imaging, including proposed benchmarks for AB-MR imaging. We will review the basics of performing an audit, including possible strategies to implement if benchmarks are not being met, with case-based examples.

TECHNIQUE
Background

The concept of an abbreviated protocol for breast MR imaging was first introduced in 2014 by Kuhl, whereby T2-weighted imaging (T1WI) precontrast and postcontrast sequences were obtained in less than 3 minutes with 2 sets of derived images, including a First contrast-enhanced Acquisition SubTracted (FAST) sequence and maximum intensity projections (MIP). Her study demonstrated a significantly decreased study interpretation time of ~30 seconds while maintaining diagnostic accuracy equivalent to FP-MR imaging.[2] This paved the way for others to explore the utility of AB-MR imaging, which included variations of the FAST protocol using diffusion-weighted imaging (DWI) and T2-weighted imaging (T2WI).[6–10]

Acquisition Time

As the name suggests, AB-MR imaging has a shortened protocol and, therefore, a shorter acquisition time than FP-MR imaging.[2] Given variations in AB-MR protocols and institutional practices, there is a resultant variation in the time to acquisition for AB-MR imaging, with a meta-analysis reporting a range from 180 to 264 seconds.[2,11–13] A systematic review by Hernandez[14] determined an average acquisition time of 5.88 minutes. This was still much faster than that reported for FP-MR imaging, which ranged from 1024 to 1440 seconds. When all scan-related activities are considered, such as postprocessing and other technologist-related tasks, patient throughput increased by 38% compared with FP-MR imaging, which was less than predicted based on scan times. It was noted that during FP-MR imaging, many of the scan-related activities could be performed at idle times during the scan but this was not the case with AB-MR imaging due to the very short scan time.[14]

Kinetics

The original description of AB-MR imaging by Kuhl in 2014[11] only included one postcontrast sequence, and most authors have used this definition. However, some studies have added later postcontrast sequences.[15–17] This may increase the scanning time to less than 10 minutes without significantly affecting table time (<15 minutes).[15] Choudhery[17] added 2 postcontrast sequences every 60 to 75 seconds up to 180 to 205 seconds, allowing time–intensity curves to be generated. The addition of kinetic information to AB-MR imaging may enhance the radiologist's confidence in their diagnosis[15] (**Fig.** 1A–E) and could affect sensitivity and specificity, as discussed later.

Interpretation Time

AB-MR imaging consistently requires less time to interpret than FP-MR imaging, with a meta-analysis providing a range of 42 to 144 seconds for the interpretation of AB-MR images compared with 192 to 396 seconds for the interpretation of FP-MR images.[2,12,13,18] In a study assessing training radiologists to read AB-MR images, comparing radiologists who had FP-MR image reading experience with those with only mammography reading experience, the median interpretation time of AB-MR images for the MR image readers versus that of mammography images for the mammography radiologists was 98 versus 113 seconds. This decreased to 78 versus 102 seconds after the second set of images was provided for an overall average of 89 seconds.[19] The average interpretation time for AB-MR images provided by Hernandez[14] was 3.38 minutes, which excluded the time needed to review the patient's chart and prior imaging.

IMPLEMENTATION
Benefits

The use of AB-MR imaging offers reduced complexity and cost compared with FP-MR imaging[11] by decreasing image acquisition and interpretation times.[5] AB-MR imaging also reduces patient time spent in the magnet, which increases patient acceptability of the examination while improving access to the modality.[11]

Barriers

Potential barriers to expanding AB-MR imaging use relate to knowledge gaps, workforce issues, and cost. Additional training is required for radiologists to be competent in interpreting AB-MR images. However, existing research supports that current mammogram readers require less than a day of training to interpret AB-MR images accurately.[19]

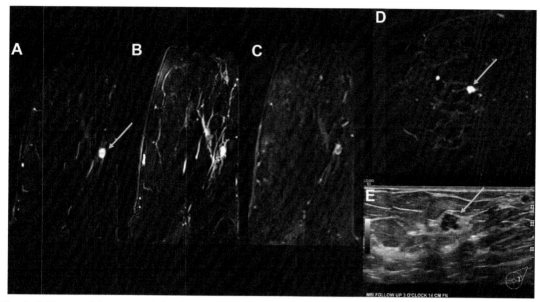

Fig. 1. A 39-year-old woman. High-risk screening examination demonstrates an irregular mass on (*A*) 2-min axial postcontrast subtraction and (*B*) axial T2WI fat suppression images with (*C*) type-III kinetics (*arrows*). (*D*) Irregular morphology is better assessed on the 2-min subtracted isotropic multiplanar sagittal reformats (*arrow*) (*E*). Although a lymph node remains in the differential, a second look ultrasound and subsequent biopsy confirmed a high-grade IDC.

Breast MR imaging screening has high direct and indirect costs[7] but is cost-effective in women with a high lifetime risk for breast cancer.[11] Additionally, studies assessing cost have determined that MR imaging screening for women with increased breast density is feasible[14,20,21] and the 2022 European guidelines recommend MR imaging screening for women with dense breasts.[22] When evaluating cost, it is essential to consider all scan-related (table time) and nonscan-related activities.[14]

Protocol

The American College of Radiology (ACR) has requirements for performing an FP-MR imaging, including T2WI, precontrast T1, early phase postcontrast T1 and delayed phase postcontrast T1 (within 4 minutes of injection), slice thickness of 3 mm or lesser, and in-plane pixel (phase and frequency) of 1 mm or lesser.[23] There is no formal definition or single standardized protocol for AB-MR imaging (**Table 1**). In general, AB-MR imaging is accepted as having a protocol that evolved from the initial prospective trial by Kuhl, which did not include a T2 sequence,[11] acquisition time of less than 10 minutes,[24] and an overall scan time of 1 to 18 minutes.[2,24,25] Based on published literature and a recent survey of the Society of Breast Imaging members,[24–26] the required sequences are listed in **Table 2**, ideally, with a resolution of

Table 1	
Abbreviated breast MR protocol definitions	
Dynamic contrast-enhanced MR imaging	Sensitive for breast cancer detection, with morphologic and kinetic (vascular) information regarding lesions
Multiparametric MR imaging	Incorporates additional functional imaging techniques, such as DWI and spectroscopy
AB-MR imaging	Although no formal definition, typically an acquisition time of <10 min is considered accepted, similar to EA1141 trial (4)
Ultrafast MR imaging	Not a required component of AB-MR imaging but may be included in AB-MR imaging protocols. Exploits early contrast wash-in characteristics. This is done by rapid sequential imaging within the first 2 min, to establish a "wash-in" kinetic curve. Techniques and protocols related to this are beyond the scope of this review

Table 2 Comparison of sequences between dynamic full-protocol breast MR and abbreviated breast MR imagings		
	FP-MR Imaging	Abbreviated MR Imaging
Scout localizer	X	X
T1, precontrast	X	X
T1, postcontrast, first pass	X	X
T1, postcontrast, second pass	X	Optional
T1, postcontrast, third pass	X	Optional
T1, postcontrast, fourth pass	X	—
T1, postcontrast, first pass SUB	X (post-processing)	X (post-processing)
T2-weighted sequence	X	Optional
Kinetics map	X	Optional

1 mm or lesser and a section thickness of 3 mm or lesser.[25]

The accepted variation for AB-MR protocols results in differences in available diagnostic information due to the specific sequences obtained. For example, if only a single contrast-enhanced sequence is obtained, kinetic calculations cannot be performed but derived images such as subtraction and MIP images can still be generated (**Fig. 2**A–D). For this reason, the inclusion of the otherwise lengthy T2WI has been suggested because it can allow the downgrading of otherwise indeterminate lesions in the absence of kinetic information (**Fig. 3**A–D).[24,26]

Additional factors to consider when implementing an AB-MR protocol are that the total scan duration will be shorter than the FP-MR protocol, even with the inclusion of subtraction and MIP sequences, because the postprocessing does not affect scan time. Finally, the AB-MR protocol should reflect the institution's FP-MR protocol to promote acceptance and understanding among technologists and interpreting radiologists.[26]

AUDITING MR IMAGING
Auditing/Outcomes

A breast imaging audit is a quality assurance process used in radiology to evaluate the accuracy and efficacy of breast imaging techniques, including mammography, ultrasound, and MR imaging. Performing a basic audit allows radiologists to assess their overall performance of breast imaging interpretation in relation to established benchmarks. We will describe the basics of an audit and review relevant statistical terms. Additionally, we will discuss proposed benchmarks for AB-MR imaging, review practical tips on how to perform an audit with case-based examples and discuss the clinical implications of the results of an audit.

Audit Basics

In simple terms, a breast-imaging audit involves reviewing a sample of studies for a specific modality, for example, screening mammograms, and calculating statistical metrics, which typically include cancer detection rate (CDR), sensitivity,

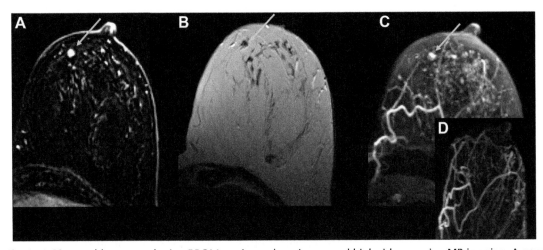

Fig. 2. A 66-year-old woman who is a BRCA1 carrier undergoing annual high-risk screening MR imaging. A new 4 mm solitary enhancing focus in the inner left breast on axial 2-min CE subtracted images (*A*), appears hypointense on axial T2WI (*B*) (*arrows*). A comparison of the current (*C*) and prior (*D*) 2-min CE subtracted MIP confirms this is new from the prior study. Subsequent MR-guided biopsy revealed IDC, pT1a N0, ER+, and Her-2-.

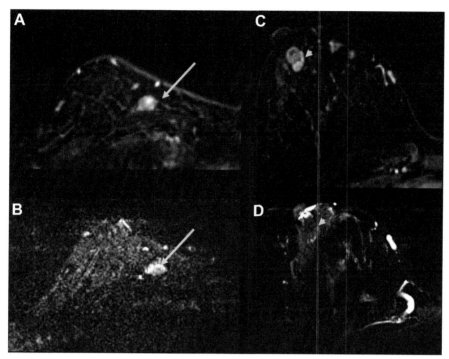

Fig. 3. A 38-year-old woman. Axial CE subtracted 2 min sequence (*A*) demonstrates a circumscribed mass (*arrow*) with dark internal septations and T2 hyperintensity (*B*). This was classified as BI-RADS 3, with interval stability, consistent with a fibroadenoma. In another 45-year-old woman, (*C*) MR imaging demonstrates a similar-appearing circumscribed enhancing mass on axial CE subtracted 2-min images (*arrowhead*) without T2 hyperintensity, classified as BI-RADS 4A (*D*). Percutaneous ultrasound-guided biopsy was diagnostic for a fibroadenoma. BI-RADS, breast imaging reporting and data system.

and specificity, among others. These measures can then be compared with established benchmarks, a standard put in place to help measure performance and the effectiveness of the screening program. The goals of a breast-screening audit are to help radiologists detect a high percentage of breast cancers in the population at an early stage when they are more curable.[27] Additionally, it is essential to diagnose breast cancers within an acceptable range of recommended additional imaging (recalls) and tissue diagnosis to minimize cost and patient morbidity, as outlined in the benchmarks. Performing audits help radiologists identify areas for improvement in their practice while working toward the goals of breast cancer screening. There are currently audit benchmarks in place for mammography, screening ultrasound, and MR imaging[27,28] but owing to its emerging use, there is not yet an established benchmark for AB-MR imaging.

Statistical Measures of an Audit

An audit of AB-MR imaging practice should include several key statistical terms. Therefore, it is helpful to understand these concepts because they apply to breast imaging and AB-MR imaging.

These terms are summarized in the BI-RADS manual[27] Glossary of Statistical Terms, with the most relevant measures outlined below (**Table 3**).

Performing a Basic Audit

Completing a basic audit requires collecting a considerable amount of data and calculating several metrics—which is more than what is legally mandated by the Food and Drug Administration.[27] Having more metrics available for comparison with benchmarks allows for a more holistic evaluation of the breast imaging program and individual interpreting physicians. Data are collected and analyzed in 12-month increments to allow sufficient time to assess patient outcomes. When collecting the data, it is important to maintain separate datasets for screening and diagnostics examinations because outcomes and corresponding benchmarks for these examinations are different.[27,29–31] When screening and diagnostic data cannot be separated, a combined analysis may be performed, and the results must be interpreted carefully. Many current electronic medical records (EMRs), such as EPIC, provide audit data in the Mammography Quality Standards Act (MQSA) module.

Table 3
Summary of statistical terms and definitions

Statistical Measures	Definition	Formula
Positive predictive values (PPVs)	PPVs are calculated based on definitions recommended by the American College of Radiology, with 3 separate definitions[23]	
	PPV_1 is the percentage of all positive screening examinations that result in a tissue diagnosis of cancer within 1 y. Given that a positive screening for breast MR imaging involves a BI-RADS 4 or 5 assessment, the PPV_1 for MR imaging is essentially the same as a PPV_2	PPV_1 = true positive/(number of positive screening examinations)
	PPV_2 is the percentage of all diagnostic or screening examinations recommended for tissue diagnosis or a surgical consultation resulting in a tissue diagnosis of cancer within 1 y	PPV_2 = TP/(number of screening or diagnostic examinations recommended for tissue diagnosis)
	PPV_3, also known as biopsy yield of malignancy, is the percentage of all known biopsies done due to a positive diagnostic examination that resulted in a tissue diagnosis of cancer within 1 y	PPV_3 = TP/(number of biopsies)
Sensitivity	Sensitivity is the probability of interpreting an examination as positive when cancer exists. This is measured as the number of positive examinations with a tissue diagnosis of cancer within 1 y of imaging divided by all cancers present in a population examined within 1 y	Sensitivity = TP/(TP + FN)
False negative	The number of cancer cases missed at imaging	
Specificity	It is the probability of interpreting an examination as negative when cancer is not present. This is measured as the number of negative examinations where there is no tissue diagnosis of cancer within 1 y of examination divided by all examinations for which there is no tissue diagnosis of cancer within 1 y	Specificity = TN/(TN + FP)
Cancer detection rate	The number of cancers detected at imaging per 1000 patients examined. This should be calculated separately for screening and diagnostic examinations	Cancers detected/screening examinations
Abnormal interpretation rate	Abnormal interpretation rate (AIR) is the percentage of examinations that are interpreted as positive. For screening examinations, positive examinations include BI-RADS 3, 4, and 5 for breast MR imaging	Abnormal interpretation rate = positive examinations/all examinations

The Importance of Quality Benchmarks

Quality benchmarks play a crucial role in comparison and improvement, providing a standard against which organizations can measure their performance and identify areas of strength and weakness. Benchmarks can improve processes, practices, and outcomes and help set realistic and achievable goals. Quality benchmarks provide a means to objectively evaluate performance and help determine how well organizations meet expectations. Quality benchmarks provide valuable information for decision-making processes, continuous improvement, accountability, and transparency and are essential for maintaining high-performance standards.

Origin of MR Screening Benchmarks

The BI-RADS performance benchmarks for mammography were first established in 1995 and were updated to include screening MR imaging in 2013.[27] Although the performance benchmark for mammography is based on the Breast Cancer Surveillance Consortium (BCSC)[32] data, those for MR imaging screening are based on 5 prospective high-risk screening trials[33–37] performed at academic centers in women with genetic mutations placing them at risk for breast cancer.

AUDITING ABBREVIATED BREAST MR

Cancer Detection Rate

The FP-MR in the BI-RADS lexicon recommends a CDR of 20 to 30 per 1000,[27] including in situ and invasive cancers. The BCSC screening MR study found a CDR of 17 out of 1000.[38] For screening MR imaging, the CDR varies with the population being screened. In a study of screening MR imaging of 5170 screening examinations in 2637 women in one center, 87% with prior MR imaging screens, CDR was highest in the women who had a genetic mutation or history of chest irradiation (26/1000), intermediate for those with a personal history of breast cancer (12/1000) and history of high-risk lesions (15/1000), and lowest for those with a family history of breast cancer (8/1000).[39] Additionally, CDR is higher for prevalence (baseline) than incidence (subsequent) screening, and the DENSE trial for women with extremely dense breasts found incremental CDRs of 16.5 out of 1000 in the first round of MR imaging screening[40] and 5.9 out of 1000 in the second round.[41] Other studies show similar results.[41]

There are a few published rates of CDR using AB-MR imaging, summarized in **Table 4**. The ECOG-ACRIN trial found CDR of 15.2 out of 1000[24] for above-average risk women. Systematic review of screening AB-MR imaging found a high CDR of 17.8 out of 1000.[42–44] Kwon's AB-MR imaging study of 1975 women found CDRs of 11.7 out of 1000 in the prevalence and 3.8 out of 1000 in the incidence rounds, highest in high-risk compared with intermediate-risk women (CDR 28.7/1000 vs 7.4/1000).[45] Heacock and colleagues did not find that adding T2WI changed the CDR, although it increased lesion conspicuity.[9]

The Median Size of Invasive Cancers

Although the established benchmark in screening for the median size of invasive cancers is 14 mm for mammography and 10 mm for breast ultrasound, this has not yet been determined for screening MR imaging.[27] Published MR imaging screening studies have found a median tumor size of invasive cancers of 10 to 15 mm.[12,28,38,44] With AB-MR imaging, in 2 studies, the median size of invasive cancers was 10.5 mm (range 4–48 mm)[24] and 17 mm (range 9–30 mm).[45] Given the similar resolution of AB-MR and FP-MR imagings, a similar benchmark for the median size of invasive cancers could be used.

Percentage of Node-negative Invasive Cancers

The ACR benchmark for FP-MR imaging is that greater than 80% of invasive cancers should be node-negative.[27] With FP-MR imaging, reported rates are 62%[38] to 88% node-negative cancers.[44] With AB-MR imaging, node-negative cancers are reported from 83.3%[45] to 96%.[24] Therefore, similar benchmarks of greater than 80% could be used for both AB-MR and FP-MR imagings.

Percentage Minimal Cancer

Minimal cancer is defined as invasive cancer of 10 mm or lesser or ductal carcinoma in situ (DCIS).[27] The BI-RADS lexicon indicates that greater than 50% of cancers should be minimal cancer with screening MR imaging.[27] The BCSC reported FP-MR imaging detected 69% minimal cancers,[32] and another center detected 70.6%.[44] With AB-MR imaging, 62.5%[24,] and 79%[45] minimal cancers were found, showing similar performance to FP-MR imaging.

Abnormal Interpretation Rate

AIR is the number of positive interpretations divided by the number of screening examinations. With screening MR imaging, this included BI-RADS 0, 3, 4 and 5,[38,44] although the use of BI-RADS 0 is discouraged with MR imaging in the BI-RADS lexicon.[45] AIR for screening FP-MR has a wide reported range from 9.5% to 25.9%.[28,38,40,43,44,46] As with all screening modalities, AIR varies

Table 4
Summary of principal abbreviated breast MR studies

	Screening Examinations (AB-MR Imaging) Number	Cancer Detection Rate (per 1000 Examinations)	PPV$_2$ (%) Biopsy Recommendation	PPV$_3$ (%) Biopsy Performed	Sensitivity (%)	Specificity (%)
ACR BI-RADS Benchmark (FP-MR imaging)[27]		20–30	≥15	20–50	>80	85–90
Kuhl et al,[11] 2014	606	18.2	24.4	N/A	100	94.3
Moschetta et al,[16] 2016	470	N/A	N/A	N/A	89	91
Harvey et al,[12] 2016	568	12.3	5.1	N/A	100	96.1
Chen et al,[18] 2017	478	31.4	21.7	N/A	92.9–93.8	86.5–88.3
Panigrahi et al,[13] 2017	1052 (651)	13.3	N/A	30.4	81.8	97.2
Park et al,[49] 2020	1045	9.9	35	N/A	70	98
Comstock et al,[24] 2020	1444	15.2	31.0	19.6	95.7	86.7
Geach et al,[2] 2021[a]	3251	17.8	N/A	N/A	94.8	94.6
Kwon et al,[45] 2021	3037	6.9–10.7	31.6–63.2[b]	N/A	75–80[b]	93.5–94.1[b]
Naranjo et al,[48] 2022	427	49	14–20[c]	N/A	92–90[c]	71–83[c]

Table. Summary of relevant studies included in this review listed by author, date, and reference.
[a] Please note systematic review (reference 2) includes references 11, 12, 18, and 13, listed above.
[b] Refers to the range for year 1 to year 3 of screening.
[c] The first value is for AB-MR without T2, and the second is with T2WI.

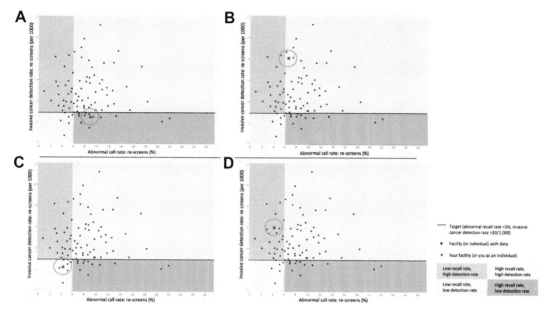

Fig. 4. Screening Quality Report: Categorization of interpretative performance. This figure represents a facility's performance compared with other facilities for screening MG imaging. This could be adapted for use with AB-MR screening. The same can be generated to depict an individual radiologist's performance (*green circles*) compared with other radiologists. The goal is to have a low AIR and high CDR (*dark green quadrant*) (*A*). (*B*) Shows one with high AIR and high CDR, (*C*) shows one with a low AIR and low CDR, while (*D*) has high AIR and low CDR (*orange*). Interpretation of facility/individual results in the context of other facilities/individual results is more helpful than interpretation of results in isolation.

considerably with prevalence and incidence screening. It decreased from 9.5% on the first screen in the DENSE trial[40] to 3.2% on the second round.[41] AIR is variable depending on the population screened, and higher CDRs will be linked to higher recall rates. Sippo and colleagues found that the AIR was higher in women with *BRCA* mutations (11%) versus those with a high-

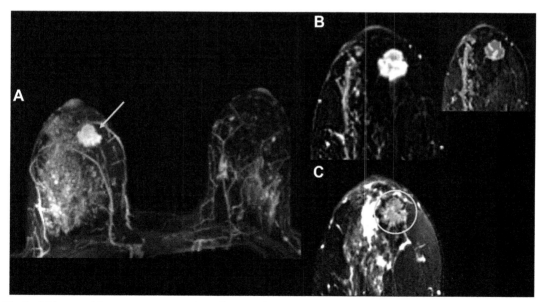

Fig. 5. A 31-year-old woman. BRCA2 positive, baseline high-risk screening MR imaging, normal mammograms. CE subtracted sequences, MIP (*A*) and axial (*B*) demonstrate an irregular, heterogeneously enhancing mass (*arrow*) with type III kinetics (*inlay*) and T2 hypointensity (*C, circled*), BI-RADS 5. Ultrasound-guided biopsy revealed a 1.7 cm grade 3 IDC, ER/PR+, and Her-2–.

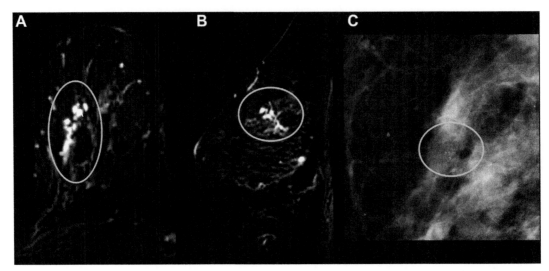

Fig. 6. A 52-year-old woman. High-risk screening MR imaging demonstrates heterogeneous, clumped, nonmass enhancement on 2-min CE subtracted sequences (*A*, axial; *B* isotropic sagittal reformat) (*circles*), classified as BI-RADS 4B. Corresponding calcifications are seen on mammogram (*C*), which were biopsied with stereotactic guidance revealing high nuclear grade DCIS.

risk lesion (9%) or personal history of breast cancer (6%).[39] With AB-MR imaging, Comstock found a recall rate of 15% on baseline MR imaging screen.[24] Kwon's AB-MR imaging study reported AIR 7.1% (62 out of 871) in year 1, which decreased slightly to 6.9% (77 out of 1121) in year 3.[45] Therefore, no clear AIR benchmark for FP-MR or AB-MR imaging is yet available.

Positive Predictive Value 2 (Recommendation for Tissue Diagnosis) and Positive Predictive Value 3 (Biopsy Performed)

ACR BI-RADS for screening MR imaging suggests a PPV_2 of 15%, and a PPV_3 of 20% to 50%.[27] In studies, PPV_2s for FP-MR imaging range from 19% to 24%, and PPV_3s from 21% to 27%,[28,38,44] meeting ACR's benchmarks. In Sippo's study, PPV_3s were not different among the high-risk groups screened with MR imaging at an average PPV_3 of 41% but were lower among those with a family history as the only risk factor with PPV_3 of 14%.[39]

There are no specific benchmarks for AB-MR imaging but one AB-MR imaging study found PPV_3 of 19.6%[24] and Kwon found PPV_3 of 31.6% in year 1 increased to 63.2% in year 3,[45] meeting the ACR benchmark for FP-MR imaging.

Sensitivity and Specificity

If measurable, that is, if outcomes data are linked to a regional tumor registry, the sensitivity should be greater than 80% for screening MR imaging, and the specificity should be 85% to 90%.[27] The

BCSC centres had a sensitivity of 81% and specificity of 83%.[38] In a systematic review of 11 AB-MR imaging studies published from 2014 to 2019, Gao and Heller found that the mean pooled sensitivity of FP-MR imaging was 96.5% and

Table 5
Typical BI-RADS MR imaging findings

BI-RADS	MR Imaging Findings and Enhancement Patterns
BI-RADS 1	Normal BPE/fibroglandular enhancement
BI-RADS 2	Lymph node, biopsy-proven benign mass, and fat necrosis
BI-RADS 3	Probable fibroadenoma (High T2, circumscribed mass, and nonenhancing septations)
BI-RADS 4	Unique NME on baseline study New unique NME New or unique mass without typically benign features (low T2)
BI-RADS 5	Spiculated mass (low T2) Rim enhancing mass (T2 may be bright at center with thick irregular enhancing walls) Type 3 (washout) kinetics if available

Abbreviations: BPE, background parenchymal enhancement; NME, nonmass enhancement.

specificity 87.3%, whereas AB-MR imaging had a slightly lower mean pooled sensitivity of 94.3% and specificity of 83.6%.[47] A more recent systematic review in 2021, including 2763 women and 3251 screening rounds, found that the overall sensitivity of AB-MR imaging was 94.8%, not significantly different from FP-MR imaging, with a similar specificity of 94.6%.[2] Naranjo's study comparing FP-MR imaging with AB-MR imaging with and without T2WI in 292 *BRCA* genetic mutation carriers found that pooled sensitivity was 94% for FP-MR imaging, 92% for AB-MR imaging, and 90% for AB-MR plus T2WI (all p values [*ps*] > .001).[48] Pooled specificity was 80% for FP-MR imaging, 71% for AB-MR imaging, and 83% for AB-MR plus T2WI (all *ps* < .001).[48]

One study showed that adding a second post-contrast sequence did not change the sensitivity and might slightly reduce the specificity of AB-MR imaging.[26] However, others found that adding postcontrast sequences improved specificity but decreased sensitivity.[49] Kwon's study using 2 postcontrast sequences and T2WI found an AB-MR imaging sensitivity of 75% to 80% and a specificity of 93.5% to 94.1% in year 1 to year 3, respectively.[45] Although BI-RADS has not yet provided benchmarks for AB-MR imaging, these data suggest that AB-MR imaging meets the same benchmarks as FP-MR imaging for PPV$_3$, sensitivity and specificity if T2WI is added.

Techniques to Improve Quality Performance for Abbreviated Breast MR After an Audit

An audit of breast screening provides feedback to facilities and radiologists about their performance relative to performance benchmarks. Once an audit has been performed, the results may be analyzed to address areas for improvement, as has been used with screening mammography (**Fig. 4**A–D). This may facilitate improvements in reader performance and improve the overall effectiveness of the screening program.[50] Radiologists should aim for as low an AIR as achievable while maximizing CDR and PPV$_3$. The key is to provide education and feedback on the audit results. Although medical audits of screening mammography are mandatory in the United States,[51] they are not required for screening MR imaging. The voluntary nature means that there are opportunities for improvement that may not be used, and efforts to do this should be facilitated to minimize the time and resources required.

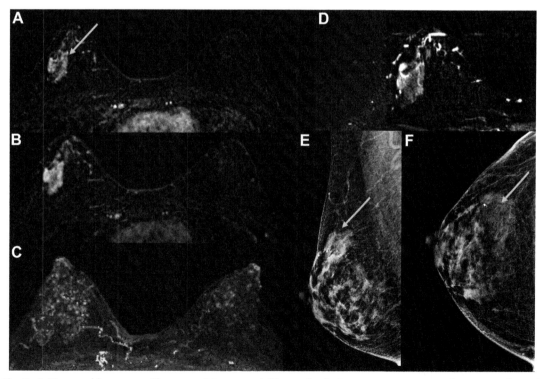

Fig. 7. A 42-year-old woman with asymmetric segmental increasing heterogenous nonmass enhancement (*arrow*) on (*A*) 2-min subtracted and (*B*) 4-min subtracted sequences with type I kinetics (*C*) MIP. Axial (*D*) demonstrates a lack of T2 hyperintensity, classified as BI-RADS 4A. The corresponding lesion is seen on mammogram (*E, F, arrows*). US-guided biopsy revealed benign pseudoangiomatous stromal hyperplasia (PASH), which was concordant.

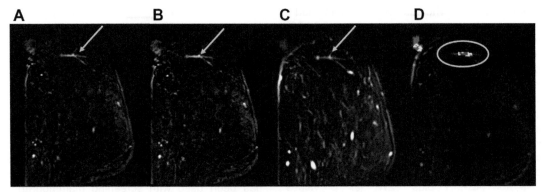

Fig. 8. A 49-year-old woman with linear-branching nonmass enhancement (*A*) demonstrates type III kinetics on delayed-phase imaging (*B, D*) with mild T2 hyperintensity (*C*) (*arrows*) and washout Type III kinetics (*oval*) (D) . Given the suspicious morphology and kinetics (BI-RADS 4B), the patient underwent an MR imaging-guided biopsy revealing an intraductal papilloma without atypia.

The MQSA module in the EMR is one way to provide the audit to radiologists in a readily available format. This may also be used by facilities to illustrate areas for improvement. It is crucial to ensure that radiologists meet the minimum volume requirement of MR imaging reads per year (the ACR recommends 500 MR imagings in subspeciality to be read in 36 months).[23] Some radiologists with low CDRs may require interventions to improve their cancer detection. Case reviews of cancers detected with AB-MR imaging (**Figs. 5A–C** and **6A–C**) may help to educate them, with typical examples (**Table 5**). Other radiologists with high AIRs and CDRs may benefit from education in ways to reduce AIR. This may include a review of anonymized consecutive recalled cases that should be recalled (**Figs. 7A–F** and **8A–D**) and not be recalled (**Fig. 9**). Double reading MR imagings may also help to reduce AIR without compromising CDR or PPV₃. Chan and colleagues found that double reading cases being considered for MR imaging biopsy reduced the percentage of cases referred for biopsy from 8.6% to 5.5%[52] with no change in CDR. A reader training study of AB-MR imaging found AIR of 20% decreased to 6% with the use of a second reader.[53] Given the current workforce shortages of breast radiologists and technologists and the cost of MR imaging biopsy, reducing the AIR will have a positive impact on valuable resources. In addition, promising options include artificial intelligence, which has been shown to improve radiologists' performance in reading breast MR imaging[54] and to avoid benign biopsies by 20%.[55]

Barriers to the implementation of AB-MR included knowledge gaps, workforce issues, and costs. Jones and colleagues[19] demonstrated that some knowledge gaps and workforce issues could be addressed with less than a day of training for current mammogram readers. Furthermore, breast MR imaging has been shown to be cost-effective in women with a high lifetime risk for breast cancer,[11] which is a point that can be emphasized when considering costs.

A framework was established by the Canadian Partnership Against Cancer to improve the performance of screening mammography and to reduce AIR. This consisted of peer review and mentorship, education, standardized report cards (audits), minimum reading volumes, double reading, and

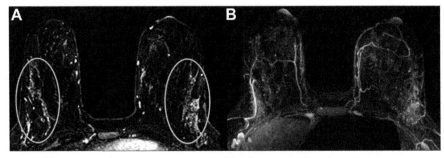

Fig. 9. A 36-year-old woman with a typical appearance of background parenchymal enhancement (*oval*) seen on high-risk screening MR imaging (*A*, 2-min CE subtracted; *B*, 2-min MIP). If unilateral or focal, it may need further assessment; otherwise, it can be dismissed.

batch reading.[56] Similar principles should be considered for screening AB-MR reading.

SUMMARY

AB-MR imaging has evolved during the last decade with potential for many benefits to patients, organizations, and providers. Assessment of performance metrics is a key component in breast imaging quality assurance, particularly when initiating new/novel imaging tools. Carefully reviewing institutional and individual audit data and comparing it to those proposed or established allows an opportunity for continual quality improvement, as has been demonstrated in mammography and FP-MR imaging. Although there are no established criteria currently for AB-MR imaging, ensuring the metrics meet or exceed those of FP-MR imaging will ensure any proposed AB-MR program is on the correct trajectory.

CLINICS CARE POINTS

- Higher CDR is linked to higher AIR; the population being screened partly determines AIR, with higher CDRs found among women at the highest risk for breast cancer.

- PPV₃ should meet expected benchmarks for breast MR of 20% to 50%.

- Comparison to prior examinations, education, and double reading AB-MR all may help to reduce AIR while maintaining high CDR.

- Benchmarks provide a valuable tool to facilitate performance improvement of individual radiologists and institutions.

DISCLOSURE

The authors have nothing to disclose.

REFERENCES

1. Stewart BW, World Health O, Stewart BW, Wild C, International Agency for Research on C and World Health O. World cancer report 2014. Lyon, France: International Agency for Research on Cancer; 2014.
2. Geach R, Jones LI, Harding SA, et al. The potential utility of abbreviated breast MRI (FAST MRI) as a tool for breast cancer screening: a systematic review and meta-analysis. Clin Radiol 2021;76(2). 154. e11-154.e22.
3. Saadatmand S, Obdeijn IM, Rutgers EJ, et al. Survival benefit in women with BRCA1 mutation or familial risk in the MRI screening study (MRISC). Int J Cancer 2015;137(7).
4. Monticciolo DL, Newell MS, Moy L, et al. Breast Cancer Screening for Women at Higher-Than-Average Risk: Updated Recommendations From the ACR. J Am Coll Radiol 2023. https://doi.org/10.1016/j.jacr.2023.04.002.
5. Baxter GC, Selamoglu A, Mackay JW, et al. A meta-analysis comparing the diagnostic performance of abbreviated MRI and a full diagnostic protocol in breast cancer. Clin Radiol 2021;76(2).
6. Chhor CM, Mercado CL. Abbreviated MRI protocols: Wave of the future for breast cancer screening. Am J Roentgenol 2017;208(2).
7. Greenwood HI. Abbreviated protocol breast MRI: The past, present, and future. Clin Imag 2019;53: 169–73.
8. Mango VL, Morris EA, David Dershaw D, et al. Abbreviated protocol for breast MRI: Are multiple sequences needed for cancer detection? Eur J Radiol 2015;84(1):65–70.
9. Heacock L, Melsaether AN, Heller SL, et al. Evaluation of a known breast cancer using an abbreviated breast MRI protocol: Correlation of imaging characteristics and pathology with lesion detection and conspicuity. Eur J Radiol 2016;85(4):815–23.
10. Grimm LJ, Soo MS, Yoon S, et al. Abbreviated Screening Protocol for Breast MRI. A Feasibility Study. Acad Radiol 2015;22(9):1157–62.
11. Kuhl CK, Schrading S, Strobel K, et al. Abbreviated breast Magnetic Resonance Imaging (MRI): First postcontrast subtracted images and maximum-intensity projection - A novel approach to breast cancer screening with MRI. J Clin Oncol 2014; 32(22):2304–10.
12. Harvey SC, Di Carlo PA, Lee B, et al. An Abbreviated Protocol for High-Risk Screening Breast MRI Saves Time and Resources. J Am Coll Radiol 2016;13(11).
13. Panigrahi B, Mullen L, Falomo E, et al. An Abbreviated Protocol for High-risk Screening Breast Magnetic Resonance Imaging: Impact on Performance Metrics and BI-RADS Assessment. Acad Radiol 2017;24(9):1132–8.
14. Hernández ML, Osorio S, Florez K, et al. Abbreviated magnetic resonance imaging in breast cancer: A systematic review of literature. Eur J Radiol Open 2021;8. https://doi.org/10.1016/j.ejro.2020.100307.
15. Dogan BE, Scoggins ME, Son JB, et al. American College of Radiology–Compliant Short Protocol Breast MRI for High-Risk Breast Cancer Screening: A Prospective Feasibility Study. Am J Roentgenol 2018;210(1):214–21.
16. Moschetta M, Telegrafo M, Rella L, et al. Abbreviated Combined MR Protocol: A New Faster Strategy for Characterizing Breast Lesions. Clin Breast Cancer 2016;16(3):207–11.

17. Choudhery S, Chou SHS, Chang K, et al. Kinetic Analysis of Lesions Identified on a Rapid Abridged Multiphase (RAMP) Breast MRI Protocol. Acad Radiol 2020;27(5):672–81.

18. Chen SQ, Huang M, Shen YY, et al. Application of Abbreviated Protocol of Magnetic Resonance Imaging for Breast Cancer Screening in Dense Breast Tissue. Acad Radiol 2017;24(3).

19. Jones LI, Geach R, Harding SA, et al. Can mammogram readers swiftly and effectively learn to interpret first post-contrast acquisition subtracted (FAST) MRI, a type of abbreviated breast MRI?: A single centre data-interpretation study. Br J Radiol 2019; 92(1104):20190663.

20. Kaiser CG, Dietzel M, Vag T, et al. Cost-effectiveness of MR-mammography vs. conventional mammography in screening patients at intermediate risk of breast cancer - A model-based economic evaluation. Eur J Radiol 2021;136. https://doi.org/10.1016/j.ejrad.2020.109355.

21. Froelich MF, Kaiser CG. Cost-effectiveness of MR-mammography as a solitary imaging technique in women with dense breasts: an economic evaluation of the prospective TK-Study. Eur Radiol 2021;31(2). https://doi.org/10.1007/s00330-020-07129-5.

22. Mann RM, Athanasiou A, Baltzer PAT, et al. Breast cancer screening in women with extremely dense breasts recommendations of the European Society of Breast Imaging (EUSOBI). Eur Radiol 2022; 32(6):4036–45.

23. Mann RM, Athanasiou A, Baltzer PAT, et al. Breast cancer screening in women with extremely dense breasts recommendations of the European Society of Breast Imaging (EUSOBI). Eur Radiol 2022; 32(6):4036–45.

24. Comstock CE, Gatsonis C, Newstead GM, et al. Comparison of Abbreviated Breast MRI vs Digital Breast Tomosynthesis for Breast Cancer Detection Among Women With Dense Breasts Undergoing Screening. JAMA 2020;323(8):746–56.

25. Grimm LJ, Conant EF, Dialani VM, et al. Abbreviated Breast MRI Utilization: A Survey of the Society of Breast Imaging. Journal of breast imaging (Online) 2022;4(5):506–12.

26. Grimm LJ, Mango VL, Harvey JA, et al. Implementation of Abbreviated Breast MRI for Screening: AJR Expert Panel Narrative Review. Am J Roentgenol (1976) 2022;218(2):202–12.

27. D'Orsi CJ, Sickles EA, Mendelson EB, et al. American College of radiology BI-RADS® Atlas, breast imaging reporting and data system. Reston, VA: American College of Radiology; 2013. Published online.

28. Niell BL, Gavenonis SC, Motazedi T, et al. Auditing a breast MRI practice: performance measures for screening and diagnostic breast MRI. J Am Coll Radiol 2014;11(9).

29. Dee KE, Sickles EA. Medical audit of diagnostic mammography examinations: Comparison with screening outcomes obtained concurrently. Am J Roentgenol 2001;176(3).

30. Sardanelli F, Podo F. Breast MR imaging in women at high-risk of breast cancer. Is something changing in early breast cancer detection? Eur Radiol 2007; 17(4).

31. Rosenberg RD, Yankaskas BC, Abraham LA, et al. Performance benchmarks for screening mammography. Radiology 2006;241(1).

32. Ballard-Barbash R, Taplin SH, Yankaskas BC, et al. Breast Cancer Surveillance Consortium: a national mammography screening and outcomes database. Am J Roentgenol 1997;169(4):1001–8.

33. Zhang Z. Detection of Breast Cancer With Addition of Annual Screening Ultrasound or a Single Screening MRI to Mammography in Women With Elevated Breast Cancer Risk. JAMA 2012;307(13): 1394.

34. Kriege M, Brekelmans CTM, Boetes C, et al. Efficacy of MRI and Mammography for Breast-Cancer Screening in Women with a Familial or Genetic Predisposition. N Engl J Med 2004;351(5).

35. Warner E, Plewes DB, Hill KA, et al. Surveillance of BRCA1 and BRCA2 mutation carriers with magnetic resonance imaging, ultrasound, mammography, and clinical breast examination. JAMA 2004;292(11).

36. Leach MO, Brindle KM, Evelhoch JL, et al. The assessment of antiangiogenic and antivascular therapies in early-stage clinical trials using magnetic resonance imaging: issues and recommendations. Br J Cancer 2005;92(9):1599–610.

37. Kuhl CK, Schrading S, Leutner CC, et al. Mammography, Breast Ultrasound, and Magnetic Resonance Imaging for Surveillance of Women at High Familial Risk for Breast Cancer. J Clin Oncol 2005;23(33): 8469–76.

38. Lee JM, Ichikawa L, Valencia E, et al. Performance Benchmarks for Screening Breast MR Imaging in Community Practice. Radiology 2017;285(1):44–52.

39. Sippo DA, Burk KS, Mercaldo SF, et al. Performance of Screening Breast MRI across Women with Different Elevated Breast Cancer Risk Indications. Radiology 2019;292(1):51–9.

40. Bakker MF, de Lange SV, Pijnappel RM, et al. Supplemental MRI Screening for Women with Extremely Dense Breast Tissue. N Engl J Med 2019;381(22): 2091–102.

41. Veenhuizen SGA, de Lange SV, Bakker MF, et al. Supplemental Breast MRI for Women with Extremely Dense Breasts: Results of the Second Screening Round of the DENSE Trial. Radiology 2021;299(2): 278–86.

42. Sung JS, Stamler S, Brooks J, et al. Breast Cancers Detected at Screening MR Imaging and Mammography in Patients at High Risk: Method of Detection

Reflects Tumor Histopathologic Results. Radiology 2016;280(3):716–22.

43. Kuhl CK, Strobel K, Bieling H, et al. Supplemental breast MR imaging screening of women with average risk of breast cancer. Radiology 2017; 283(2).

44. Strigel RM, Rollenhagen J, Burnside ES, et al. Screening Breast MRI Outcomes in Routine Clinical Practice: Comparison to BI-RADS Benchmarks. Acad Radiol 2017;24(4).

45. Kwon MR, Choi JS, Won H, et al. Breast cancer screening with abbreviated breast MRI: 3-year outcome analysis. Radiology 2021;299(1):73–83.

46. Berg WA, Sechtin AG, Marques H, et al. Cystic Breast Masses and the ACRIN 6666 Experience. Radiol Clin 2010;48(5):931–87.

47. Gao Y, Heller SL. Abbreviated and Ultrafast Breast MRI in Clinical Practice. Radiographics 2020;40(6): 1507–27.

48. Naranjo ID, Sogani J, Saccarelli C, et al. MRI Screening of BRCA Mutation Carriers: Comparison of Standard Protocol and Abbreviated Protocols With and Without T2-Weighted Images. Am J Roentgenol 2022;218(5):810–20.

49. Park KW, Han SB, Han BK, et al. MRI surveillance for women with a personal history of breast cancer: comparison between abbreviated and full diagnostic protocol. Br J Radiol 2020;93(1106): 20190733.

50. Linver MN, Paster SB, Rosenberg RD, et al. Improvement in mammography interpretation skills in a community radiology practice after dedicated teaching courses: 2-year medical audit of 38,633 cases. Radiology 1992;184(1):39–43.

51. United States. Congress. Senate. Committee on Health EL, Pensions. Mammography Quality Standards Reauthorization Act of 2003 : report (to accompany S. 1879). Washington, D.C: U.S. G.P.O. : For sale by the Supt. of Docs., U.S. G.P.O., Congressional Sales Office; 2003.

52. Chan J, Seely J, Lau J. Does Double Reading of Screening Breast MRI Scans Impact Recall Rates and Cancer Detection? Can Assoc Radiol J 2023; 74(2):398–403.

53. Jones LI, Marshall A, Elangovan P, et al. Evaluating the effectiveness of abbreviated breast MRI (abMRI) interpretation training for mammogram readers: a multi-centre study assessing diagnostic performance, using an enriched dataset. Breast Cancer Res 2022;24(1):1–55.

54. Jiang Y, Edwards AV, Newstead GM. Artificial Intelligence Applied to Breast MRI for Improved Diagnosis. Radiology 2021;298(1):38–46.

55. Witowski J, Heacock L, Reig B, et al. Improving breast cancer diagnostics with deep learning for MRI. Sci Transl Med 2022;14(664).

56. Framework for addressing abnormal call rates in breast cancer screening – Canadian Partnership Against Cancer, Toronto: Canadian Partnership Against Cancer; 2020. Pan-Canadian Framework for Action to Address Abnormal Call Rates in Breast Cancer Screening (pcdn.co) Accessed January 13, 2024.

Clinical Integration of Artificial Intelligence for Breast Imaging

Louise S. Wilkinson, BA, BM, BCh, FRCR[a],*,
J. Kevin Dunbar, MBChB, MPH, FFPH[b],
Gerald Lip, MB BCH, BAO (Ireland), MRCS (Ireland), FRCR (London)[c]

KEYWORDS

- Breast screening • Mammography • AI • Integration

KEY POINTS

- Research indicates that artificial intelligence is approaching readiness for use in clinical practice.
- There are challenges to integration with existing information technology systems.
- Successful integration requires a multidisciplinary team approach.
- Monitoring is essential to prove efficacy and identify inequalities.
- Communication with service users is necessary to engender trust.

INTRODUCTION

Breast screening is seen as an ideal candidate for the application of artificial intelligence (AI) because it involves large volumes of image data and a simple outcome: a cancer is either present or not. As more trials of AI products demonstrate accuracy comparable with human readers, it is impossible to ignore the pressure to adopt AI. But even if we agree that AI is ready for breast screening, we still need to ask whether the services that deliver breast screening are ready for AI.

AI products that reliably associate features on images with certain conditions or diseases are now feasible because modern computing power allows machine learning techniques to be applied to many thousands of digital images in a short period of time. These products are now translating from research into daily clinical practice, and organisations will need to embrace the change wisely in order to adopt new functionality safely and fairly without inadvertently introducing inequalities.

This article does not describe how these AI products are trained and validated. Instead we assume that regulator-approved products are available, and we use our personal expertise and experience to explore the practicalities of integrating one into a service that uses digital mammography to deliver breast screening to a community. The topics covered include: mapping the existing breast screening pathway and information technology (IT) systems in use; choosing which AI product to consider; procurement and implementation; validation and ongoing monitoring; and required governance around introducing "non-human" decision makers into the workflow (**Fig. 1**).

KEY DEFINITIONS

- AI product: The algorithm(s) that are added into the workflow to support decision-making
- End-to-end workflow: The essential elements that make up the delivery of a breast screening program
- Breast screening service: An organization/team that delivers breast screening program to a community

[a] Oxford Breast Imaging Centre, Churchill Hospital, Old Road, Headington, Oxford OX3 7LE, UK; [b] Regional Head of Screening Quality Assurance Service (SQAS) - South, NHS England, England, UK; [c] North East Scotland Breast Screening Service, Aberdeen Royal Infirmary, Foresterhill Road, Aberdeen AB25 2XF, UK
* Corresponding author.
E-mail address: louise.wilkinson11@outlook.com

Radiol Clin N Am 62 (2024) 703–716
https://doi.org/10.1016/j.rcl.2023.12.006

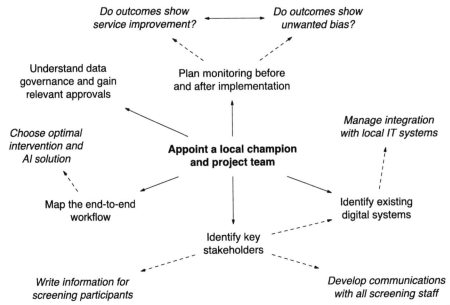

Fig. 1. Key themes for safe implementation of AI for mammography image interpretation into the breast-screening pathway.

- Users: People who deliver the service and people who use the service.

IMAGINING AI IN BREAST SCREENING: WHAT COULD A SUCCESSFUL INTEGRATION LOOK LIKE?

The new generation AI products promise to improve accuracy and efficiency in clinical decision-making but we need to be clear about how they fit into the clinical environment. In the management of breast cancer, the current focus is on AI products that assist with image interpretation, but AI products could be usefully applied at many different points in the diagnostic pathway (**Fig. 2**). Adoption of AI will be more successful if we consider the teams, systems, and processes that make up the whole breast screening service, and how each of these parts will be affected.

Above all, the transition to an AI-supported service will require a team that can acquire the necessary expertise and new skills.[1,2] Radiologists need to learn how to make the best use of AI[3] and develop data science skills to assess the quality of the data used in AI products.[4,5]

In some countries, breast screening is delivered as a national screening program, which may be an easier environment in which to manage organizational change and implement monitoring at scale. Sophisticated measurement of the impact of introducing AI will be limited in smaller organizations with a less-systematic approach to screening, in which case measurement of outcomes and planning for implementation of AI may require additional monitoring to be introduced. Any overarching data analysis that incorporates multiple organizations should specify data fields such as algorithm and version to be captured alongside numbers of cases examined and outcomes and other variables such as modality and postprocessing, which may affect algorithm performance. Regardless of the local organization of screening, successful implementation requires integration of AI products with existing technology. Screening workflow depends on a mature landscape of digital systems and will be substantially complicated by the introduction of AI. Where and how AI products should fit into the existing IT landscape will be a complex challenge requiring clinical, technical, governance, and business expertise.[6] Regular monitoring is crucial to demonstrate that the analysis and reporting workflow remains timely, stable, and comprehensive.

Clinicians should be aware that AI products will interpret a mammogram in new ways. When performed by human readers, image interpretation is heterogenous with some natural variation between readers. Experienced readers try to balance sensitivity (the detection of as many abnormalities as possible) against specificity (limiting the number of women recalled for further tests). In any given service, the readers will have different strengths and weaknesses for identifying key features such as calcifications or distortions but these will tend

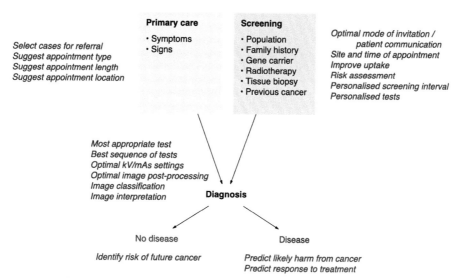

Fig. 2. Opportunities for AI to improve early diagnosis in the breast cancer pathway.

to balance out across the service as a whole. In contrast, AI products will offer more homogenous and consistent image interpretation such that, if presented with the same set of mammograms on multiple occasions, the AI product should generate the same response every time. This consistency might be welcome but it is important to consider not only how it might change the existing balance of reading within a service but also what could be missed.

The output of any mammogram interpretation, by human or AI, is impacted by a wide range of variables associated with, for example, breast (size, density, parenchymal texture, and feature type) and mammography machine (image acquisition parameters, postprocessing, and manufacturer). There is a risk that the mechanical consistency of an AI product might systematically miss features on some images that would have been picked up by at least one human reader in a service. The impact will depend on variations in the population screened, the equipment, the image data, and how the AI product and the human readers perform. If an AI product is deployed in a relatively small screening service, such variability may not be obvious. However, as the scale of the intervention increases with larger programs or multiple sites, any latent deficiencies in an AI product will become significant. Therefore, a successful clinical integration will need to monitor outcomes such as sensitivity and specificity very closely and will need to identify the variables that affect screening results. Variation in performance will be easier to identify by monitoring at scale in centralized organizations rather than by fragmented evaluation in smaller screening services

but even in the smallest organizations, monitoring of recall rate, cancer detection rate, and cancers not identified by reader or AI are essential to ensure that an AI-enhanced workflow is operating within acceptable parameters. Our case study discussed later indicates that such monitoring is best performed at modality level.

The data-driven nature of AI image interpretation risks widening inequalities. Without careful monitoring, increased usage of an AI product could negatively affect groups who happen to be underrepresented in the training data.[7] Successful integration therefore requires continuous monitoring of the AI product's performance analyzed by relevant subgroups, and services should work to establish the impact of an AI product on different groups of the population.

PREPARING FOR IMPLEMENTATION: UNDERSTANDING YOUR END-TO-END WORKFLOW

To prepare for implementation, you need to start with a clear and in-depth understanding of your service's end-to-end workflow, considering all the elements that contribute to running your service and how each one might be impacted by introducing an AI product. This will help develop a clear vision of your service's unique needs, where AI products can be integrated most effectively for you, and how to tailor AI solutions to local practices and effectively evaluate their impact. Analysis of the end-to-end workflows in your breast-screening services can be structured by thinking about the processes involved, the users, and the digital systems and what data they need.

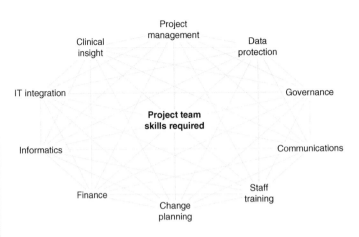

Fig. 3. Skills required in the project team.

Processes

Screening processes describe the steps and timing of the screening pathway, including invitation (or communication of screening recommendation), scheduling, image acquisition, reporting, further assessment, documentation, and monitoring of outcomes. Documentation of processes should identify areas of practice where there is room for improving efficiency, accuracy, or turnaround times. AI products could be introduced at any of these stages, and adoption of AI at one stage may influence performance at other stages of the workflow—careful consideration should be given to what the unintended consequences of introducing AI might be.

Users

Service delivery depends on more than just a clinical team. It encompasses all the disciplines that support and manage infrastructure, such as operational managers, IT experts, procurement and finance teams, and others. The implementation of an AI product requires a multidisciplinary team with active involvement of all relevant stakeholders (**Fig. 3**). Over time, it is likely that team members will become more multiskilled: radiologists will need to learn data science skills and AI product owners will need to understand software development as well as clinical priorities. Although AI is likely to reduce the workload of human readers, the uncertainty of AI delivery in the early days of deployment means that sufficient workforce should be retained to manage reversion to conventional reading if needed.

Screening participants also need to be considered, with planned communications to address issues of trust, reliability, data ownership, privacy, and consent.

Data and Digital Systems

The data and digital systems supporting breast screening are mature and complex, with wide variation between institutions, and include local patient registers (electronic patient record), radiology information system, picture archiving and communications (PACS), imaging acquisition modalities, and more. The pre-implementation mapping will need to identify where relevant data is stored, interface options, and the reliability and consistency of the data.[8] Several reviews have described the heterogeneity of routinely stored data, the multiple systems, and nonstandard formats that are barriers to implementation.[9,10] Data that are curated with structured data formats will be easier to analyze, and application of the FAIR (Findability, Accessibility, Interoperability, and Reusability) principles[11] will support data flows and monitoring.

Integrated data and digital systems can be used to establish a baseline of performance before the integration of AI. Monitoring can then be modified to assess the influence of AI. Examining the service's workflow and anticipating the influence of AI products on performance can help define the key metrics to measure and monitor.

IMPLEMENTATION: REALIZING THE VISION

The planning and implementation of AI should be rooted in this clear and in-depth understanding of the service's end-to-end workflow, which gives clarity to what a service's specific needs are, where the most advantageous point of intervention is, and where the potential pitfalls may lie. The planning process should be undertaken by a multidisciplinary team with a wide range of perspectives on topics such as integration into existing digital systems, ongoing monitoring processes, and the impact on service users.

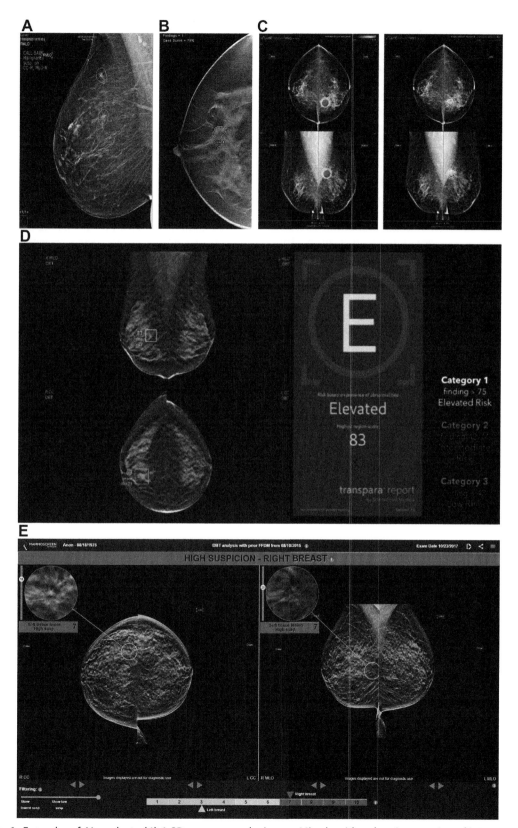

Fig. 4. Examples of AI products. (*A*) A 2D mammography image, Mia algorithm showing a region of interest and recall opinion. (*B*) A 3D mammography image, Profound AI algorithm showing a region of interest, number of

This team can help to decide the most appropriate AI intervention to support the workflow, considering current evidence for effectiveness. For example, AI products could be introduced as triage to separate cases into low (single reading) and high (double reading) probability of cancer[12]; as a reader aid to highlight areas of potential abnormality and likelihood of cancer (akin to computer-aided diagnosis); to substitute a human read in a multireader workflow; or any combination of these. One option is for the AI product to direct the reading workflow, another option is for the output to be returned to PACS (eg, image overlay or secondary DICOM capture) with the screening images to support interpretations made and transcribed by a human reader. In a single reader workflow, AI could be tuned to give readers confidence to improve specificity by classifying images as extremely low likelihood of abnormality. A study on retrospective US and UK data by McKinney[13] demonstrated an improvement in specificity and specificity. There is potential for automating AI output into structured reporting systems. Examples of current commercially available AI products are seen in **Fig. 4**.

Choosing a vendor and product is complex. Procurement should consider the vendor's earlier experience of implementing AI and include independent discussion with existing customers. Implementation will be made more complex by the number of sites, AI products, and degree of automation. An AI product may include a single algorithm or an ensemble of algorithms, and the performance may change when versions are updated. Decision-makers should consider that this is a rapidly evolving market, and there is likely to be a shift from a multitude of diverse incompatible applications to a smaller number of established vendors offering platforms that interact across devices and systems.[14]

Choosing a product should start from an understanding of the AI training dataset and how the product performed in external validation. Dataset bias in AI products might introduce or widen inequalities in screening services, and although efforts to quantify dataset bias are in progress,[15] services need to be aware that AI products may not perform uniformly across populations. Running an AI product initially on retrospective case sets which reflect the local population, and then in silent mode for a trial period will give an indication of real-world resilience before active implementation. AI products may dismiss nonstandard cases such as women with augmented breasts, previous surgery, or without the standard number of images. The challenges for implementation of AI for digital breast tomosynthesis have been discussed by Taylor and colleagues.[16]

The pilot period is an opportunity to confirm that sensitivity and specificity targets will be achieved. Vendors and service users will need to work together to ensure that the chosen product is "tuned" to existing performance, which includes setting an operating point to maintain the existing balance of sensitivity and specificity within the reading process and to avoid undue disruption to workload or accuracy.[17] AI output can then be monitored against anticipated performance. In the current naïve epoch of introducing AI in image interpretation, lessons are being learnt about how AI should be implemented, how operating points should be set and what degree of change in performance can be tolerated. It is to be hoped that openness and sharing local experience by service users will contribute to developing standard approaches.

There are several options for deploying AI products, either on site or in a cloud environment and images may be transferred directly from the acquisition modality for analysis or retrieved from PACS but images that are not analyzed locally may need to be pseudonymised before external transfer.[18] Leiner[19] explores the issues of how to apply AI products to image data, highlighting the challenges of multiple stand-alone point solutions and recommending a dedicated platform for the deployment of AI. Guidance on risk management in the implementation of Health IT systems has been described by NHS Digital.[20]

As with all IT systems, a robust set of service management disciplines should be drawn up (**Fig. 5**) and contingency plans for unanticipated downtime should be defined to ensure that there is a recovery plan in the event of failure of the AI-supported system. The deployment plan should include model retraining, updating, or replacing algorithms with minimal disruption and downtime, and there should

findings, and overall case score. (*C*) A 2D mammography image and AI algorithm showing a region of interest with a heatmap option with darker red showing increasing suspicion or contour lines with percentage score with a higher score indicating increasing suspicion. (*D*) A 3D mammography image, Transpara AI algorithm showing a region of interest with exam risk score. (*E*) 3D mammography image, AI algorithm showing a region of interest with lesion descriptor, incorporating information from prior images. (Image Courtesy: [*A*] courtesy of Kheiron Medical Technologies [*B*] Image courtesy of iCAD Inc. [*C*] courtesy of Lunit Insight [*D*] Image courtesy of ScreenPoint Medical [*E*] courtesy of Therapixel.)

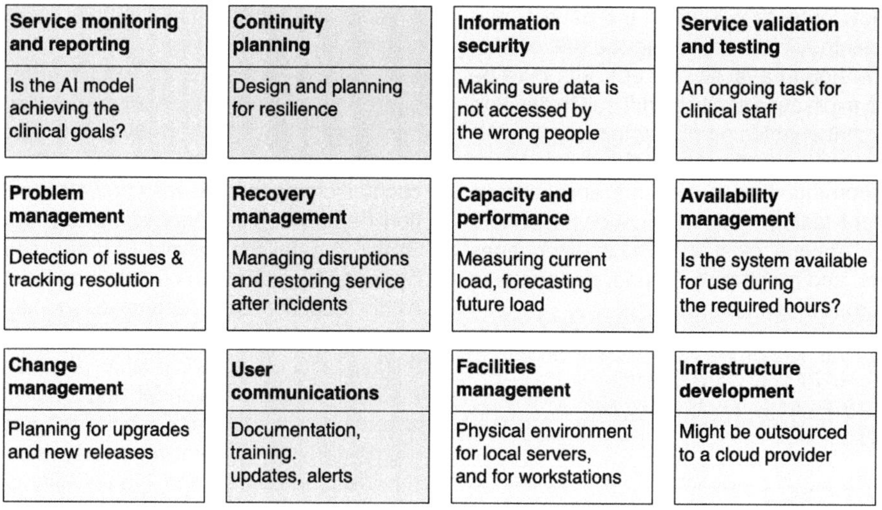

Service monitoring and reporting	Continuity planning	Information security	Service validation and testing
Is the AI model achieving the clinical goals?	Design and planning for resilience	Making sure data is not accessed by the wrong people	An ongoing task for clinical staff

Problem management	Recovery management	Capacity and performance	Availability management
Detection of issues & tracking resolution	Managing disruptions and restoring service after incidents	Measuring current load, forecasting future load	Is the system available for use during the required hours?

Change management	User communications	Facilities management	Infrastructure development
Planning for upgrades and new releases	Documentation, training. updates, alerts	Physical environment for local servers, and for workstations	Might be outsourced to a cloud provider

Fig. 5. Service management disciplines for IT systems.

also be consideration of future changes, for example, changing from two-dimensional (2D) to three-dimensional (3D) mammography, replacement of 2D with 3D + synthetic views, and what happens when initial contract ends. All IT systems eventually become obsolete, so it is also vital to plan in good time for the future replacement of the AI product and other dependent systems.

The impact of introducing AI products on users needs consideration. It is important to engender trust with service users by being open and having good quality evidence that the planned change has been properly considered and the benefits are clear. Barriers to adoption of AI include concern about inconsistent technical performance, unstructured implementation processes, uncertain clinical value, and variance in acceptance but it is recognized that it may relieve cost pressures and add clinical value.[21] All staff should engage positively to get the best out of AI products, and initial mapping of service users, including clinical teams and screening participants, provides an opportunity to discuss any concerns and aspirations.

Given that there is a diversity of AI products and outputs, staff will require training on the function and use of the systems adopted locally.

Various AI products have received approval for breast cancer screening in the United States[22] but it has been highlighted that there are gaps in the validity of training and monitoring.[23] The US Food and Drug Administration is actively assessing how regulatory and safety concerns[24] should be addressed. In the European Union, the Medical Device Regulations have been enforced, mandating deeper scrutiny of software as a medical device,[25] and in the United Kingdom, the AI and Digital Regulations Service[26] maps out the regulatory and health technology assessment pathway for AI and digital technologies.

At present, there is little understanding how humans interact with AI outcomes to reach a final decision,[27] and concerns have been raised about automation bias, where readers favor suggestions from automated decision-making systems, or the reverse. The work of Dratch[28] showed that less-experienced radiologists were more likely to be influenced by an AI prompt but even experienced radiologists may be influenced, although to a lesser degree. Regular, ongoing feedback and open discussion may help human readers to understand how AI is arriving at an outcome and to develop an appropriate level of trust. A change in diagnostic pathways may be required if lesions identified by AI cannot be perceived by the human reader.[10] With time, AI may take over a substantial proportion of image interpretation workload, changing the type and distribution of images seen by clinicians and making it potentially difficult to maintain some competencies through routine practice. At present, it is likely that a human reader will always be the final arbiter of the AI supported workflow.[29]

The attitudes of screening participants should be addressed. A review of public attitudes to AI products showed a lack of trust in their data privacy, patient safety, technological maturity, and the possibility of full automation; however, education on AI capabilities made AI more acceptable to the public.[30] Currently, there is no accepted consensus on requirements for informing patients about the use of AI, and details will be specific to the local jurisdiction, the AI product, and the service. Consent to screening could include information about the use of AI, including the purpose of the AI, risks it poses, how outputs will affect the patient, and what choices they have regarding the use of AI in their care. Although a facility for opt out could be considered, in practice it may be difficult to develop a workflow that enables participants to decline AI-supported image interpretation. Services should work with communities to evaluate and improve their patient-facing communications, ensure appropriate options exist in relevant languages and formats, and monitor the impact on uptake of services across patient populations.

AVOIDING HARM: MONITORING, GOVERNANCE, AND TRUST AFTER IMPLEMENTATION
Monitoring

The purpose of monitoring an AI-supported workflow is to ensure that AI is enhancing clinical care and not undermining it. For all their potential, AI products for image interpretation are still immature, and there is limited experience of how to integrate them into established clinical workflows. Monitoring of AI-supported systems is therefore an essential part of every clinical implementation, the responsibility of the AI vendor and the healthcare organization, and of the relevant legal and governance processes.[31] Monitoring should demonstrate that the AI product is performing as expected, producing consistent results, and not creating or widening inequalities.

To ensure AI products are operating as expected, the end-to-end workflow for each mammography unit should be monitored on a daily basis to demonstrate stability and timeliness, and identify cases where the AI product has not returned a result. The AI output and human performance should reflect the outcomes specified before implementation, including recall rate, positive predictive value of recall, cancer detection rate, and the missed cancer rate. The frequency of reporting monitored outcomes will vary by parameter and by the volume of workload. For example, recall rate should be measured frequently, and variation may prompt adjustment of either the algorithm operating point or the behavior of the human readers. Cancer detection rate will necessarily be monitored at longer intervals and missed (interval) cancers should be actively identified and scrutinized routinely. A recent external validation of an AI tool[32] discusses the difficulty of evaluating and monitoring AI in more detail.

Monitoring should be designed to identify unanticipated bias and inequality. Diagnostic outcomes can be compared with variables of population (prevalent or incident screen, breast size and density, age, and ethnicity), of image data (modality, exposure, and postprocessing), and in the AI

product itself (algorithm changes, software upgrades). The procurement process should ensure that data on variables that could affect AI outcomes is available to support detailed analysis and monitoring. The sensitivity and specificity of AI may drift over time due to external factors such as changes in disease prevalence or population demographics. Anomalies may be identified earlier if detailed analysis is performed at scale by central organizations rather than independently within local services. Automated monitoring using visualization dashboards can provide real-time intelligence for changes in positive and negative predictive values and the underlying recall and cancer detection rate.[33] Formal monitoring can be supplemented by patient-reported and clinician-reported outcomes and high-quality surveys to identify challenges, uncertainties, and health policy gaps.[34]

The nature of the cancers detected by any AI product should be routinely analyzed. If AI preferentially identifies slow growing cancers, impact on mortality will be limited. If AI is to save lives, it will need to diagnose potentially fatal cancers. In 2012, an independent review of breast screening[35] concluded that one death was prevented for about every 3 overdiagnosed cases identified and treated. There is potential for training AI to select out the most significant cases with the aim of reducing mortality but this requires analysis of large volumes of image data with long-term follow-up, highlighting the importance of a systematic and coordinated approach to monitoring.

Live monitoring of AI is essential for incident identification. Audit of algorithmic performance may be necessary when gross errors are noted. This can be complex and may require computational, bioinformatics, and statistical skills.[36] However, improving explainability by reliably predicting how AI will perform in specified scenarios will support shared decision-making and increase trust. AI will not always work as advertised,[37] so contingency plans are needed in case monitoring demonstrates a substantial change in AI performance such that the AI-supported service is deemed unacceptable. Thresholds of acceptable performance should be defined in advance with alerts built into the monitoring system, and monitoring should be sufficient to demonstrate the root cause of changes in AI output and allow affected screening cases to be identified. This will allow services to apply corrective action, which might include restoring updated software to previous versions, retuning the AI output to meet sensitivity and specificity targets, switching AI algorithm, or removal of AI support from the screening workflow.

Governance and Trust

Beyond monitoring, effective governance is needed—a "system of rules, practices, processes, and technological tools" that ensure that ethical and legal commitments are met.[38] At its core, effective governance should assure fairness, transparency, trustworthiness, and accountability, which is made more challenging by the "black-box" nature of AI. AI product performance depends on training data sets,[39] and the decision-making process may be complex, opaque, and hard to explain.[40] Governance requires that the product works effectively when implemented, that it continues to operate as expected, that patients and clinicians can trust it, and that any risks to patients can be mitigated. Governance should encompass a range of issues including consent, data privacy, and legal indemnity. Implementation of AI will need to acknowledge and adhere to local regulations and data processing agreements on information and data governance, especially where personal health data is concerned. Contracts should be established with local legal input but it is essential they ensure patient data rights are respected and roles in response to errors, incidents, and ongoing evaluation are defined. This can take a significant amount of time.

The use of AI has raised concerns about the security and privacy of data.[41] The staff responsible for service delivery should ensure that patient data is kept safe through administrative, physical, and technical measures. They should understand the flow of patient data and ensure that they can explain to patients what the data is used for, the level of identifiability of data used, where it is processed, how it is kept safe, and any relevant rights for their legal jurisdiction—including if/how patients can opt out of automated data processing. Participation in care using AI cannot be taken as consent for any other data processing related to an AI product. For example, where images are retained for future validation and testing, either by the service or by the company providing the AI product, this should be made clear and explicit consent should be obtained. Information should be available to patients to enable them to make decisions about whether their data can be used for these purposes, including how they can change their minds in future.

Services should be aware of the potential need to support postmarket surveillance activities that regulators demand of manufacturers,[42] which may include provision of relevant information to test ongoing accuracy and to investigate errors and incidents. Legal and regulatory arrangements are changing[43] and should be reviewed periodically.

Services should ensure they understand any implications for indemnity cover when using an AI product. Because this is a developing field, the legal implications of patient harm stemming from use of an AI product are not yet clear. Basic principles of clinical care apply, and the responsible clinicians must be able to explain and justify their decisions. Due to the complex interaction between human and AI, both vendors and clinicians have obligations when patient harm occurs. Services should ensure they have relevant local advice on where legal accountability lies and what they may be asked to demonstrate in the event of a patient coming to harm.

CASE STUDY: INITIAL EVALUATION OF PHASED INTRODUCTION OF IMAGE INTERPRETATION ARTIFICIAL INTELLIGENCE INTO A UK BREAST SCREENING PROGRAM

This case study outlines a project to evaluate use of AI into a UK screening service.[44] The service contributes to a population-screening program with high workflow of normal cases and low number of cancers and conforms to national standards including a 3-year screening interval. The study is limited by regulatory approval[45] requiring double reading with arbitration/consensus.[46] In this study, cases were double read as per standard practice and any cases not identified at double reading but flagged as suspicious by AI underwent further review to ensure that suspicious lesions had not been overlooked.

The project was led by a clinical champion who established a multidisciplinary team supported by the host organization. Members of the project board included leads from the national digital board, public health, the developers of the underlying IT system, e-health, project management, and patient champions. The project team mapped out all elements of the screening pathway and documented the essential IT infrastructure (Fig. 6). A project plan was developed, which considered how the AI would be used in clinical practice, proposed a scheme for monitoring AI output for drift, performance, and uptime, and a plan for dealing with changes in performance.

Extensive outreach with training days and regular information sessions was arranged with all service staff, including the administration and radiology team, breast surgeons, and oncologists. During start-up, the project team worked with clinical users to train them in use of the AI output and how the information contributed to the overall outcome of the screening decision. Members of the public helped to co-develop the letters and information that would be sent out to the screening participants.

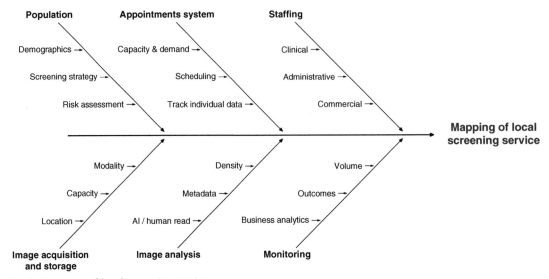

Fig. 6. Mapping of local screening service.

The Introduction of Artificial Intelligence Was Phased

Phase 1—Test whether the AI product performed as predicted with the local population: Two sets of representative test images were created. The first set, enriched with cancers, was used to assess whether the AI needed calibration to conform to current sensitivity and specificity of the screening service. The project specified that the algorithm performance was set to detect and rule out cancer cases at a predefined threshold. The second validation set was used to assess if the calibration had the desired effect on recall rate and cancer detection.

Phase 2—Run in silent mode: AI was set up to work alongside normal workflow for a short period[47] to establish that the system was working as predicted. The center performs 2000 screening examinations per month, and 3 months was allocated for connectivity testing and also to fit into the "pipeline" of selecting eligible participants, allocating appointments, sending invitations, and marking attendance for screening. This connection phase was key to confirm that IT connectivity was robust, to measure uptime and stability of the model in the clinical environment, to determine whether it can analyze all the images presented, to check whether the output messages are being sent and received consistently, and to document any loss in the process.

A key aspect of this connect phase was to link the AI messages to the existing quality assurance measures and reports, resulting in an almost-live dashboard. Reports on recall rate, AI versus reader opinion, discordant, and concordant outcomes were reviewed in the same fashion as existing normal human performance reports.

Phase 3—Live implementation of third read by AI: All cases that were highlighted by AI were

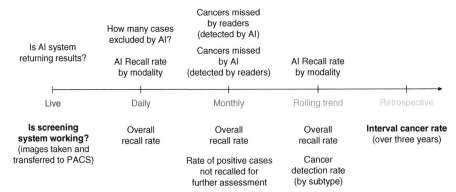

Fig. 7. Examples of parameters for monitoring of AI-supported breast-screening workflow (the monitoring cycle may vary depending on the volume of cases included in the workflow).

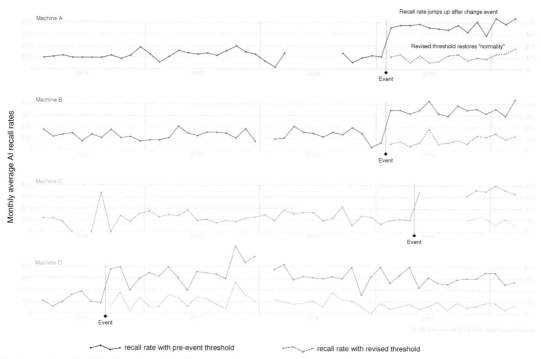

Fig. 8. As described by de Vries and colleagues, observations of 4 different machines across 4 years, show that AI recall rates jump after software change events. Clinical thresholds need to be adjusted to restore "normality."

allocated to an additional human reader arbitration/consensus step, such that human reader(s) made the final decision to call for further assessment.

Fig. 7 shows the parameters that are being systematically monitored. **Fig. 8** demonstrates how a routine remote update of postprocessing algorithm on the mammogram image changed the performance of a breast-screening AI to recall more patients without any change in human performance. This was an unanticipated outcome and demonstrates that changes in any part of the hardware or software environment may cause significant destabilizing change in AI output. The servicing and upgrade schedules vary between mammography units, accounting for the time difference in performance changes. The change occurred while the system was running in silent mode, and there was no impact on reader behavior or screening outcomes.

This case study has demonstrated that it is possible to integrate a single vendor AI into a breast screening service interface and establish effective systematic monitoring. The case study revealed the need to monitor performance in near real time at each site. With increasing use, optimal thresholds could be specified for each modality and AI combination, adjusted for the prevalence of cancer in the population screened. Recall rate and cancer detection rate are currently being

monitored but considerably more experience is required to evaluate how the type of cancers that are being detected compare to current practice.

SUMMARY

We have described an approach to integrate AI products for image interpretation in breast screening, ensuring that the choice of algorithm(s) and deployment is based on an understanding of the local breast screening pathway. This is the beginning of a new era of image interpretation, and there is much to learn as the technology moves from research and evaluation into routine clinical use. We believe that success depends on having a multidisciplinary team approach to planning and implementing technology, supported by careful monitoring of the impact of introducing a "nonhuman reader." Services should also be mindful of complying with local legislation and governance principles and must work proactively to avoid introducing or widening inequalities.

It is likely that the early benefit of AI in breast screening will be an improved workflow (eg, reduced reporting times and lower false-positive rates) but ultimately the goal should be for AI to improve early diagnosis of fast-growing cancers that have the potential to be fatal. More accurate classification of lesions at diagnosis may inform treatment options and improve outcomes.[48] Radiologists must contribute to the development of integrated systems, gaining expertise in data science to ensure they understand and support the quality of the data used in AI, with new roles for individuals with both clinical qualifications and understanding of IT.

CLINICS CARE POINTS

- Understand your workflow before you start, plan interventions accordingly and define thresholds for acceptable performance.
- Ensure engagement of relevant stakeholders, including staff, screening participants, and existing IT system owners.
- Plan your monitoring and think about how you will identify inconsistency and inequality.
- Define how AI result will be adopted into your reporting system and plan audit to ensure all cases have been managed appropriately.
- Allow sufficient time to understand data-protection issues and meet local legal and governance requirements.
- Implement with a phased approach including retrospective case sets, silent mode, and go live.
- Contingency planning for failure of AI supported workflow, change in local IT systems, and end of contract.

DISCLOSURE

Dr G. Lip has received funding from the NHS for research work with Kheiron Medical Technologies. He is supported by a grant form the Chief Scientist Office of Scotland and has received speaker and panel fees from Bayer, Hologic and General Electric.

REFERENCES

1. Bajwa J, Munir U, Nori A, et al. Artificial intelligence in healthcare: transforming the practice of medicine. Future Healthc J 2021;8(2):e188–94.
2. Topol E. Preparing the healthcare workforce to deliver the digital future. NHS Health Education England. 2019 Available at: https://topol.hee.nhs.uk/ Accessed August 14, 2023.
3. European Society of Radiology (ESR). What the radiologist should know about artificial intelligence - an ESR white paper. Insights Imaging 2019 4; 10(1):44.
4. Miller DD. The medical AI insurgency: what physicians must know about data to practice with intelligent machines. npj Digital Medicine 2019;2:62.
5. Finlayson SG, Subbaswamy A, Singh K, et al. The Clinician and Dataset Shift in Artificial Intelligence. N Engl J Med 2021;385:283–6.
6. Bizzo BC, Dasegowda G, Bridge C, et al. Addressing the Challenges of Implementing Artificial Intelligence Tools in Clinical Practice: Principles From Experience. J Am Coll Radiol 2023;20(3): p352–60.
7. Obermeyer Z, Powers B, Vogeli C, et al. Dissecting racial bias in an algorithm used to manage the health of populations. Science 2019;366(6464): 447–53.
8. Koh DM, Papanikolaou N, Bick U, et al. Artificial intelligence and machine learning in cancer imaging. Commun Med 2022;2:133.
9. Shaikh FA, Kolowitz BJ, Awan O, et al. Technical Challenges in the Clinical Application of Radiomics. JCO Clin Cancer Inform 2017;1:1–8.
10. Zheng D, He X, Jing J. Overview of Artificial Intelligence in Breast Cancer Medical Imaging. J Clin Med 2023;12(2):419.
11. Wilkinson M, Dumontier M, Aalbersberg I, et al. The FAIR Guiding Principles for scientific data management and stewardship. Sci Data 2016;3:18.
12. Lang K, Josefsson V, Larsson A-M, et al. Artificial intelligence-supported screen reading versus standard double reading in the Mammography Screening with Artificial Intelligence trial (MASAI): a clinical safety analysis of a randomised, controlled, non-inferiority, single- blinded, screening accuracy study. Lancet Oncol 2023;24(8):936–44.
13. McKinney SM, Sieniek M, Godbole V, et al. International evaluation of an AI system for breast cancer screening. Nature 2020;577:89–94.
14. Alexander A, Jiang A, Ferreira C, et al. An Intelligent Future for Medical Imaging: A Market Outlook on Artificial Intelligence for Medical Imaging. J Am Coll Radiol 2020;147(1 pt B):165–70.
15. Ganapathi S, Palmer J, Alderman JE, et al. Tackling bias in AI health datasets through the STANDING Together initiative. Nat Med 2022;28:2232–3.
16. Taylor CR, Monga N, Johnson C, et al. Artificial Intelligence Applications in Breast Imaging: Current Status and Future Directions. Diagnostics 2023;13(12): 2041.
17. Dembrower K, Salim M, Eklund M, et al. Implications for downstream workload based on calibrating an artificial intelligence detection algorithm by standalone-reader or combined-reader sensitivity matching. J Med Imaging 2023;10(Suppl 2):S22405.
18. Kaissis GA, Makowski MR, Rückert D, et al. Secure, privacy-preserving and federated machine learning in medical imaging. Nat Mach Intell 2020;2:305–11.

19. Leiner T, Bennink E, Mol CP, et al. Bringing AI to the clinic: blueprint for a vendor-neutral AI deployment infrastructure. Insights Imaging 2021;12(1):11.

20. NHS75 Digital. DCB0160: Clinical Risk Management: its Application in the Deployment and Use of Health IT Systems. 2018. Available at DCB0160: Clinical Risk Management: its Application in the Deployment and Use of Health IT Systems - NHS Digital Accessed August 14, 2023.

21. Strohm L, Hehakaya C, Ranschaert ER, et al. Implementation of artificial intelligence (AI) applications in radiology: hindering and facilitating factors. Eur Radiol 2020;30(10):5525–32.

22. ACR Data Science Institute AI Central. Available at: https://aicentral.acrdsi.org/. Accessed October 6, 2023.

23. Potnis KC, Ross JS, Sanjay A, et al. Evaluation of FDA Device Regulation and Future Recommendations. JAMA Intern Med 2022;182(12):1306–12.

24. US Food and Drug Administration. Proposed Regulatory Framework for Modifications to Artificial Intelligence/Machine Learning (AI/ML)-Based Software as a Medical Device (SaMD) Available at: https://www.fda.gov/files/medical%20devices/published/US-FDA-Artificial-Intelligence-and-Machine-Learning-Discussion-Paper.pdf. Accessed October 6, 2023.

25. Medical Devices – New regulations - Overview. European Commission. Medical Devices – New regulations - Overview. 2022. Available at: Overview (europa.eu). Accessed August 14, 2023.

26. NHS England - Transformation Directorate. The AI and Digital Regulations Service. Available at: AI and digital regulations service - AI Regulation - NHS Transformation Directorate (england.nhs.uk) Accessed August 14, 2023.

27. Kerschke L, Weigel S, Rodriguez-Ruiz A, et al. Using deep learning to assist readers during the arbitration process: a lesion-based retrospective evaluation of breast cancer screening performance. Eur Radiol 2022;32(2):842–52.

28. Dratsch T, Chen X, Rezazade Mehrizi M, et al. The Impact of Artificial Intelligence BI-RADS Suggestions on Reader Performance. Radiology 2023;307:4.

29. Topol EJ. High-performance medicine: the convergence of human and artificial intelligence. Nat Med 2019;25:44–56.

30. Chew HSJ, Achananuparp P. Perceptions and Needs of Artificial Intelligence in Health Care to Increase Adoption: Scoping Review. J Med Internet Res 2022;24(1):e32939.

31. Carter SM, Rogers W, Win KT, et al. The ethical, legal and social implications of using artificial intelligence systems in breast cancer care. Breast 2020;49:25–32.

32. Cushnan D, Young KC, Ward D, et al. Lessons learned from independent external validation of an AI tool to detect breast cancer using a representative UK data set. Br J Radiol 2023;96(1143):20211104.

33. de Vries CF, Colosimo SJ, Staff RT, et al. Impact of Different Mammography Systems on Artificial Intelligence Performance in Breast Cancer Screening Radiology. Artif Intell 2023;5:3.

34. Gilbert S, Pimenta A, Stratton-Powell A, et al. Continuous Improvement of Digital Health Applications Linked to Real-World Performance Monitoring: Safe Moving Targets? Mayo Clin Proc: Digital Health 2023;1(3):276–87.

35. Independent UK Panel on Breast Cancer Screening. The benefits and harms of breast cancer screening: an independent review. Lancet 2012;380(9855):1778–86.

36. Liu X, Glocker B, McCradden M, et al. The medical algorithmic audit. The Lancet Digital Health 2022;4(5):e384–97.

37. Clark P, Kim J, Aphinyanaphongs Y. Marketing and US Food and Drug Administration Clearance of Artificial Intelligence and Machine Learning Enabled Software in and as Medical Devices: A Systematic Review. JAMA Netw Open 2023;6(7):e2321792.

38. Mäntymäki M, Minkkinen M, Birkstedt T, et al. Defining organizational AI governance. AI Ethics 2022;2:603–9.

39. Reddy S, Allan S, Coghlan S, et al. A governance model for the application of AI in health care. J Am Med Inform Assoc 2020;27(3):491–7.

40. Shin D. The effects of explainability and causability on perception, trust, and acceptance: Implications for explainable AI. Int J Hum Comput Stud 2021;146:102551.

41. Young AT, Amara D, Bhattacharya A, et al. Patient and general public attitudes towards clinical artificial intelligence: a mixed methods systematic review. Lancet Digit Health 2021;3(9):e599–611.

42. AI and Digital Regulations Service. Post-market surveillance of medical devices. 2023 Available at: Post-market surveillance of medical devices - AI regulation service - NHS (innovation.nhs.uk). Accessed August 14, 2023.

43. Medicines and Healthcare products Regulatory Agency. Software and AI as a Medical Device Change Programme – Roadmap. 2023. Available at Software and AI as a Medical Device Change Programme - Roadmap - GOV.UK (Available at: www.gov.uk) Accessed August 14, 2023.

44. Seedat F, Taylor Phillips S. Guidance for using AI in Breast Screening. 2022. Available at: https://nationalscreening.blog.gov.uk/2022/08/01/guidance-on-evaluating-ai-for-use-in-breast-screening/. Accessed August 14, 2023.

45. Gemini. AI-assisted breast screening. Available at: https://www.nhsgrampian.org/about-us/innovation-h

ub/our-projects/current-projects/gemini/. Accessed October 18, 2023.

46. NHS England. Breast Screening Guidance for Image Reading. 2023 Available at: https://www.gov.uk/government/publications/breast-screening-guidance-for-image-reading/breast-screening-guidance-for-image-reading. Accessed August 14, 2023.

47. Langlotz CP. Will Artificial Intelligence Replace Radiologists? Radiol Artif Intell 2019;1(3):e190058.

48. Varoquaux G, Cheplygina V. Machine learning for medical imaging: methodological failures and recommendations for the future. npj Digit Med 2022;5: 48.

Patient Communication Innovations in Breast Imaging

Shadi Aminololama-Shakeri, MD, FSBI*, Kaitlin M. Ford, MD

KEYWORDS

• Patient-centered care • Patient-physician communication • Breast radiology communication

KEY POINTS

- Innovative methods and timely communication with patients are essential in the setting of increased access to health information.
- Formal training and effective communication skills for radiologists can lead to better patient outcomes and reduce physician burnout.
- Patient-focused education is key in improving shared decision-making.

INTRODUCTION

The patient–physician relationship is at the heart of breast radiology, a subspecialty, which has been at the leading edge of radiology practice in the arena of patient communication. Decades before the widespread recognition of the importance of structured reporting and patient-centered care practices in radiology, mammography reporting and patient communication standards were codified as a pillar of practice by the Mammography Quality Standards Act[1] and the Breast Imaging Reporting and Data System.[2–4] Effective communication influences overall patient experience, well-being, and adherence to medical recommendations while concurrently reducing patient-perceived pain and anxiety.[5,6] Breast radiologists play a pivotal role not only in conveying diagnostic findings but also in engaging patients in comprehensive discussions about their care and management. Increasingly, breast radiologists are the health professionals who engage in conversation when a patient's breast malignant diagnosis is confirmed or excluded.[7] In our academic institution, as in many other breast radiology practices, the verbal discussion of a new breast cancer diagnosis with the patient has been incorporated into our daily practice. In fact, in California, Senate Bill 1419 sponsored by the California Medical Association permits a delay in the electronic release of a potentially life-changing test result, such as a cancer diagnosis, specifically to allow time for physicians to interpret this information.[8] The added layer of direct patient communication and consultation has had many implications ranging from effects on trainee education to physician wellness and burnout. Another impetus for more widespread modifications in practice has been the coronavirus disease 2019 (COVID-19) pandemic, which required adaptations in communication practices in breast radiology. This worldwide crisis introduced a new and unique set of challenges for breast radiologists, necessitating inventive strategies to establish rapport and meet patients' emotional needs within the constraints of limited contact and personal protective equipment.[9] These unusual circumstances further highlighted the indispensable role of communication during crisis and the demand for innovative approaches to enhance patient communication.[10] In this review, we aim to discuss salient patient communication opportunities in breast imaging and describe innovative approaches that can serve as a model for other areas in radiology.

Department of Radiology, University of California Davis, 4860 Y Street, Suite 3100, Sacramento, CA 95817, USA
* Corresponding author.
E-mail address: sshakeri@ucdavis.edu

Radiol Clin N Am 62 (2024) 717–724
https://doi.org/10.1016/j.rcl.2024.01.004

PATIENT ACCESS TO HEALTH INFORMATION

With increased patient access to health information via electronic medical records (EMRs), and the twenty-first Century Cures Act, a federal mandate for the release of personal health information without delay, radiologists are in the midst of a shift in how best to report and communicate imaging findings.[11] Internet-based systems have been shown to empower patients to access their medical images and reports, promoting health literacy, and active participation in decision-making.[12] In addition, more patients are using online platforms through patient portals or smartphone applications to access their health information, particularly their radiology reports. In one study of 61,131 patients with at least one radiology report available on the online patient portal access, more than 50% (31,308) of patients with web portal access reviewed their radiology reports in comparison to only 30% (1971 out of 5731) reviewed their clinical notes.[13–15] This trend is even more pronounced in breast imaging, where a cancer diagnosis has been shown to increase online information-seeking behavior.[16] These changes necessitate breast radiologist adaptation and accommodation to varying patient preferences and changing expectations. For example, in a survey to evaluate patients' perceptions and communication preferences regarding risk assessment results, when faced with a hypothetical scenario of elevated lifetime risk of breast cancer (>20%) patients were 10 times more likely to prefer oral communication of risk assessment than if their lifetime risk was less than 20%.[17] This is divergent from the results for patients with a hypothetical risk less than 20%, as patients were more amenable to written communication.

INNOVATIONS IN REPORTING
Patient Communication

A prominent area of innovation in improving radiologist communication in breast cancer care revolves around innovations in radiology report generation. This includes the integration of image-rich reports and the inclusion of relevant key images. Emerging image-processing software is currently being tested to automate the incorporation of pertinent images in radiology reports. For example, some programs can create visual timelines illustrating breast cancer disease progression using images from serial studies. Another program being explored harnesses natural language processing to identify and compare summary statements from previous radiology reports.[13,14,18]

A pioneering effort by the New York University (NYU) Grossman School of Medicine involves creating concise video radiology reports, prepared by radiologists, which seamlessly integrate into the patient information portal.[19] These videos act as tools to aid both patients and referring providers in understanding imaging results. A survey conducted by NYU assessing the patient's overall experience and ability to comprehend their imaging test results revealed that 91% of respondents preferred this combined approach, desiring both written and video radiology reports. The integration of multimedia reports, key images, and interactive interfaces within patient portals and radiology reports enhances patient comprehension and engagement, ultimately improving patient–physician communication.[13]

Provider Communication

The radiology report often includes information for the referring provider as well as the patient. Many different approaches have been devised to keep the ordering physician in the communication loop of findings, recommendations, and necessary follow-up action items. There is no current standardized method for this type of information exchange and the interactions may include a phone call, dictated reports, mobile the Health Insurance Portability and Accountability Act (HIPAA) compliant collaborative messaging platforms, and rarely, physical mailing or faxing of printed reports. Direct messaging through the EMRs may be used as well. One area in breast imaging that requires clear communication with the referring provider is postbiopsy recommendations. As the physicians who perform radiology-pathology concordance evaluation after breast interventions, we find it best at our institution to document the next step recommendations in a standardized addendum to the procedural report. Included in that documentation is the mode of informing the patient, typically a prearranged telephone encounter, as well as the means of informing the ordering provider, typically via messaging through the EMRs.

BEYOND THE RADIOLOGY REPORT: CHALLENGES AND INNOVATIONS IN DIRECT COMMUNICATION

The radiology report has evolved beyond its traditional role as a method of communication between the referring physician and the radiologist; now, it also serves as a platform for direct patient communication.[13,18] This shift necessitates radiologist preparation for engagement with patients who are equipped with a greater understanding of medical information. Radiologists have had to proactively adapt to these changing dynamics, ensuring their communication skills encompass both accurate diagnostic explanations and effective handling of patient queries and concerns. Breast radiologists have shown enthusiasm toward increasing efforts at the personal and practice level to improve their modes of communication and skills.[20] Although face-to-face consultations with patients are already routine in breast imaging, online patient inquiries about imaging results and clinical implications are anticipated to increase, particularly from screening patients who typically do not have in person consultation at the time of the examination. With widespread adoption of online portals offering efficient and convenient access to medical data, adjustments in radiology workflows have resulted. In a survey of 1000 patients by the American Medical Association, 65% expressed that they would want to speak with their physician first in the event of receiving life-changing test results. In keeping with these results, as described above, legislators in California have passed a law, which counters the immediate electronic release of sensitive radiology and other test results until a physician has discussed this with the patient.[21] As physicians seeking opportunities to deliver patient-centered and family-centered care, radiologists and more specifically, breast radiologists are poised to have these conversations.[3] In fact, some practices already incorporate contact information within the imaging report for access to a radiologist in response to the American College of Radiology (ACR) Imaging 3.0 and the Radiological Society of North America (RSNA) Radiology Cares campaigns for patient-centered care.[3,22,23] Other institutions have taken proactive measures vis-à-vis these patient requests by establishing formal radiology consultation clinics. These venues, which may be comprised of both in-person and remote video consultations, are established with the purpose of reviewing imaging findings directly with patients. This approach has proven successful and demonstrated higher patient satisfaction and understanding.[24–27] Breast radiology practices may emulate this model and initiate structured consultations with radiologists/radiologist extenders. Consultations not only serve to explain various screening modalities but also may help direct high-risk patients to genetic counseling and oncology services.[13,28] This type of clinical service can enhance patient-centered care, facilitate referrals, and optimize the utilization of supplemental screening for those with a high lifetime risk of breast cancer.[13]

Timing of Communication

The ease of access to radiology reports through online patient portals has also elevated patient expectations and demands for timely and comprehensive communication.[29] Recent studies reveal that patient satisfaction is closely tied to speedy delivery of results rather than to the type of physician providing the result. This highlights the necessity of timely patient communication to alleviate patient stress and anxiety.[30–33] To address this, some breast imaging centers even offer same-day breast screening slots for real-time interpretation.[34]

Challenges to Communication

The shrinking radiology workforce and increasing demands for imaging may make it challenging to meet the demand of direct patient communication.[35,36] Yet at the same time, there is demand for a tailored approach to meet individual patient preferences and needs, especially as patients are increasingly motivated to engage in shared decision-making regarding their health. Yet studies have shown that individualized communication is lacking even when desired by patients, for example, in the setting of risk assessment. A 2015 study that surveyed women undergoing screening or surveillance mammography at 2 urban academic outpatient breast imaging centers in the United States[17] found that although 86% of women expressed interest in learning their estimated lifetime risk of breast cancer, only 8% had undergone formal risk assessment. Potential large-scale approaches include incorporating breast cancer risk models into screening mammography reports, using augmented intelligence-based tools, and incorporating patient-reported data at the time of imaging to identify candidates who may benefit from referral for formal risk assessment.[28,37]

Adding to the complexities of dealing with workforce shortages are the seismic practice changes caused by the COVID-19 pandemic. In the aftermath of the pandemic, breast cancer and lung cancer screening rates have remained low among Medicare enrollees.[38] This is particularly concerning in terms of further widening existing disparities in breast cancer screening and outcomes. A recent study, for example, found that the already decreased rates of screening in low-income patients, and those from historically marginalized groups, have not rebounded.[38] Our evolving role as radiologists practicing in patient-centered and family-centered care delivery environments requires flexibility, nimble responsiveness, collaboration, and trust-building in an increasingly patient-engaged health-care landscape.[39] One means of achieving this is through patient education.

EMPOWERING PATIENTS THROUGH EDUCATION

Amplifying science-based, educational messages to decrease breast cancer disparities needs to be prioritized. The use of visual aids, educational pamphlets, multimedia, and patient-centered language can enhance patient knowledge. A recent study providing patients with educational handouts about biopsy markers before procedures demonstrated significant improvements in self-assessed patient knowledge and comfort scores.[40] Incorporating educational videos that can supplement or even replace traditional informed consent for procedures also merits exploration and has been performed successfully in other specialties. The use of educational videos has been reported as equivalent to standard verbal informed consent in several studies and may also lead to improved patient recall of core aspects of the consent as well as higher patient satisfaction.[41,42]

Implementing workstations or portable tablets in clinics for showing key patient images can facilitate discussions about procedures, follow-up, or biopsy recommendations. This approach may aid patients in structuring focused questions that are best addressed by the radiologist as well as improve clinician workflow efficiency in the clinic. Empowering patients through education, including the use of additional online resources and handouts, supports informed decision-making and has been shown to increase patient involvement and enhance satisfaction with treatment options.[43] The American Cancer Society (ACS), Society of Breast Imaging, and the ACR, for example, offer various online resources that radiologists can reference during discussion about breast pathology results, helping counteract information retention challenges. Multipronged information reinforcement is particularly important because patients may retain a fraction of the information conveyed during conversations with their physicians. Additionally, patient recall and processing of information has been shown to decrease following biopsy recommendations or in the setting of difficult diagnoses.[43,44]

Patient-focused education through the use of social media has gained popularity along with calls for wider physician engagement.[45,46] Although professional societies are embracing this movement with production of accessible material for patients, there is great variability in the quality of information available through digital media.[47,48]

Assessment of all educational materials for barriers to patient comprehension such as readability and grade level are important. The use of non-English language versions of presented materials is also crucial for adequate communication with non-English speaking patients.[49–51] This is of particular importance given the numerous obstacles non-English speakers face in the clinical setting. One recent study reported remarkable barriers for non-English speakers when seeking information regarding cancer care services including a high mean readability grade level of patient education articles greater than or equal to that of 10th graders.[52]

Artificial intelligence (AI)-based tools may be integrated into the radiologist's workflow for patient communication and education. Large language models, such as ChatGPT, could be used to translate reports into patient-friendly language.[53] Although countless applications of AI may be helpful in breast radiology practice, it is not yet known how receptive patients will be to AI-assisted communication tools particularly in the setting of a potential cancer diagnosis.[54] Additionally, although AI applications are promising, they still need rigorous evaluation for quality and accuracy.[55,56]

Other Preventive Services

The breast imaging community has yet to fully explore the potential for educational opportunities that could be offered to women routinely presenting for their screening mammograms. The breast radiology clinic is an optimal platform for introducing and reinforcing education regarding healthy lifestyle choices including referrals to other preventive services such as lung cancer screening or even cardiovascular wellness programs (see supplement Figs. 1 and 2 for sample educational materials). Initial efforts by radiologists seeking to offer these services are currently underway.[57]

RADIOLOGIST EDUCATION

Experience and training are pivotal for effective communication. Research demonstrates that physicians with more experience and training in patient communication foster improved healthcare outcomes and higher patient adherence rates.[6] Conversely, physicians lacking proficient communication skills are more susceptible to litigation.[58] Consequently, the Accreditation Council for Graduate Medical Education (ACGME), American Board of Radiology (ABR), and Society of Breast Imaging (SBI) have collectively highlighted the significance of cultivating communication skills. The ACGME and ABR have integrated communication skills as a core competency and graduation requirement for radiology residents. Similarly, the breast imaging fellowship curriculum and SBI have reemphasized proficiency in patient interactions and communication skills training to not only improve patient health-care outcomes and satisfaction but also to augment radiology's value.[59,60] Nonetheless, a recent survey conducted among SBI fellowship directors revealed that only a minority of programs, accounting for 32% of respondents, offer formal communication skills training.[61] The majority of programs primarily rely on feedback based on observed fellow-patient interactions.[61] To better prepare future breast radiologists, it is imperative for fellowship programs to include formal communication skills training using the variety of methodologies available including simulation-based training.[62] Insights from other specialties where management of complex patient interactions are prevalent, illuminate the efficacy of implementing communication skills boot camps, simulations, didactic courses, and group sessions. Such programs, such as surgery, neurosurgery, and obstetrics and gynecology, have even introduced practical laminated cards with useful phrases that their trainees can refer to in-patient discussions.[61,63,64] Reports on the effectiveness of such programs have demonstrated that continuous education effectively safeguards against decline of skills over time. Furthermore, they affirm that regular training sessions, in contrast to singular didactic modules, yielded enhanced skill acquisition and improved retention.[61] Although an iterative approach to formal communication skills training is favored, even an isolated module may be helpful as demonstrated by one academic program.[65] A dedicated hour-long evidence-based lecture tutorial to breast imaging fellows delivered as part of their weekly core curriculum lectures included tutorials on specific scenarios. A presurvey and postsurvey demonstrated improved confidence in specific challenging patient-centered communication scenarios. Trainees' understanding of the importance of medical error disclosure was also improved. Although there is mounting evidence that simulation-based communication training is a highly efficacious methodology for lower resourced, smaller training programs, even a single lecture-based tutorial seems to have a role and can be effective.

Adept patient–physician communication has a profound impact on both patient experience and outcomes and radiologist well-being. Delivering distressing news has been shown to generate significant stress on physicians, sometimes with lasting effects, underscoring the need for refined communication skills to manage such situations.[66] Proficient communication holds significance for radiologist well-being because it reduces perceived stress, enhances comfort in patient interactions, and mitigates the risk of burnout.[67] Building a strong rapport with patients results in heightened personal satisfaction and overall work gratification for radiologists, consequently reducing the likelihood of burnout.[10]

AUDITING THE PATIENT EXPERIENCE

Monitoring patient feedback is essential to see if breast radiologists are meeting patient expectations and providing a satisfactory patient experience. This allows radiology departments to assess areas where changes can be made to improve patient experience.[68] Previous studies have identified barriers to a positive patient experience, including clinician discomfort with angry patients, suboptimal practice settings to incorporate communication into the radiologist workflow and loss of revenue because it takes the radiologist's time away from relative value unit-generating activities. In the same study, most breast radiologists reported willingness to undertake additional training to increase patient satisfaction.[20]

SUMMARY

Effective patient communication within radiology is important for enhancing patient experience and cultivating patient-centered care. Radiology must embrace the evolving landscape of available technologies while also remaining adaptable to dynamic patient needs and fostering deeper patient engagement. Whether implementing a comprehensive approach using image-rich reports, establishing formal radiology consultation clinics, enhancing educational resources, or augmenting radiologist training in communication techniques, providing clear and accurate information that patients can understand is key. Amid the changing landscape, regular patient feedback will continue to be indispensable not only for highlighting areas of improvement but also for ensuring good patient-centered practices.

Key Innovative Communication Aids: Patient portals

Technological advances in generating reports: image rich reports, visual timelines, and video reports

Patient consultation clinics: in-person and virtual

Educational Resources: visual aids, education videos, online resources, and patient handouts

Integration of AI-based tools: language models

Links to Additional Communication Related Content:

1. ACS—online resource for patient information: https://www.cancer.org/cancer/types/breast-cancer.html

2. Society of Breast Imaging—Updated Fellowship Training Curriculum for Breast Imaging: https://academic.oup.com/jbi/article/3/4/498/6067554?login=false

3. ACGME—Program requirements. For Graduate Medical Education in Diagnostic Radiology—Communication skills on page 28/70 https://www.acgme.org/globalassets/pfassets/programrequirements/420_diagnosticradiology_2022.pdf

4. ACR Imaging 3.0—Patient and Family Centered Care: https://www.acr.org/Practice-Management-Quality-Informatics/Patient-Family-Centered-Care

5. RSNA—Patient-centered care: https://www.rsna.org/practice-tools/patient-centered-care

CLINICS CARE POINTS

- Building a strong rapport with patients results in heightened personal satisfaction and overall work gratification for radiologists, consequently reducing the likelihood of burnout.[10]

- Proficiency in patient interactions and communication skills training not only improves patient health-care outcomes and satisfaction but also augments radiology's value.[59,60]

- Amplifying science-based, educational messages to patients in the aftermath of the pandemic to decrease breast cancer disparities need to be prioritized more urgently.

- Formal training in communication skills during breast imaging fellowship with frequent reinforcement is recommended.

- AI-based solutions for improving patient communication of imaging findings are promising but testing for accuracy is still needed.

DISCLOSURE

The authors have no relevant financial disclosures.

SUPPLEMENTARY DATA

Supplementary data related to this article can be found online at https://doi.org/10.1016/j.rcl.2024.01.004.

REFERENCES

1. Fed Regist Vol. 88, No. 47/Rules and Regulations. 2023, Available at: https://www.govinfo.gov/content/pkg/FR-2023-03-10/pdf/2023-04550.pdf.(Accessed September 1 2023.

2. Reporting and Data Systems (RADS). 2023. Available at: https://www.acr.org/Clinical-Resources/Reporting-and-Data-Systems. [Accessed 1 September 2023].

3. Imaging 3.0, Available at: https://www.acr.org/Practice-Management-Quality-Informatics/Patient-Family-Centered-Care. Accessed September 1, 2023.

4. Burnside ES, Sickles EA, Bassett LW, et al. The ACR BI-RADS experience: learning from history. J Am Coll Radiol 2009;6:851–60.

5. Miller LS, Shelby RA, Balmadrid MH, et al. Patient Anxiety Before and Immediately After Imaging-Guided Breast Biopsy Procedures: Impact of Radiologist-Patient Communication. J Am Coll Radiol 2016;13:e62–71.

6. Zolnierek KB, Dimatteo MR. Physician communication and patient adherence to treatment: a meta-analysis. Med Care 2009;47:826–34.

7. Adler DD, Riba MB, Eggly S. Breaking bad news in the breast imaging setting. Acad Radiol 2009;16:130–5.

8. California Senate Bill No. 1419 Health information, Available at: https://leginfo.legislature.ca.gov/faces/billTextClient.xhtml?bill_id=202120220SB1419, 2022. Accessed September 1, 2023.

9. Oppenheimer DC, Harvey JA. Remote Radiology: Point—Enhance Efficiency, Promote Work-Life Balance, and Ameliorate Staffing Issues. Am J Roentgenol 2023;221:1–2.

10. Milch V, Nelson AE, Austen M, et al. Conceptual Framework for Cancer Care During a Pandemic Incorporating Evidence From the COVID-19 Pandemic. JCO Glob Oncol 2022;8:e2200043.

11. 21st Century Cures Act. 2016. 2023. Available at: https://www.congress.gov/114/bills/hr34/BILLS-114hr34enr.pdf. [Accessed 1 September 2023].

12. Greco G, Patel AS, Lewis SC, et al. Patient-directed Internet-based Medical Image Exchange: Experience from an Initial Multicenter Implementation. Acad Radiol 2016;23:237–44.

13. Lee CI, Lee JM. Maximizing Value Through Innovations in Radiologist-Driven Communications in Breast Imaging. AJR Am J Roentgenol 2017;209:1001–5.

14. Arnold CW, McNamara M, El-Saden S, et al. Imaging informatics for consumer health: towards a radiology patient portal. J Am Med Inf Assoc 2013;20:1028–36.

15. Miles RC, Hippe DS, Elmore JG, et al. Patient Access to Online Radiology Reports: Frequency and Sociodemographic Characteristics Associated with Use. Acad Radiol 2016;23:1162–9.

16. Bass SB, Ruzek SB, Gordon TF, et al. Relationship of Internet health information use with patient behavior and self-efficacy: experiences of newly diagnosed cancer patients who contact the National Cancer Institute's Cancer Information Service. J Health Commun 2006;11:219–36.

17. Amornsiripanitch N, Mangano M, Niell BL. Screening Mammography: Patient Perceptions and Preferences Regarding Communication of Estimated Breast Cancer Risk. AJR Am J Roentgenol 2017;208:1163–70.

18. Lee CI, Langlotz CP, Elmore JG. Implications of Direct Patient Online Access to Radiology Reports Through Patient Web Portals. J Am Coll Radiol 2016;13:1608–14.

19. Recht MP, Westerhoff M, Doshi AM, et al. Video Radiology Reports: A Valuable Tool to Improve Patient-Centered Radiology. Am J Roentgenol 2022;219:509–19.

20. Aminololama-Shakeri S, Soo MS, Grimm LJ, et al. Radiologist-Patient Communication: Current Practices and Barriers to Communication in Breast Imaging. J Am Coll Radiol 2019;16:709–16.

21. Preventing patient harm, Available at: https://www.ama-assn.org/system/files/patient-privacy-survey-results-preventing-patient-harm.pdf. Accessed September 1, 2023.

22. Available at: http://www.rsna.org/radiology_cares/. Accessed September 1, 2023.

23. Kemp J, Gannuch G, Kornbluth C, et al. Radiologists Include Contact Telephone Number in Reports: Experience With Patient Interaction. AJR Am J Roentgenol 2020;215:673–8.

24. Mangano MD, Bennett SE, Gunn AJ, et al. Creating a Patient-Centered Radiology Practice Through the Establishment of a Diagnostic Radiology Consultation Clinic. AJR Am J Roentgenol 2015;205:95–9.

25. Daye D, Joseph E, Flores E, et al. Point-of-Care Virtual Radiology Consultations in Primary Care: A Feasibility Study of a New Model for Patient-Centered Care in Radiology. J Am Coll Radiol 2021;18:1239–45.

26. Panagides JC, Achuck E, Daye D. Synchronous Virtual Patient Consultations in Radiology. AJR Am J Roentgenol 2022;219:164–5.

27. Mohan SK, Hudgins PA, Patel MR, et al. Making Time for Patients: Positive Impact of Direct Patient Reporting. AJR Am J Roentgenol 2018;210:W12–7.

28. Aminololama-Shakeri S, Soo MS, Grimm LJ, et al. Screening Guidelines and Supplemental Screening Tools: Assessment of the Adequacy of Patient–

Provider Discussions. Journal of Breast Imaging 2019;1:109–14.

29. Becker CD, Kotter E. Communicating with patients in the age of online portals—challenges and opportunities on the horizon for radiologists. Insights into Imaging 2022;13:83.

30. Basu PA, Ruiz-Wibbelsmann JA, Spielman SB, et al. Creating a patient-centered imaging service: determining what patients want. AJR Am J Roentgenol 2011;196:605–10.

31. Bull AR, Campbell MJ. Assessment of the psychological impact of a breast screening programme. Br J Radiol 1991;64:510–5.

32. Mathioudakis AG, Salakari M, Pylkkanen L, et al. Systematic review on women's values and preferences concerning breast cancer screening and diagnostic services. Psycho Oncol 2019;28:939–47.

33. Shah BA, Staschen J, Pham N, et al. Communicating Mammography Results: By What Method and How Quickly Do Women Want Their Screening Mammogram Results? J Am Coll Radiol 2019;16:928–35.

34. Shah BA, Mirchandani A, Abrol S. Impact of same day screening mammogram results on women's satisfaction and overall breast cancer screening experience: a quality improvement survey analysis. BMC Wom Health 2022;22:338.

35. Bluth EI, Frush DP, Oates ME, et al. Medical workforce in the United States. J Appl Clin Med Phys 2022;23(Suppl 1):e13799.

36. Kalidindi S, Gandhi S. Workforce Crisis in Radiology in the UK and the Strategies to Deal With It: Is Artificial Intelligence the Saviour? Cureus 2023;15:e43866.

37. Rupert DJ, Squiers LB, Renaud JM, et al. Communicating risk of hereditary breast and ovarian cancer with an interactive decision support tool. Patient Educ Couns 2013;92:188–96.

38. Doan C, Li S, Goodwin JS. Breast and Lung Cancer Screening Among Medicare Enrollees During the COVID-19 Pandemic. JAMA Netw Open 2023;6:e2255589.

39. Larson DB, Langlotz CP. The Role of Radiology in the Diagnostic Process: Information, Communication, and Teamwork. AJR Am J Roentgenol 2017;209:992–1000.

40. Kutay E, Milch H, Sayre J, et al. Fear of the Unknown: The Benefits of a Patient Educational Handout on Breast Biopsy Markers. Journal of Breast Imaging 2022;4:285–90.

41. Penn JP, Nallani R, Dimon EL, et al. Educational Informed Consent Video Equivalent to Standard Verbal Consent for Rhinologic Surgery: A Randomized Controlled Trial. Am J Rhinol Allergy 2021;35:739–45.

42. Padival R, Harris KB, Garber A, et al. Video Consent for Colonoscopy Improves Knowledge Retention and Patient Satisfaction: A Randomized Controlled Study. J Clin Gastroenterol 2022;56:433–7.

43. Castleton K, Fong T, Wang-Gillam A, et al. A survey of Internet utilization among patients with cancer. Support Care Cancer 2011;19:1183–90.

44. Soo MS, Shelby RA, Johnson KS. Optimizing the Patient Experience during Breast Biopsy. Journal of Breast Imaging 2019;1:131–8.

45. Attai DJ, Cowher MS, Al-Hamadani M, et al. Twitter Social Media is an Effective Tool for Breast Cancer Patient Education and Support: Patient-Reported Outcomes by Survey. J Med Internet Res 2015;17:e188.

46. Seidel RL, Jalilvand A, Kunjummen J, et al. Radiologists and Social Media: Do Not Forget About Facebook. J Am Coll Radiol 2018;15:224–8.

47. Lee SC, Monga AK, Kawashita T, et al. Analyzing the quality of mammography-related YouTube videos. Breast J 2020;26:2327–8.

48. Available at: https://urlisolation.com/browser?clickId=2F105ADB-12C2-4EA0-8971-42936F79A4CA&traceToken=1694542743%3Bnshs_hosted%3B https%3A%2Fwww.youtube.com%2Fplaylist%3F&url=https%3A%2F%2Fwww.youtube.com%2Fplaylist%3Flist%3DPLO4LWAjSkEXU-huq0-AG8nWCelegh_a2U. [Accessed 1 September 2023].

49. Rubin GD, Krishnaraj A, Mahesh M, et al. Enhancing Public Access to Relevant and Valued Medical Information: Fresh Directions for RadiologyInfo.org. J Am Coll Radiol 2017;14:697–702 e4.

50. Bange M, Huh E, Novin SA, et al. Readability of Patient Education Materials From RadiologyInfo.org: Has There Been Progress Over the Past 5 Years? AJR Am J Roentgenol 2019;213:875–9.

51. Novin SA, Huh EH, Bange MG, et al. Readability of Spanish-Language Patient Education Materials From RadiologyInfo.org. J Am Coll Radiol 2019;16:1108–13.

52. Chen DW, Banerjee M, He X, et al. Hidden Disparities: How Language Influences Patients' Access to Cancer Care. J Natl Compr Cancer Netw 2023;21:951–959 e1.

53. Lyu Q, Tan J, Zapadka ME, et al. Translating radiology reports into plain language using ChatGPT and GPT-4 with prompt learning: results, limitations, and potential. Vis Comput Ind Biomed Art 2023;6:9.

54. Derevianko A, Pizzoli SFM, Pesapane F, et al. The Use of Artificial Intelligence (AI) in the Radiology Field: What Is the State of Doctor-Patient Communication in Cancer Diagnosis? Cancers 2023;15.

55. Butte AJ. Artificial Intelligence-From Starting Pilots to Scalable Privilege. JAMA Oncol 2023. https://doi.org/10.1001/jamaoncol.2023.2867.

56. Chen S, Kann BH, Foote MB, et al. Use of Artificial Intelligence Chatbots for Cancer Treatment Information. JAMA Oncol 2023. https://doi.org/10.1001/jamaoncol.2023.2954.

57. Sandler KL, Haddad DN, Paulson AB, et al. Women screened for breast cancer are dying from lung cancer: An opportunity to improve lung cancer screening in a mammography population. J Med Screen 2021;28:488–93.

58. Huntington B, Kuhn N. Communication gaffes: a root cause of malpractice claims. SAVE Proc 2003;16:157–61. discussion 61.

59. Katzen JT, Grimm LJ, Brem RF. The American College of Radiology/Society of Breast Imaging Updated Fellowship Training Curriculum for Breast Imaging. Journal of Breast Imaging 2021;3:498–501.

60. Radiology program requirements, Available at: https://www.acgme.org/Specialties/Overview/pfcatid/23/Radiology. Accessed September 1, 2023.

61. Dodelzon K, Katzen J. State of Communication Training During the Breast Imaging Fellowship Year. Journal of Breast Imaging 2023;5:80–4.

62. Sarkany D, DeBenedectis CM, Brown SD. A Review of Resources and Methodologies Available for Teaching and Assessing Patient-Related Communication Skills in Radiology. Acad Radiol 2018;25:955–61.

63. Haglund MM, Rudd M, Nagler A, et al. Difficult conversations: a national course for neurosurgery residents in physician-patient communication. J Surg Educ 2015;72:394–401.

64. Chung EH, Truong T, Jooste KR, et al. The Implementation of Communication Didactics for OB/GYN Residents on the Disclosure of Adverse Perioperative Events. J Surg Educ 2021;78:942–9.

65. Dodelzon K, Reichman M, Askin G, et al. Effect of a communication lecture tutorial on breast imaging trainees' confidence with challenging breast imaging patient interactions. Clin Imag 2020;65:143–6.

66. Ptacek JT, Ptacek JJ, Ellison NM. "I'm sorry to tell you ..." physicians' reports of breaking bad news. J Behav Med 2001;24:205–17.

67. Parikh JR, Sun J, Mainiero MB. What Causes the Most Stress in Breast Radiology Practice? A Survey of Members of the Society of Breast Imaging. J Breast Imaging 2021;3:332–42.

68. Kapoor N, Yan Z, Wang A, et al. Improving Patient Experience in Radiology: Impact of a Multifaceted Intervention on National Ranking. Radiology 2019;291:102–9.

Moving?

Make sure your subscription moves with you!

To notify us of your new address, find your **Clinics Account Number** (located on your mailing label above your name), and contact customer service at:

Email: journalscustomerservice-usa@elsevier.com

800-654-2452 (subscribers in the U.S. & Canada)
314-447-8871 (subscribers outside of the U.S. & Canada)

Fax number: 314-447-8029

Elsevier Health Sciences Division
Subscription Customer Service
3251 Riverport Lane
Maryland Heights, MO 63043

*To ensure uninterrupted delivery of your subscription, please notify us at least 4 weeks in advance of move.

Printed and bound by CPI Group (UK) Ltd, Croydon, CR0 4YY

08/05/2025

01864748-0020